T0276182

Networks of the Brain

Networks of the Brain

Olaf Sporns

The MIT Press
Cambridge, Massachusetts
London, England

First MIT Press paperback edition, 2016

© 2011 Massachusetts Institute of Technology

All rights reserved. No part of this book may be reproduced in any form by any electronic or mechanical means (including photocopying, recording, or information storage and retrieval) without permission in writing from the publisher.

This book was set in Syntax and Times Roman by Toppan Best-set Premedia Limited.

Library of Congress Cataloging-in-Publication Data

Sporns, Olaf.
Networks of the brain / Olaf Sporns.
  p.; cm.
Includes bibliographical references and index.
ISBN 978–0-262–01469–4 (hardcover: alk. paper), 978-0-262-52898-6 (pb)
1. Neural networks (Neurobiology) I. Title.
[DNLM: 1. Brain—physiology. 2. Nerve Net. WL 300 S764n 2011]
QP363.3.S56   2011
612.8—dc22

2010006957

For Anita

Contents

Preface

We live in the age of networks. For most of us, networks are an integral part of our daily social and intellectual lives, connecting us at an ever accelerating pace and transforming the way we communicate, learn, create, work, and play. The importance of networks has long been realized in the social sciences, resulting in a rich literature that capitalizes on quantitative network analysis to understand the web of social relations, cooperation and conflict among individuals and organizations. More recently, networks have become of central interest in the natural sciences, particularly in the study of complex biological systems, including the brain. Modern network approaches are beginning to reveal fundamental principles of brain architecture and function. This book highlights the many emerging points of contact between neuroscience and network theory.

With this book I wanted to introduce networks to neuroscientists and make neuroscience appealing to all those working on theoretical network models. I also wanted to give a real sense of how broadly and deeply network thinking applies to neuroscience. I attempted to strike a balance between providing a broad overview of the many areas of neuroscience where network approaches have begun to make a difference and exploring at least some of these areas in sufficient detail to illustrate the substance and direction of the field. This balance requires a compromise between breadth and depth. Rather than focusing on a single "model system" or level of analysis, I chose to emphasize how networks connect levels of organization in the brain and how they help us link structure to function. In order to keep the book accessible and focus more of the discussion on the relevance of network approaches to many areas of neuroscience, I opted for an informal and nonmathematical treatment of the subject. Readers interested in the statistical and computational underpinnings of network science can find more formal and analytic treatments in numerous monographs and review articles.

In each section of the book, I attempted to provide substantial discussion of open research questions, in order to give a sense of the many controversies and uncertainties that still pervade the field. I wanted to document the rapid pace of discovery and innovation in brain networks while also exposing the historical roots of the field. Not all areas of neuroscience have been equally covered. In the past, much of my own work has focused on the structure and dynamics of large-scale brain networks, and thus research in this area is discussed at some length. Other areas—for example, the burgeoning field of cellular network analysis and modeling or exciting developments in the study of invertebrate nervous systems—are not treated in as much detail. While the book contains many scholarly references, they necessarily represent only a selection, and I am afraid that some relevant areas have not been discussed or cited. I sincerely apologize to all who believe that their work has been overlooked.

This book would not have been possible without a network of colleagues and friends. I am deeply grateful to Paul Layer, who many years ago took me on as an undergraduate research assistant and who opened my eyes to the wonders and mysteries of the brain. My PhD advisor, Gerald Edelman, had an enormous impact on my thinking, and it was a privilege to be a part of the unique intellectual environment he created at the Neurosciences Institute in New York and San Diego. Many years of working with Giulio Tononi have been invaluable for developing key ideas about complexity and networks. Interactions with Rolf Pfeifer, Esther Thelen, and Linda Smith sharpened my appreciation of dynamics and developmental change. Working with Barry Horwitz, Randy McIntosh, and Rolf Kötter shaped my ideas about the link between structure and function in the brain. The work of my students Chris Honey and Jeff Alstott was instrumental for formulating many of the key ideas of the book—and I thank them for encouraging me to write it and for cheering me on as I toiled in my office. I also greatly appreciate the many interactions with my colleagues at Indiana University, whose integrative, cross-disciplinary, and forward-looking way of approaching complex scientific questions I admire.

Many friends have given freely of their time to read and critique early drafts of the book. I especially thank Mika Rubinov, who provided significant scientific and editorial input to several chapters. I also thank Dani Bassett, Diarmuid Cahalene, Barb Finlay, Chris Honey, Barry

Horwitz, Marcus Kaiser, Rolf Kötter, Rolf Pfeifer, Anne Prieto, and Larry Yaeger for reading portions of the text. Their comments have helped to improve the book—any remaining imperfections or errors are, of course, my own responsibility. I am grateful to all those who provided original images for the book's many illustrations—my special thanks to Alfred Anwander, Christian Beaulieu, Kevin Briggman, John Chen, Peter Franssen, Gaolang Gong, Patric Hagmann, Biyu He, Shun Iwasawa, Hans Meinhardt, Michael Nonet, Rolf Pfeifer, James Rilling, Emmanuelle Tognoli, Arjen van Ooyen, Larry Yaeger, and Malcolm Young. Bob Prior and Susan Buckley at MIT Press gave important and helpful advice, and I thank them for their enthusiasm and encouragement. Finally, I thank my wife, Anne Prieto, for her love and support and for patiently putting up with a higher than usual level of restlessness and distraction.

1 Introduction: Why Networks?

What can network science tell us about the brain? This question, in a nutshell, is the subject of this book. The book describes the ways in which the integrative nature of brain function may be usefully addressed from a complex network perspective. In doing so, the book brings together two rapidly expanding fields that until now have been largely pursued in isolation—neuroscience and the emerging science of complex networks.

Over the last decade, the study of complex networks has dramatically expanded across diverse scientific fields, ranging from the social sciences to physics and biology. This expansion reflects modern trends and currents that have changed the way scientific questions are formulated and research is carried out. Increasingly, science is concerned with the structure, behavior, and evolution of complex systems such as cells, brains, ecosystems, societies, or the global economy. To understand these systems, we require not only knowledge of elementary system components but also knowledge of the ways in which these components interact and the emergent properties of their interactions. The increasing availability of large data sets and powerful computers makes it easier than ever before to record, analyze, and model the behavior of systems composed of thousands or millions of interacting elements. All such complex systems display characteristic diverse and organized patterns. These patterns are the outcome of highly structured and selective coupling between elements, achieved through an intricate web of connectivity. Connectivity comes in many forms—for example, molecular interactions, metabolic pathways, synaptic connections, semantic associations, ecological food webs, social networks, web hyperlinks, or citation patterns. In all cases, the quantitative analysis of connectivity requires sophisticated mathematical and statistical techniques.

Why should we take advantage of modern network approaches to study the brain? Primarily, because these approaches can provide fundamental insights into the means by which simple elements organize into dynamic patterns, thus greatly adding to the insights that can be gained by considering the individual elements in isolation. Virtually all complex systems form networks of interacting components. Interactions of even very simple components, such as water molecules, can generate complex patterns, such as eddies in the flow of an oceanic stream or the beautiful symmetries of snow crystals. Very different systems can generate strikingly similar patterns—for example, the motions of particles in a fluid or gas and the coordinated movements of bacterial colonies, swarms of fish, flocks of birds, or crowds of commuters returning home from work. The brain is a complex system par excellence whose complex components continually create complex patterns. The collective actions of individual nerve cells linked by a dense web of intricate connectivity guide behavior, shape thoughts, form and retrieve memories, and create consciousness. No single nerve cell can carry out any of these functions, but when large numbers are linked together in networks and organized into a nervous *system*, behavior, thought, memory, and consciousness become possible. Understanding these integrative functions of the brain requires an understanding of brain networks and the complex and irreducible dynamic patterns they create.

Brain networks span multiple spatial scales, from the microscale of individual cells and synapses to the macroscale of cognitive systems and embodied organisms. This architecture is also found in other complex systems—for example, in the multiscale arrangement of social networks, ranging from interpersonal relations and cohesive social groups, to local communities and urban settlements, all the way to national economies and global political organizations.[1] In multiscale systems, levels do not operate in isolation—instead, patterns at each level critically depend on processes unfolding on both lower and higher levels. The brain is a case in point. We cannot fully understand brain function unless we approach the brain on multiple scales, by identifying the networks that bind cells into coherent populations, organize cell groups into functional brain regions, integrate regions into systems, and link brain and body in a complete organism. In this hierarchy, no single level is privileged over others. The notion that brain function can be fully reduced to the operation of cells or molecules is as ill-conceived as the complementary view that cognition can be understood without making reference to its biological substrates. Only through multiscale network interactions can molecules and cells give rise to behavior and cognition. Knowledge about network interactions on and across multiple levels of organization is crucial for a more complete understanding of the brain as an integrated system.

The study of brain connectivity has already opened new experimental and theoretical avenues in many areas of neuroscience. Connectivity plays an important role in neuroanatomy, neurodevelopment, electrophysiology, functional brain imaging, and the neural basis of cognition. The analysis of network architecture and connectivity illuminates a number of problems that concern integrative brain function:

• Nervous systems are composed of vast numbers of neural elements that are interconnected by synapses and axonal pathways. Quantitative methods of network science can probe for architectural principles that shape brain anatomy.

• Single neurons engage in complex physiological responses. These responses result from network interactions among a great number of individual nerve cells connected in local circuits as well as between brain regions.

• Distinct sensory features within and across modalities are represented in different portions of the cerebral cortex. Their integration as part of a coherent perceptual or cognitive state is the outcome of distributed network processes involving large parts of the brain.

• When a person is cognitively at rest, quietly awake and alert, the brain engages in a characteristic pattern of dynamic neural activity. The spatiotemporal profile of this pattern is molded by an intricate structural network of nerve fibers and pathways.

• Changes in sensory input or cognitive task result in highly specific patterns of brain activation. These patterns are the effects of dynamic perturbations of a complex and continually active network.

• The outcomes of brain trauma and disease include significant and long-lasting neurological deficits. These insults result in structural network damage, and the extent and location of the disturbance can inform predictions about the nature and severity of cognitive dysfunction as well as the potential for recovery and compensatory response.

• Cognitive performance exhibits significant variation across healthy individuals. The analysis of brain connectivity is beginning to draw links between individual variations in behavior/cognition and variations in brain networks.

• Behavior and cognition change over development and the entire life span. The growth and maturation of anatomical connections in the brain modify the range of neural responses and cognitive capacities.

• Brain and body are dynamically coupled through continual cycles of action and perception. By causing bodily movement, brain networks can structure their own inputs and modulate their internal dynamics.

These and other key questions of neuroscience can be productively addressed from the perspective of complex networks, and they form the central subject matter of the book. We have a lot of ground to cover. We will begin by defining brain networks and network measures. In the next two chapters, we introduce neuroscientists to some of the basic concepts and methods of network theory, and network scientists to some of the fundamentals in brain connectivity. Chapter 2 provides an intuitive survey of some of the quantitative tools and concepts from network science that are important in studies of the brain. Chapter 3 describes some fundamental techniques and approaches used to extract brain networks from neuroscience data. The next four chapters primarily consider anatomical networks of cells and brain regions. Chapter 4 offers a network perspective on the relationship between brain anatomy and function, while chapter 5 outlines modern neuroanatomical techniques that promise to extract structural brain networks of unprecedented quality and resolution. Chapter 6 reviews some of the key architectural principles of anatomical networks known so far, while chapter 7 attempts to illuminate their functional meaning and evolutionary origin. The next four chapters of the book are primarily devoted to network dynamics. Chapter 8 discusses functional networks generated by spontaneous activity in neural systems, while chapter 9 attempts to draw links between brain networks and cognition. Chapter 10 outlines our knowledge of brain network disruptions in neurological and psychiatric disease. Chapter 11 focuses on the growth, development, and aging of brain networks across the life span. The final three chapters of the book address different aspects of network complexity. Chapter 12 makes the case for diverse and flexible neural dynamics as a prerequisite for efficient computation, and chapter 13 traces the origin of complex dynamic patterns to structural patterns of network connectivity. Finally, chapter 14 broadens the subject of brain connectivity further by examining the role of the body in shaping the functioning of brain networks.

What exactly are networks? How can we define them and measure their properties? The next chapter will try to answer these questions and illustrate some of the quantitative methods and tools that allow us to characterize the networks of the brain.

2 Network Measures and Architectures

In addition to that branch of geometry which is concerned with magnitudes, and which has always received the greatest attention, there is another branch, previously almost unknown, which Leibniz first mentioned, calling it the geometry of position. This branch is concerned only with the determination of position and its properties; it does not involve measurements, nor calculations made with them. It has not yet been satisfactorily determined what kind of problems are relevant to this geometry of position, or what methods should be used in solving them. Hence, when a problem was recently mentioned, which seemed geometrical but was so constructed that it did not require the measurement of distances, nor did calculation help at all, I had no doubt that it was concerned with the geometry of position [...].[1]
—Leonhard Euler, 1736

Euler's problem was a popular puzzle involving seven bridges across the river Pregel in the East Prussian city of Königsberg (today's Kaliningrad). These bridges spanned the two main branches of the river and linked four separate parts of the city including a small island (see figure 2.1). The problem was to find a path by which a person could cross each of these bridges exactly once and return to the starting point. Popular opinion held that this was impossible, but there was no proof that such a path could not be found. Euler provided a mathematical treatment of the problem in an article published in the Proceedings of the Petersburg Academy in 1736 (Euler, 1736). Euler proved that the Königsberg path did not exist and found a general solution that could be applied to an arbitrary arrangement of bridges and landmasses. More importantly, he realized that the problem could be resolved by solely taking into account the relative position of bridges and landmasses and that precise geographical position or physical distance was unimportant. In doing so, Euler is generally credited with founding the field which he referred to as the "geometry of position" (*geometria situs*) and which is now known as graph theory.[2]

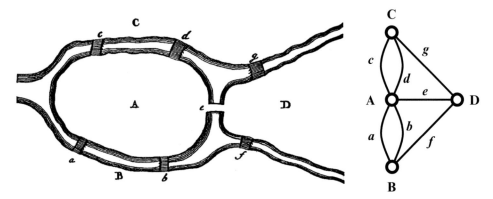

Figure 2.1
Euler's solution to the Königsberg bridge problem. The illustration on the left is from
Euler's original paper and shows the river Pregel and its seven bridges joining four landmasses. The illustration on the right is the graphical representation of the problem—
landmasses have been replaced by nodes and bridges by edges. Euler showed that a path
that traverses all bridges exactly once and leads back to the point of origin is impossible.

Graph theory is the mathematical study of networks, or graphs. While
some of graph theory falls under pure mathematics and has no immediate applications, the use of graph theoretical formalism is often invaluable in the treatment of real-world problems, such as the Königsberg
bridge puzzle. Two nineteenth-century examples from physics and chemistry further illustrate this point. While looking for ways to compute
voltage and current flow in electrical networks, the physicist Gustav
Kirchhoff represented these networks as graphs and formulated several
original theorems that laid the foundation of circuit theory in electrical
engineering. Kirchhoff's contemporary, the mathematician Arthur
Cayley, applied graph theoretical concepts to the problem of enumerat-
ing chemical isomers, molecules that contain the same number of atoms
bonded together in different ways. This approach allowed the complete
characterization of various groups of hydrocarbons as families of chemical graphs.[3]

Today, graph theory is one of the most active branches of mathematics.
Its applications are everywhere, ranging from structural mechanics,
urban planning, and scheduling and routing of air traffic to electronic
communications, polymer chemistry, and social sciences. However, until
recently, most studied networks were relatively small. For instance, social
scientists focused on analyses of small network structures (such as circles
and chains) and on identification of conspicuous network elements, such
as influential people in social networks (Wasserman and Faust, 1994;

Borgatti et al., 2009). Over the last decade, the study of networks has expanded to include the statistical descriptions of much larger systems. This novel approach, sometimes called a "new network science," aims to characterize the structure and the dynamics of complex networks and consequently make predictions of their global functionality. Over the last few years this approach has revealed commonalities and differences in local and global organization of real-world networks from social, biological, technological, and other domains (Strogatz, 2001; Albert and Barabási, 2002; Newman, 2003; Amaral and Ottino, 2004; Watts, 2004; Barabási and Oltvai, 2004; Boccaletti et al., 2006; Costa et al., 2007; Börner et al., 2007; Barabási, 2009).[4]

This chapter introduces the basic terminology and methodology of network science and its most important mathematical foundation, graph theory. I start by defining some basic terms and concepts frequently encountered in network studies. I then survey network measures of particular importance to neuroscience. I informally describe each measure and discuss its neuroscientific relevance and interpretation. I then describe the major classes of network architectures and discuss their main structural features and neuroscientific relevance. I will return to a more in-depth discussion of these network measures and architectures throughout the book—here the emphasis is on providing the reader with the necessary basic concepts and terminology, as well as an intuitive and conceptual understanding of how networks are organized.

There are no equations in this book. To assist the reader in translating network science terminology to neural applications, I provide a "Network Glossary" at the end of the volume. The glossary contains brief definitions of terms which are frequently used in network studies and throughout the book. Exact mathematical definitions of all measures can be found in relevant review articles (e.g., Rubinov and Sporns, 2010). There are also many textbooks on graph theory, including the classic treatments by Harary (1969), Bollobás (1979), and Chartrand (1985), as well as more specialized surveys focusing on algorithms and practical applications.

Graphs and Networks: Definitions

A graph is a mathematical representation of a real-world network[5] or, more generally, of some system composed of interconnected elements. A simple graph comprises a set of nodes and a set of edges. Nodes represent the fundamental elements of the system, such as people in social networks. Edges represent connections between pairs of nodes, such as friendships between pairs of people. Edges can be undirected or directed from origin to destination. Independently, edges can be binary or can be associated with a weight. It is useful to distinguish graphs based on the types of edges they contain: for instance, undirected graphs contain only undirected edges, while directed graphs contain only directed edges. All four types of binary/weighted and undirected/directed graphs are important for describing networks of the brain. The distinction between undirected and directed graphs is especially important, as most graph measures are defined and computed slightly differently for these two major classes of graphs. Most of the classical work in graph theory has been carried out for binary undirected graphs, and in-depth treatments of directed or weighted graphs can be found in more specialized text-books (e.g., Chartrand and Lesniak, 1996; Bang-Jensen and Gutin, 2001). All graph-based approaches discussed in this book can be applied to networks that are binary or weighted, directed or undirected, provided that all edges represent single dyadic (pairwise) relationships, and none of the edges have negative weights. While more specialized applications of graph theory allow for the mathematical treatment of graphs that include multiple as well as negative edges, these methods have not yet been widely applied in neuroscience.[6]

One of the most elementary representations of a graph is the adjacency matrix, also called the connection matrix. The adjacency matrix defines the topology of the graph by representing nodes as matrix rows and columns and representing edges as binary or weighted matrix entries. Nodes that are linked by an edge are called neighbors. The adjacency matrix allows the derivation of one of the most fundamental graph measures, the degree. In an undirected graph the degree of a node is the number of edges connected to that node. In directed graphs the indegree and outdegree correspond to the number of incoming and outgoing edges, respectively. In weighted graphs, the sum of all edge weights of a node gives the node strength, which is analyzed similarly to node degree. Degrees of all nodes together form the degree distribution of the network, which shows whether the network contains nodes with approximately equal degrees or whether node degrees vary over a broader range. Node degrees are fundamental because they have a significant impact on most other network measures described in this chapter, and the degree distribution can be highly informative about the graph's network architecture (see below). Another simple measure based on degree is the assortativity (Newman, 2002), defined as the correlation coefficient for the degrees of neighboring nodes. Positive assortativity indicates that edges tend to link nodes of similar degree, while negative assortativity indicates that high-degree nodes preferentially connect with low-degree nodes. In brain networks, node degree and node strength may be simply viewed as a measure of direct interaction: high-degree or high-strength nodes can be interpreted to directly interact with a large number of other nodes. A node with high indegree is influenced by many other nodes, while a node with high outdegree has many potential functional targets. The balance of node indegree and outdegree is an indication of the way the node is embedded in the overall network; for example, this balance specifies whether the node primarily sends or receives information (see chapter 4).

Nodes can be linked directly by single edges or indirectly by sequences of intermediate nodes and edges. Ordered sequences of unique edges and intermediate nodes are called paths, while sequences of nonunique edges are called walks. Many graph analyses of brain networks are based on paths. Paths can connect a node to itself, in which case the path is called a cycle. If a finite path between two nodes exists, then one node can be reached by traversing a sequence of edges starting at the other node. If all pairs of nodes are linked by at least one path of finite length, the graph is said to be connected (or strongly connected). In binary graphs, the length of a path is equal to the number of edges it contains. In weighted graphs, path lengths are computed using edge weights, such that paths composed of stronger edges span shorter lengths. The distance between two nodes is the length of the shortest path linking the nodes and is often of particular interest. All pairwise distances in a graph may be represented in the distance matrix. The global maximum of the distance matrix is also called the graph diameter. It is important to note that distance in graphs is a topological concept that does not refer to the spatial separation of nodes in geographical or metric units.

The adjacency and distance matrices have fairly straightforward interpretations, at least in the context of anatomical brain networks. Network nodes represent neural elements, such as cells, cell populations, or brain regions, while network edges represent connections between nodes, such as anatomical synapses or pathways (other types of connections are described in chapter 3). The structure of the adjacency and distance matrices together describes the pattern of communication within the network. The presence of an edge linking two nodes indicates that the two nodes can communicate directly. Paths of various lengths record possible ways by which signals can travel indirectly between two nodes. Longer paths are likely to have less of an effect than shorter paths.

Most analyses focus on shortest possible paths (distances) between nodes since these paths are likely to be most effective for internode communication.

Most of the measures discussed in the remainder of this chapter and the book are derived from the adjacency and distance matrices. Exemplar measures are schematically displayed in figure 2.2. I divide the discussion of these measures into several sections. I begin with measures that quantify the properties of local topological neighborhoods of individual nodes. I then consider measures that capture global network communication and signaling. Finally, I discuss how local and global measures of centrality allow us to determine the influence of nodes or edges within a network and thus quantify contributions of each indi-

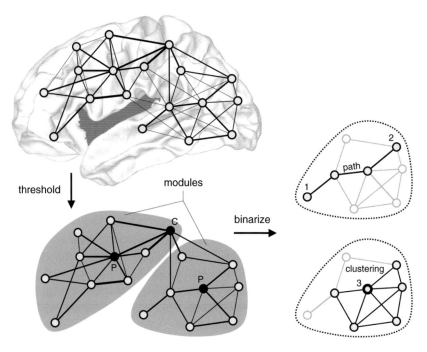

Figure 2.2
Basic concepts of graph theory. The schematic diagram shows an undirected weighted network before (top) and after (bottom) applying a threshold that removes weak connections. The network consists of two modules, linked by a connector hub (labeled "C"), and each module contains one provincial hub ("P"). Diagrams on the right show one of the modules after the connections have been binarized, and illustrate a path of minimal length (3 steps) between nodes 1 and 2 (top) and clustering around node 3 (bottom). Node 3 has 5 neighbors, and these neighbors have 5 out of 10 possible undirected connections between them, for a clustering coefficient of 0.5.

vidual element to the network's structural integrity and information flow. In introducing these measures I will give a general idea about their functional roles—much more detailed discussions are found in later chapters.

Local Segregation: Clustering and Modularity

In many networks, the effective strength of functional interactions diminishes as nodes become topologically more remote. Hence, it is often a realistic assumption that a large number of processing characteristics and functional contributions of a node are determined by its interactions within a local neighborhood. Importantly, this neighborhood is defined in terms of topological distance and does not necessarily imply close physical proximity. Several measures of local connectivity evaluate the extent to which the network is organized into densely coupled neighborhoods, also known as clusters, communities, or modules. One of the most elementary measures of local segregation is the clustering coefficient (Watts and Strogatz, 1998). The clustering coefficient of an individual node measures the density of connections between the node's neighbors. Densely interconnected neighbors form a cluster around the node, while sparsely interconnected neighbors do not. The average of the clustering coefficients for each individual node is the clustering coefficient of the graph. The clustering coefficient may be disproportionately influenced by nodes with low degree. A collectively normalized variant of the clustering coefficient, the transitivity (e.g., Newman, 2003), circumvents this potential problem. Clustering coefficient and transitivity have been generalized for weighted and directed networks (Onnela et al., 2005; Fagiolo, 2007).

Different local neighborhoods or clusters may engage in different patterns of interactions—for example, in order to carry out different processing tasks. To aid in the analysis of connection patterns in local neighborhoods, large networks or graphs can be decomposed into smaller "building blocks" or "networks-within-networks." Such subgraphs, or motifs (Milo et al., 2002; 2004a), form a basic structural alphabet of elementary circuits. For example, three nodes may be connected with directed edges in 13 distinct ways (see figure 6.4). Every network can be uniquely decomposed into a set of motifs, and the number and distribution of individual motifs reflect some functional characteristics of the network. In order to assess the significance of a given motif distribution, it is important to compare motifs derived from an empirical network to a population of randomly constructed networks that serve as a "null hypothesis." Motif analysis can be extended to weighted networks (Onnela et al., 2005), and motif composition can be evaluated for individual nodes, yielding a node-specific profile of local processing capacity (Sporns and Kötter, 2004; Sporns et al., 2007).

Networks with high levels of clustering are often (but not always) composed of local communities or modules of densely interconnected nodes. These modules are segregated from each other, such that most edges link nodes within modules, and few edges link nodes between modules. The balance of the density of within-module and between-modules connections defines a measure of network modularity (Girvan and Newman, 2002; Newman, 2006).[7] Optimization algorithms are needed to identify the partitioning scheme for which the modularity measure is maximized. Various such algorithms have been developed, such as an algorithm based on the graph's spectral properties (Newman, 2006) or an algorithm that can detect a hierarchy of smaller modules nested within larger modules (Blondel et al., 2008). Most modularity algorithms partition the network into nonoverlapping modules. Other approaches allow the detection of modules that overlap—for example, due to nodes that are central to more than one community (Palla et al., 2005).

Clustering, motifs, and modularity capture aspects of the local connectivity structure of a graph. In many cases, the information provided by these measures significantly overlaps. For example, a connectivity pattern with high clustering is also likely to simultaneously exhibit an overabundance of densely connected motif classes. This is because, in its simplest formulation, the clustering coefficient is equivalent to the fraction of fully connected three-node motifs, which are simply triangles. Highly modular graphs often consist of densely clustered communities, but high clustering alone does not necessarily indicate the existence of modules or communities (see, e.g., regular graphs, below). Despite their partial redundancy, each measure of local connectivity also provides some unique information about the way individual nodes are locally embedded (clustering, motifs) and about their community structure (modularity).

Clustering is significant in a neurobiological context because neuronal units or brain regions that form a densely connected cluster or module communicate a lot of shared information and are therefore likely to constitute a functionally coherent brain system. We will return to this important point in much more detail in later chapters. Conversely, neuronal units that belong to different clusters or modules do not share as much information and remain functionally segregated from each other. Thus, measures of clustering and modularity highlight a particular aspect of the functional organization of the brain, its tendency to form segregated subsystems with specialized functional properties. The identification of modules in brain networks is an important first step toward the characterization of these subsystems.

Global Integration: Path Length and Efficiency

While clustering, motifs, and modularity evaluate local connectivity and the segregation of the network into communities, another set of measures captures the capacity of the network to engage in more global interactions that transcend the boundaries of modules and enable network-wide integration. Many of these measures are based on paths and distances between nodes. As defined earlier, path lengths in binary graphs correspond to the number of distinct edges (or "steps along the path"), while path lengths in weighted networks correspond to the sum of the edge lengths. Edge lengths are inversely related to edge weights since edge weights express the coupling strength and thus the proximity between nodes, not their distance. To compute path lengths for weighted graphs, one must first transform edge weights to lengths.

One of the most commonly used measures of integration in brain networks is the characteristic path length (or "path length" in short), usually computed as the global average (or median) of the graph's distance matrix (Watts and Strogatz, 1998). A short path length indicates that, on average, each node can be reached from any other node along a path composed of only a few edges. However, the absolute value of the path length varies greatly with the size and density of individual graphs and, hence, provides only limited information on integration in the network. The network path length should therefore be compared to path lengths of appropriately constructed random networks (see the example below). The path length can also be significantly influenced by a small number of disconnected or remote nodes. A related and often more robust measure, the global efficiency (Latora and Marchiori, 2001), is computed as the average of the inverse of the distance matrix. A fully connected network has maximal global efficiency since all distances are equal to one (all pairs of nodes are linked by an edge), while a fully disconnected network has minimal global efficiency since all distances between nodes are infinite.

A low path length or a high efficiency indicates that pairs of nodes, on average, have short communication distances and can be reached in a few steps. Path length and efficiency are global measures of network integration. Both measures take into account only short paths, while alternative but longer paths and the total number of short paths are neglected. Other measures of global connectivity take these alternative routes into account. One example is the communicability, a measure of global information flow based on the number of walks between nodes (Estrada and Hatano, 2008), a measure that can be applied to binary and weighted networks (Crofts and Higham, 2009).

The measures discussed in this section all capture the capacity of the network to pass information between its nodes, and they are therefore of significance in a neurobiological context. For instance, structural paths that are shorter or are composed of fewer steps generally allow signal transmission with less noise, interference, or attenuation. Given two networks of equal size and density of connections, shorter path length or greater efficiency is likely to reflect better overall communication in the corresponding network. It will also be the network with the greater efficiency, another metric that is of significance in the context of brain networks. Efficiency is less sensitive to the presence of "outliers," disconnected or very weakly connected nodes, than the path length. In neural terms, a network with high efficiency places all its nodes at short distances from each other, which enables them to interact more directly, thus promoting high functional integration.

Segregation and integration place opposing demands on the way in which networks are constructed. Optimal clustering and modularity are inconsistent with high integration, since highly segregated communities will engage in very little cross talk. On the other hand, optimal efficiency or integration is only achieved in a fully connected network that lacks any differentiation in its local processing. This tension between local and global order is one of the main themes of this book, as both segregation and integration turn out to be essential for structural and functional organization of brain networks. However, before we examine the relationship between local and global connectivity in different network architectures, we need to consider the heterogeneous contributions made by individual nodes and edges.

Influence and Centrality

In most real-world settings, individual nodes or edges differ in their impact on the overall functioning of the network. Some nodes are more essential, or more influential, than others. Some edges carry more traffic, or their loss is more disruptive to the rest of the network. "Important" nodes are often more highly or densely connected to the rest of the network, facilitate global integrative processes, or play a critical compensatory role when the network is damaged. Such nodes are often referred to as "hubs," a term that is widely used yet often imprecisely defined. Hubs can be identified on the basis of several different criteria, including the degree, participation in modular connectivity, or centrality. Of these measures, the simplest indicator of a node's importance is its degree. The degree (or strength) can be highly informative in networks with very inhomogeneous degree distributions. In such networks, nodes with high degree are often essential for maintaining global connectedness. The degree is less informative about node importance in networks with fairly homogeneous degree distributions.

In networks that are composed of local communities or modules, within-module and between-modules connectivity can provide information about the specific contributions of individual nodes. Once a partition of the network into modules has been identified, the diversity of between-modules connections can be assessed with a measure called the participation coefficient (Guimerà and Amaral, 2005; Guimerà et al., 2007). High-degree nodes that maintain a diverse set of between-modules connections have a high participation coefficient. Such nodes, called connector hubs, are likely to facilitate intermodular communication and integration. On the other hand, high-degree nodes that have few or less diverse between-modules connections have a low participation index. These nodes, called provincial hubs, mostly participate in interactions within their own module and thus promote the cohesion of a single community.

Several measures of centrality are based on the notion of shortest paths. Of these, the closeness centrality and the betweenness centrality are based on the idea that a node is central if it has great control over the flow of information within the network and that this control results from its participation in many of the network's short paths (Freeman, 1977; 1978). The closeness centrality of an individual node is the inverse of the average path length between that node and all other nodes in the network. A node with high closeness centrality can reach all other nodes via short paths and may thus exert more direct influence over the nodes. The betweenness centrality of an individual node is defined as the fraction of all shortest paths in the network that pass through the node. A node with high betweenness centrality can control information flow because it is at the intersection of many short paths. Betweenness centrality can be computed not only for individual nodes but also for individual edges and for directed and weighted networks (after appropriate conversion of edge weights to distances).

The use of a specific measure to characterize the influence or centrality of a node or edge necessarily makes assumptions about the nature of the flow or dynamic process occurring on the network (Borgatti, 2005). Closeness and betweenness centrality only take into account shortest paths between nodes, but network traffic occurring on longer paths also contributes to global communication patterns. Furthermore, betweenness centrality assumes that whatever flows along the shortest path between two nodes is indivisible and unaffected by patterns of divergence or convergence along the path. A different centrality measure is based on the principal eigenvector of the graph's adjacency matrix (Bonacich, 1972; 2007). Because of the way in which it is computed, eigenvector centrality takes into account interactions of different lengths and their dispersion, relying on walks rather than shortest paths. The measure captures indirect influence patterns by which nodes that are adjacent to highly central nodes become highly central themselves. Eigenvector centrality has not yet been widely applied to biological or neuroscience data sets.[8]

The identification of highly influential nodes and/or edges on the basis of graph topology is an important part of brain network analysis. It represents a step toward the classification of network elements in terms of their potential functional roles (chapter 4). In general, centrality measures identify elements that are highly interactive and/or carry a significant proportion of signal traffic. A node that is highly central in a structural network has the potential to participate in a large number of functional interactions. Conversely, a node that is not central is unlikely to be important in network-wide integrative processes. Furthermore, the loss of nodes or edges with high structural centrality tends to have a larger impact on the functioning of the remaining network.

Network Architectures

Graphs of real-world networks fall into distinct classes that have characteristic architectural features. These architectural features reflect the processes by which the graph was constructed or developed, and they have an extremely important role to play in the function of the network as a whole. We now turn to several classes of network architectures that are the object of ongoing research and are of relevance to the brain.

We first consider a simple class of networks, known as the random network, or the Erdös–Rényi graph (after the mathematicians Paul Erdös and Alfréd Rényi, who made seminal contributions to their theoretical analysis). A random network is constructed by starting with a disconnected set of nodes and connecting pairs of nodes with a uniform probability. Random networks are composed of nodes with fairly uniform degree, and so the degree distribution has a characteristic scale defined by the mean degree. Pairs of nodes in sufficiently dense random networks are typically connected by short paths. On the other hand, nodes that are directly connected maintain uncorrelated patterns of connections, and it is very unlikely for two neighbors of a node to also be neighbors of each other. As a result, random networks have short characteristic path lengths but low levels of clustering.

Another simple class of networks is known as the regular lattice graph. In contrast to random graphs, lattice graphs have an ordered pattern of connections between nodes. Examples of lattice graphs include the ring or grid lattice, where edges link nearby nodes in one or two dimensions, respectively. By their construction, lattice graphs have connections that are "locally dense." Connected nodes tend to have the same neighbors, but distances between nodes vary greatly, with some shortest paths traversing a large number of intermediate nodes. Hence, in contrast to random graphs, lattice graphs have much higher clustering but also much longer characteristic path lengths.

Random and regular graphs are idealized models and permit some very elegant formal description and analysis. However, most real-world networks, including the networks of the brain, are not well described as either random or regular graphs. For example, the connection topology of both random and regular graphs is fairly homogeneous, with all nodes having approximately the same degree and the same level of influence. In most real-world networks, the degree and influence of individual nodes varies over a wide range. Some of the earliest and most fundamental insights into the heterogeneity of real-world networks came from network studies in the social sciences. Since at least the 1950s, network models were used to describe the structure of social groups and to explain the relationship between different topologies of social networks and their collective properties. One of these collective properties, called the "small-world effect," is a phenomenon experienced by almost everyone who participates in social interactions.[9] In a very large social group, perhaps as large as the entire human population, it is often possible to connect two individuals via surprisingly short paths of contact or acquaintanceship—the world of social relationships is a "small world," much smaller than might be expected given the size of the social network. The problem was first treated mathematically in a draft paper that was widely circulated for two decades before finally being published in the inaugural issue of the journal *Social Networks* (Pool and Kochen, 1978). The authors suspected that the small-world effect was rooted in several factors that shape social relationships, from geographical proximity to social stratification and the formation of social cliques. Stanley Milgram's famous experiments conducted in the 1960s provided empirical support for the small-world effect (Travers and Milgram, 1969) and led to the popular notion that any two humans are, on average, linked by no more than "six degrees of separation." Milgram asked randomly selected individuals in Boston and Nebraska to forward a document to target people in Boston. The origin and destination participants were not acquainted, and so participants had to forward the document to other acquaintances in a manner that would bring the document closer to its intended target. The average path length for completed paths originating from the Nebraska group was 5.7. As Jon Kleinberg pointed out (Kleinberg, 2000), Milgram's central finding revealed not only the existence of surprisingly short paths in very large social networks but also the remarkable ability of individuals to identify links that collectively produce a short path to a given target location.[10]

The modern era of network studies was launched by Duncan Watts and Stephen Strogatz in 1998. Watts and Strogatz not only devised a deceptively simple network model that explained the origin of the small-world phenomenon on the basis of connectivity patterns but also discovered that these patterns are present in a broad range of natural, social, and technological networks (Watts and Strogatz, 1998). The model interpolated between a ring lattice and a random network by variation of a single parameter, the probability that an edge of the ring lattice is randomly rewired (see figure 2.3). If this probability is zero, the network is fully regular, and if it the probability is one, the network is fully random. For intermediate settings of the rewiring probability, the graph contains a mixture of regularity and randomness. Watts and Strogatz found that at a very small rewiring probability the graph combined high clustering (much greater than that of the fully random graph) with a short path length (almost as short as that of the fully random graph). The combination of these two properties gave rise to small-world topologies, in which connected nodes have highly overlapping sets of partners (high clustering) yet pairs of nodes are, on average, connected via short paths. Impor-

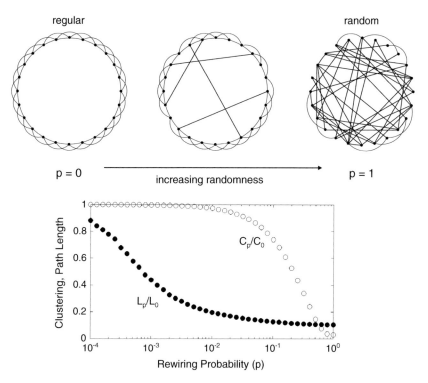

Figure 2.3
The Watts–Strogatz small-world model. Starting from a ring lattice with circular boundary conditions (upper left) connections are randomly rewired with rewiring probability p. For p = 0, the network is completely regular, for p = 1 the network is completely random. Intermediate networks consist of a mixture of random and regular connections. The plots at the bottom show the clustering coefficient C and the path length L, both normalized by their values at p = 0. Note that there is a broad parameter range where networks have clustering that is similar to that of the regular (p = 0) network and have a path length that is similar to that of the random (p = 1) network. Within this range, networks exhibit small-world attributes. Data computed following Watts and Strogatz (1998), with networks consisting of 1,000 nodes and 10,000 edges (average of 400 networks per data point).

tantly, Watts and Strogatz found that small-world attributes were present in a great variety of networks, as diverse as the electrical power grid of the western U.S. and the graph of collaborations among movie actors.

Since the original article by Watts and Strogatz (1998), networks are generally considered to have small-world architecture if they have a much higher clustering coefficient but an approximately equal path length when compared to a population of random networks with equal numbers of nodes and edges. Humphries et al. (2006; Humphries and Gurney, 2008) introduced a measure of "small-world-ness," the small-world index, which expresses the ratio of the clustering coefficient to the path length after both are normalized by corresponding values of random networks. A value of the small-world index significantly greater than one is consistent with the coexistence of the two main attributes of the small-world topology, namely, high clustering and short path length.

It is important to note that the presence of the small-world topology by itself provides only limited information about network architecture. For example, it is possible for two small-world networks to exhibit very different patterns of connectivity. One could say that there exist a number of different types of small-world architectures. Small-world architectures constructed by the algorithm of Watts and Strogatz have high clustering but are not organized into modules. A different class of small-world networks can be generated from sets of isolated modules by gradually redistributing connections from within modules to between modules (Sporns, 2006). As we will see, this class of modular small-world networks is of particular significance to the brain.

A year after the description of small-world networks, Albert-Lázló Barabási and Réka Albert reported another architecture found in many real-world networks. A defining feature of this architecture is an extremely broad and nonhomogeneous degree distribution and hence the existence of nodes with much higher degree than would be expected in a random, regular, or small-world network (see figure 2.4). A number of real-world networks, of citation data, the World Wide Web, and cellular metabolism, were found to exhibit degree distributions that followed a power law.[11] A power law implies that the probability of finding a node with a degree that is twice as large as an arbitrary number decreases by a constant factor. This relationship holds over the entire distribution. For example, if the probability of finding a node with a degree of 10 was 0.4, then doubling the degree to 20 might reduce the probability to 0.1, and doubling it again to 40 lowers the probability to 0.025 (this particular power-law distribution has an exponent of 2). Power-law degree distributions are shared across many networks and indicate a "scale-free" organization (Barabási and Albert, 1999). The term "scale-free" refers to the fact that a power-law distribution has no characteristic scale—"zooming in" on any segment of the distribution does not change its shape, and the assignment of a characteristic scale for the degree of network nodes is therefore meaningless.[12]

Barabási and Albert demonstrated that power-law degree distributions could be generated by a "preferential attachment" growth process. This growth process involves the gradual addition of nodes and the

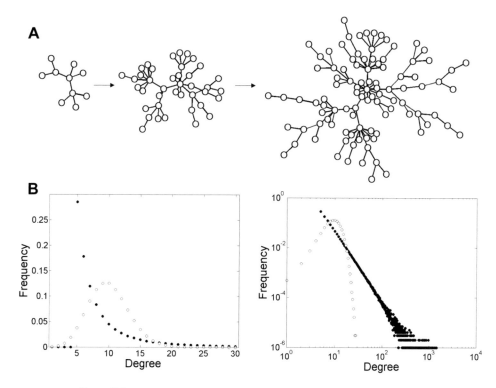

Figure 2.4
Scale-free networks, preferential attachment, and degree distribution. (A) Illustration of
the early stages of network growth by preferential attachment. Nodes are added one by
one, and a single new edge links the new node to an existing node chosen with a probability
based on node degree. The three plots show an example of a growing network at the
10-node, 20-node, and 40-node stage. (B) Degree distribution of a scale-free network (black
dots) and random network (open dots), plotted on linear (left) and double logarithmic
scales (right). Plots show average distributions for 10 networks, each with 100,000 nodes
and a mean degree of 10. Note that the distribution for the scale-free network has a slowly
decaying "heavy tail" when plotted on a linear scale and forms a straight line in the logarithmic plot, indicative of a power law. In comparison, the degrees of the random network
are distributed around a single characteristic scale.

attachment of these nodes to already existing nodes proportional to their
degree. The preferential attachment model remains a key example of
how a simple (local) growth process can shape a global statistical property of a complex network. In the simplest case, linear preferential
attachment yields scale-free networks with an exponent of 3. More
complex attachment rules that vary the "attractiveness" of nodes result
in scale-free networks with exponents anywhere between 2 and 3. If the
attachment of edges involves a cost, as is often the case in spatially

embedded networks where edges take up volume or cost energy, the degree distribution can become truncated for high degrees (Amaral et al., 2000). Such networks exhibit scale-free behavior only over a range of node degrees and are thus called broad-scale.

Random and regular, small-world and scale-free networks represent major classes of network architectures that have been the subject of extensive study and analysis in network science and graph theory. Other architectures are of interest as well but are less well studied and less clearly defined. For example, many real-world networks exhibit hierarchical connection patterns, characterized by nested levels of organization. Such hierarchical networks can combine a scale-free degree distribution and high clustering (Ravasz and Barabási, 2003). Other types of hierarchical networks may have more homogeneous degree distributions and form a small-world architecture composed of nested clusters of nodes. This hierarchical model is of special interest in the case of the brain (see chapters 9 and 12). As illustrated in figure 2.5, different classes of network architecture can be qualitatively arranged within a space of possible networks (Solé and Valverde, 2004), with each class occupying a distinct location. Each architectural class results from a different set of growth processes and enables different patterns of system dynamics. Notably, not all "niches" within this space are populated by networks that are encountered in the real world. Empty regions of this space ("exclusion zones") may be impossible to reach via realistic growth strategies, or they may generate unstable or maladaptive dynamics.

Network Analysis: An Example

Graph analysis is perhaps best illustrated by applying a set of graph measures to an example of a brain network. The example is a structural network of brain regions (nodes) and pathways (edges) covering a large portion of the macaque cerebral cortex. The network was originally derived from numerous anatomical studies and was recently described and analyzed (Honey et al., 2007; Sporns et al., 2007). The network consists of a total of 47 nodes and 505 edges.[13] All edges are binary and hence describe the presence or absence of directed anatomical connections between the nodes. Figure 2.6 shows a plot of the graph's adjacency matrix. Note that this matrix can be displayed in many different ways, depending on the ordering of the nodes along the rows and columns. Reordering the nodes does not change the structure of the graph, and all graph measures are completely invariant with respect to these per-

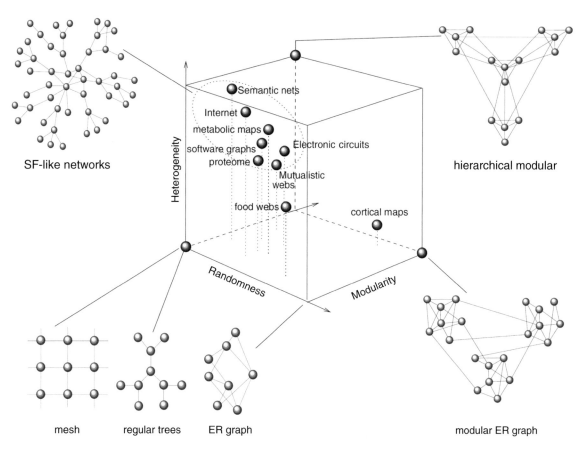

Figure 2.5
Classes of network architectures. In this schematic diagram network architectures are arranged along three major characteristics: randomness, heterogeneity (of node degrees), and modularity. "ER graphs" are Erdös–Rényi random graphs, and "SF-like networks" are networks with scale-free degree distributions. Note that "cortical maps" are placed in a separate region of this space near the location for "modular ER graphs." Reproduced from Solé and Valverde (2004) with permission.

mutations. The ordering of nodes chosen for figure 2.6 was obtained from a previous study (Honey et al., 2007) and roughly corresponds to a division of the macaque cortex into visual and sensorimotor regions. The degree distribution of the graph, also shown in figure 2.6, reveals that node degree varies rather widely within this data set, more so than would be expected in random graphs of identical size and density. Some nodes have very few connections (low-degree nodes) while others are more widely connected (high-degree nodes). The small size of the graph does

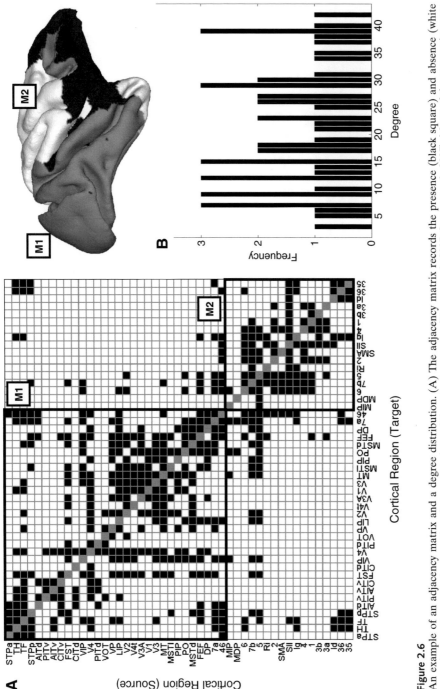

Figure 2.6

An example of an adjacency matrix and a degree distribution. (A) The adjacency matrix records the presence (black square) and absence (white square) of corticocortical connections between regions of the macaque cortex (Honey et al., 2007; Sporns et al., 2007). Many of the connections are symmetrical, and two main modules, corresponding to mostly visual (M1) and mostly somatomotor regions (M2), are indicated in the anatomical surface plot at the upper right. (B) The degree distribution (indegree plus outdegree for each node) is broad, with degrees ranging from 3 to 42. Area abbreviations (after Felleman and Van Essen, 1991): VP, ventral posterior; V1, visual area 1; MT, middle temporal; V3, visual area 3; V2, visual area 2; MSTd, medial superior temporal (dorsal); MSTl, medial superior temporal (lateral); V4, visual area 4; DP, dorsal prelunate; LIP, lateral intraparietal; VIP, ventral intraparietal; FEF, frontal eye field; FST, floor of superior temporal; PO, parieto-occipital; PIP, posterior intraparietal; V3A, visual area V3A; V4t, V4 transitional; AITv, anterior inferotemporal (ventral); PITv, posterior inferotemporal (ventral); CITv, central inferotemporal (ventral); CITd, central inferotemporal (dorsal); PITd, posterior inferotemporal (dorsal); VOT, ventral occipitotemporal; MDP, medial dorsal parietal; MIP, medial intraparietal; 46, area 46; 7a, area 7a; 5, area 5; 7b, area 7b; 6, area 6; AITd, anterior inferotemporal (dorsal); STPa, superior temporal polysensory (anterior); Ig, insular cortex (granular); STPp, superior temporal polysensory (posterior); TF, TF; TH, TH; 2, area 2; 4, area 4; 1, area 1; SII, secondary somatosensory area; SMA, supplemental motor area; 3a, area 3a; 3b, area 3b; Ri, retroinsular cortex; 35, area 35; 36, area 36; Id, insular cortex.

not allow us to reach a definite conclusion on the exact shape of the degree distribution.

Just as there are wide variations in node degree in this network, there are also significant variations in the clustering coefficient. The analysis of clustering coefficients can reveal important differences in the way individual nodes are embedded within their local neighborhoods. Figure 2.7 shows an example of how the clustering coefficient is determined. Somatosensory cortical area 3b has 5 neighbors, most of which are functionally related regions of motor or sensory cortex. These neighbors have 14 out of 20 possible connections between them. Thus, the node's clustering coefficient is 0.7, a high value which indicates that many of the neighbors of node 3b are also neighbors of each other. Across all nodes, the clustering coefficient ranges from 0.33 to 1.00, and the network average is 0.55. Some areas with very low clustering coefficient—for example, area V4—also have high node degree, which indicates that these areas communicate with a great variety of partners that are not connected to each other and thus possibly belong to different specialized communities (see also figures 4.6 and 6.8). Modularity provides complementary information about the extent to which nodes form segregated communities. An optimal modularity score of 0.33 is reached for a partition of the network into 4 modules (see figure 2.7). Each of these modules consists of regions that are functionally related and, for the most part, spatially contiguous on the cortical surface.

Figure 2.8 displays the graph's distance matrix. All entries of the distance matrix have finite values. Thus, the graph is strongly connected since all nodes can be reached from all other nodes in a finite number of steps (between 1 and 4). In functional terms, this means that all regions of the macaque cortex can communicate with all other areas. The global average of the distance matrix corresponds to the network's characteristic path length (2.05 in the current example), which is a marker of integration in the network. The shorter the path length, the "easier" it is to pass information between all pairs of nodes.

The absolute values of clustering coefficient and path length vary greatly with the number of nodes or edges in the network. A comparison with a properly constrained random model (a "null hypothesis") is essential to assess whether the clustering or the path length is significantly different from corresponding values in a population of random networks.[14] A commonly used random model consists of a population of randomly constructed networks that contain an identical number of nodes and edges, as well as identical indegrees and outdegrees for each

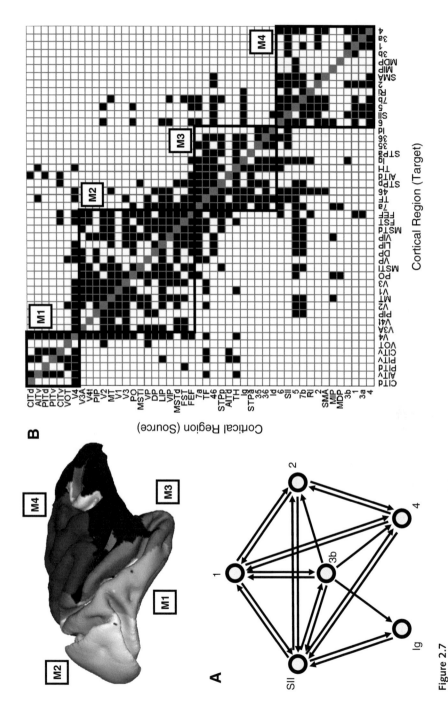

Figure 2.7
An example of clustering and modularity. (A) Connectivity in a local neighborhood around a single node, area 3b of the somatosensory cortex. The node has 5 neighbors, and 14 out of 20 possible directed connections between these neighbors exist, resulting in a clustering coefficient of 0.7. (B) Another rendering of the adjacency matrix (compare to figure 2.6), this time with nodes arranged according to their optimal modularity. Four modules (M1–M4) are indicated, and their locations are drawn in the surface plot of the macaque cortex at the upper left. For abbreviations of cortical areas see figure 2.6.

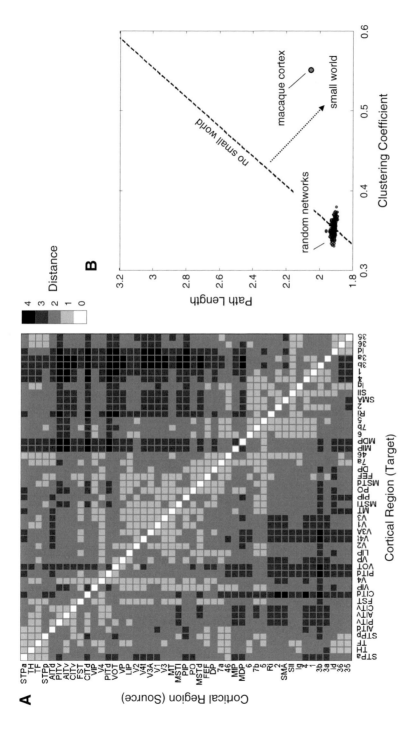

Figure 2.8

An example of a distance matrix and calculation of the small-world index. (A) The distance matrix is shown in the same node order as the adjacency matrix in figure 2.6. Pairwise distances are integers ranging from 0 (along the main diagonal) to a maximum value of 4 (the graph's diameter). (B) Clustering coefficient and path lengths of the matrix of macaque cortex and of a population of 250 random networks (with equal size, density, and degrees). Networks along the dotted line would have clustering and path length exactly proportional to the random population, and therefore a small-world index of 1 ("no small world"). Networks that fall into the region to the lower right have far greater clustering than path lengths, relative to the random population, and thus a small-world index that is much greater than 1 ("small world"). For abbreviations of cortical areas see figure 2.6.

node. Since node degrees are preserved, significant differences in graph measures are not due to the local statistics or overall distribution of node degree. Figure 2.8 shows a comparison of the average clustering coefficient and path length of the macaque cortex with corresponding measures obtained from a population of random networks with identical degrees. The macaque cortex clustering coefficient is significantly greater than the mean obtained from a random population (0.55 vs. 0.35), while its path length is approximately the same (2.05 vs. 1.91), resulting in a small-world index of 1.45. Thus, following our earlier definition, the macaque cortex appears to be a small-world network (see chapter 6).

Finally, we ask if any nodes of this network are more influential, or central, than others. As we discussed earlier, influence or centrality can be assessed on the basis of node degree, the closeness of the node to the rest of the network, or its betweenness on short paths. Figure 2.9 shows a comparison of these three measures of centrality. A set of nodes, including areas V4, FEF, 7a, 7b, 5, and 46, appear at or near the top of all three distributions, indicating that these areas are more central than other nodes. It turns out that several of these nodes correspond to brain regions that were previously classified as "association" or "integrative" centers because of their physiological responses and activations. I will discuss these areas in more detail in chapter 6.

I will have a lot more to say about the definition and interpretation of these and other network measures in coming chapters of the book. Here I wanted to demonstrate the potential of graph analysis tools and illustrate the application of these tools in a simple and intuitive example. Many additional measures can be computed on this example or any other brain network, and a variety of software packages for graph analysis and visualization are available.[15] These packages have various (and often complementary) advantages and disadvantages. Some are more suited for very large graphs (composed of thousands of nodes), while others excel in visualizing and graphically representing complex networks or provide open-access code that can be modified to fit a particular application.

Regardless of the software used in the analyses, the user of graph theoretical tools should be familiar with how graph measures are computed and be aware of their neurobiological interpretation. Several surveys of graph analysis applications to brain connectivity data are available (Sporns, 2003; Sporns et al., 2004; Stam and Reijneveld, 2007; Reijneveld et al., 2007; Bullmore and Sporns, 2009; Rubinov and Sporns,

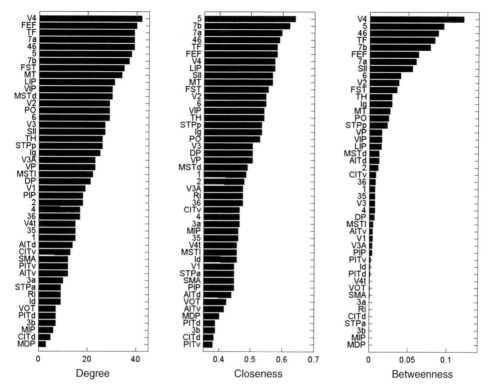

Figure 2.9
A comparison of centrality measures. Diagrams show rank-ordered distributions of degree, closeness, and betweenness for the network of macaque cortex shown in figure 2.6. The rankings of brain regions in the three plots are fairly consistent, indicating substantial overlap of these three centrality measures for this particular network. Note that this mutual agreement does not always exist—it is possible for these measures to show sharply different profiles in some network architectures. For abbreviations of cortical areas see figure 2.6.

2010). Most of these reviews provide technical details about how various graph methods are defined and computed that go beyond what is covered in this introductory chapter.

Complex Networks of the Brain

Starting with Euler's solution to the Königsberg bridge problem, graph theory and network analysis have made essential contributions to an ever wider range of the natural and social sciences. The power of graph-based approaches stems from the fact that virtually all complex systems, regardless of whether they are composed of molecules, neurons, or people, can be meaningfully described as networks.

While there is much appeal in the universality of a mathematical and statistical theory of networks, it is important to remain mindful of the distinction between a real-world system, the rich brew of mechanisms and components, and its abstract mathematical description as a graph. In order for this description to accurately model real system processes, its elementary components, nodes and edges, and their dynamic interactions must be configured in ways that are compatible with the neurobiological system under study.

Different fields have taken different approaches to the study of networks (Borgatti et al., 2009). Unsurprisingly, network theory in the physical sciences emphasized statistical descriptions of global network organization. In the social sciences, network analysis focused more on specific characteristics of nodes and edges and on the ways by which their interactions contribute to a functional outcome. These two approaches are not mutually exclusive, and I would argue that both are important in network neuroscience. Analysis of global network statistics and their association with universal classes of network architectures can provide important initial insights. These insights should be supplemented with more detailed analyses and models incorporating domain-specific knowledge about neural structure and physiology. In all cases, the use and interpretation of graph models has to be motivated by the specific functionality of the neural system at hand.

Given the importance of many of the assumptions that enter into graph descriptions and analyses, we need to gain a better understanding of the nature of brain connectivity. It turns out that there are many ways to define, measure, and represent connectivity in the nervous system. Thus, our next question must be this: What exactly are brain networks?

3 Brain Networks: Structure and Dynamics

Far from being able to accept the idea of the individuality and independence of each nerve element, I have never had reason, up to now, to give up the concept which I have always stressed, that nerve cells, instead of working individually, act together [...]. However opposed it may seem to the popular tendency to individualize the elements, I cannot abandon the idea of a unitary action of the nervous system [...][1]
—Camillo Golgi, 1906

The most fundamental concepts of the organization of the nervous system originated in the second half of the nineteenth century as the result of anatomical and physiological studies that firmly established the cellular basis of brain function. A major controversy at the time concerned two fundamentally different views of neural organization. One view, which became synonymous with the term "neuron doctrine," stated that the nerve cell, or neuron, was the anatomical, physiological, metabolic, and genetic unit of the nervous system. The opposing view rejected the idea that neurons were bounded structures and instead proposed that the thin branches of neuronal fibers formed a continuous nerve network, or "reticulum," allowing neural activity to spread freely across the brain. By the turn of the century, the controversy was settled. The neuron doctrine became, and has remained, one of the foundations of modern neuroscience.

Camillo Golgi was a strong advocate of the nerve network, and his defiant words, quoted above, were spoken on the occasion of his Nobel lecture in 1906, at a time when the neuron doctrine was already firmly established. Golgi's stance was a matter of great irritation for his rival Ramón y Cajal, with whom he shared the Nobel Prize. Cajal's work, much of which utilized a cellular stain developed by Golgi, delivered crucial evidence that neurons were individual cells and communicated through discrete junctions, later termed synapses by Charles Sherrington.

Golgi's futile insistence on a diffuse and continuous nerve network may
have been motivated by his desire to account for the more integrative
or "holistic" aspects of brain function (Shepard, 1991). Golgi was sharply
critical of the concept of functional localization, which he thought was
incompatible with a network "evidently destined to establish a bond of
anatomical and functual [sic] union between the cellular elements"
(Shepard, 1991, p. 99). Golgi could not accept the idea that neurons were
discrete anatomical and functional units of the brain because, he argued,
the functional independence of neurons could not account for the integrative action of the nervous system. Instead, he saw the reticulum as an
anatomical means to ensure functional unity. The dense plexus of fibrils
and fibers formed by neuronal processes (see figure 3.1) provided a

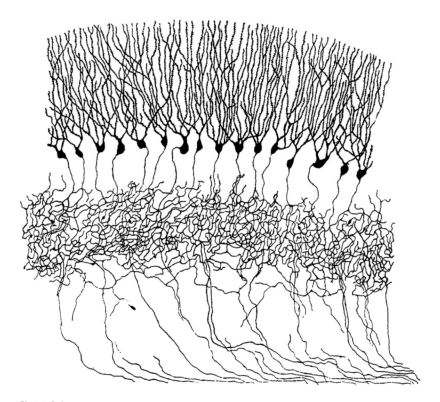

Figure 3.1
The nerve network of the hippocampus from a drawing by Camillo Golgi. At the top,
granule cells of the dentate gyrus send out fine axonal fibers that intermingle within a
"reticular zone" with input fibers arriving from the bottom of the diagram. The reticular
zone is represented as a diffuse network. The image was presented during Golgi's 1906
Nobel Lecture. Reproduced after Shepard (1991).

substrate for structural and functional continuity, and this continuity allowed nerve cells to act collectively.

Despite the victory of Cajal and the neuron doctrine, the intellectual struggle over the manner in which discrete cellular elements can achieve continuity and collective action is far from resolved.[2] A network-based approach may provide a way to address this question, because networks naturally relate the structure of a divisible material object, the brain, to the integrated and continuous flow of neural dynamics. Furthermore, the concepts and tools of complex networks can be applied to both brain structure and function and thus provide a common theoretical framework to understand their relationship. However, any such study must begin with appropriate definitions of brain networks. These definitions are not straightforward as there are many different ways to measure and construct networks from neural data sets. Network topology sensitively depends on the designation of nodes and edges, as well as on the choice of recording techniques and association measures. In this chapter, I provide a brief overview of empirical techniques for observing the brain and describe the most common measures of connectivity used to define brain networks. Throughout the chapter I distinguish three types of connectivity: structural connectivity of physical coupling, functional connectivity of statistical dependencies in neural dynamics, and effective connectivity of causal influences.

Observing the Brain

For much of the early history of neuroscience, observing the brain meant visually examining its anatomy: the convolutions of the cerebral hemispheres, the nerve fibers and gray matter regions, and the fine structure of neurons and their axonal and dendritic processes. Over 100 years ago, techniques for staining and sectioning nerve tissue were already well developed and widely applied, and anatomists such as Dejerine and Cajal had cataloged and described brain and neuronal morphology in exquisite detail. Cajal, who deduced that neurons were polarized cells and relayed signals from a receptive structure (the dendrite) to a transmissive one (the axon), annotated his meticulous ink drawings of neuronal circuits with arrows indicating the direction of signal propagation. However, the nature of the propagated signal remained obscure until later in the twentieth century as new methods for detecting electrical activity of neural tissue began to appear.

Most of the major breakthroughs regarding the nature of neuronal activity and neurotransmission were obtained with electrophysiological recordings of single neurons, carried out in the intact brain of an awake or anesthetized animal, or in an explanted piece of tissue. Such recordings provide extremely high spatial (micrometer) and temporal (millisecond) resolution and allow direct observation of electrical currents and potentials generated by single nerve cells. This high resolution comes at considerable cost, as all cellular recording techniques are highly invasive, requiring surgical intervention and placement of bulky recording electrodes within brain tissue. Nevertheless, electrophysiological recordings allow the most direct access to neural signals. Most, but not all, neurons communicate via action potentials or "spikes," and neural recordings are therefore often transformed into series of discrete spiking events that can be characterized in terms of rate and timing. Neural activity can also be recorded with a variety of optical imaging methods, based on intrinsic voltage-dependent signals and calcium- or voltage-sensitive dyes.

Less direct observations of electrical brain activity involve the recording of electromagnetic potentials generated by combined electrical currents of large neuronal populations. These techniques—electroencephalography (EEG) and magnetoencephalography (MEG)—are noninvasive as recordings are made through groups of sensors placed on, or near, the surface of the head.[3] EEG and MEG directly record signals generated by neuronal activity and consequently have a high temporal resolution. On the other hand, the spatial resolution is comparatively poor as neither technique allows an unambiguous reconstruction of the electrical sources responsible for the recorded signal. Since sources are difficult to localize in anatomical space, EEG and MEG signals are often processed in sensor space, and their analysis involves a broad range of signal processing techniques in the time and frequency domain.

Noninvasive techniques for recording neural activity at high spatial and temporal resolution do not currently exist. Positron emission tomography (PET) and functional magnetic resonance imaging (fMRI), respectively, measure metabolic and hemodynamic signals, which are only indirectly related to neural activity. Both techniques allow the reconstruction of spatially localized signals at millimeter-scale resolution across the imaged brain volume.[4] In the case of fMRI, the primary measure of activity is the contrast between the magnetic susceptibility of oxygenated and deoxygenated hemoglobin within each volume element ("voxel"), hence called the "blood oxygen level-dependent" (BOLD) signal. However, although blood oxygenation, blood volume, and flow rate are coupled to neuronal activity and cerebrovascular responses, the nature of this coupling is complex and can vary across regions of the brain. Consequently, the BOLD signal can only be viewed as an indirect measure of neural activity.[5] In addition, the slow time constants of the BOLD response result in poor temporal resolution on the order of seconds.[6] Hence, one important objective of neuroimaging data analysis is the inference of neural processes that are causally responsible for the observed data (see below).

The nature of neural signals recorded by the above techniques differs significantly in both spatial and temporal resolutions and in the directness with which neuronal activity is detected. The simultaneous use of two or more recording methods within the same experiment can reveal how different neural or metabolic signals are interrelated (Logothetis et al., 2001). Each technique measures a different aspect of neural dynamics and organization, and the interpretation of neural data sets must take these differences into account. There are several reasons why the current heterogeneity of methods and approaches is likely to persist. First, all methods for observing brain structure and function have advantages but also disadvantages that limit their range of applicability or resolution. Some methods provide great structural detail but are invasive or cover only a small part of the brain, while other methods may be noninvasive but have poor spatial or temporal resolution. Second, nervous systems are organized on multiple scales, from synaptic connections between single cells, to the organization of cell populations within individual anatomical regions, and finally to the large-scale architecture of brain regions and their interconnecting pathways. Different techniques are sensitive to different levels of organization.

This last point deserves to be emphasized. The multiscale aspect of the nervous system is an essential feature of its organization and network architecture. Descriptions of the brain at large scales should not be regarded as poorly resolved approximations of an underlying microscopic order. Instead, brain connectivity at the large scale (among regions and systems) describes neural processes that are the outcome of dynamic coordination among smaller elements, and such a description has as much validity as one that captures processes at the small scale (among individual cells and synapses). Different scales offer parallel and complementary views of brain organization and cannot be reduced to a single observational scale or method.[7] The multiscale nature of brain networks and dynamics will occupy us over most of the book (e.g., chapters 9, 12, and 13).

Defining Brain Connectivity

Given the broad range of methods for observing the brain, it is not surprising that there are also many different ways to describe and measure brain connectivity (Horwitz, 2003; Lee et al., 2003; Jirsa and McIntosh, 2007). Brain connectivity can be derived from histological sections that reveal anatomical connections, from electrical recordings of single nerve cells, or from functional imaging of the entire brain. Even when using a single recording technique, different ways of processing neural data may result in different descriptions of the underlying network.

Perhaps the most fundamental distinction is between structural connectivity as a "wiring diagram" of physical links and functional connectivity as a web of "dynamic interactions." Throughout the book we will adhere to this very basic distinction. As will become apparent in many later chapters, structural and functional connectivity are mutually interdependent, and one of the most important questions in the area of brain networks concerns the way in which structural and functional networks shape and constrain each other. A third class of brain networks defines "effective connectivity," which encompasses the network of directed interactions between neural elements. Effective connectivity attempts to go beyond structural and functional connectivity by identifying patterns of causal influence among neural elements. While the vast majority of network studies have so far been carried out on structural and functional connectivity, effective connectivity is of special interest because it attempts to reveal the causes driving observed patterns of neural activity.

Before describing individual measures of connectivity, let us define the three main types of brain connectivity more precisely:

Structural connectivity refers to a set of physical or structural (anatomical) connections linking neural elements. These anatomical connections range in scale from those of local circuits of single cells to large-scale networks of interregional pathways. Their physical pattern may be thought of as relatively static at shorter time scales (seconds to minutes) but may be plastic or dynamic at longer time scales (hours to days)—for example, during development or in the course of learning and synaptic remodeling (see chapter 4). Depending on how anatomical networks are recorded or traced (see chapter 5), the resulting structural networks may contain binary or weighted edges, and these edges may be either directed or undirected (see chapter 2).

Functional connectivity captures patterns of deviations from statistical independence between distributed and often spatially remote neuronal units (Friston, 1993; 1994). The basis of all functional connectivity is time series data from neural recordings. These data may be extracted from cellular recordings, EEG, MEG, fMRI, or other techniques. Deviations from statistical independence are generally taken to indicate dynamic coupling and can be measured, for example, by estimating the correlation or covariance, spectral coherence, or phase locking between pairs of time series. Unlike structural connectivity, functional connectivity is highly time dependent, and it can be statistically nonstationary. In many cases, functional connectivity changes on a scale of hundreds of milliseconds, and it is modulated by external task demands and sensory stimulation, as well as the internal state of the organism. Because it expresses statistical relationships, functional connectivity does not make any explicit reference to causal effects among neural elements or to an underlying structural model of the anatomy. Hence, an observed statistical dependence between two nodes does not allow the inference of a causal interaction between them.

Effective connectivity describes the network of causal effects between neural elements (Friston, 1994; Büchel and Friston, 2000), which can be inferred through time series analysis, statistical modeling, or experimental perturbations. Like functional connectivity, effective connectivity is time dependent and can be rapidly modulated by external stimuli or tasks, as well as changes in internal state. Some approaches to effective connectivity derive directed interactions from temporal precedence and are consequently "model free." Others require the specification of an explicit causal model including structural parameters, that is, anatomical pathways. The estimation of effective connectivity requires complex data processing and modeling techniques, several of which are described later in this chapter.

While these definitions provide a rough operational framework for discussing and investigating brain connectivity, the close relationship between structure and function in the brain can create some ambiguity as to whether a neural parameter is best classified as structural or functional. For example, neuronal function is profoundly constrained by biophysical properties of neurons, which in turn depend on cellular morphology as well as the expression, chemical modification, and cellular distribution of molecular components. Similarly, neuronal communication is significantly affected by axonal conduction delays, which depend on structural attributes of the axon (length, diameter, and myelination). Thus, a comprehensive representation of structural connectivity should comprise not only information about whether connections between pairs of nodes are present or absent but also about neuronal biophysical properties and axonal conduction delays. Very few of the currently available structural connectivity data sets include this information.

No single mode of brain connectivity is sufficient to fully explain how brain networks operate. It is sometimes proclaimed that the function of the brain will become apparent once we possess the brain's wiring diagram (see chapter 5). Such views are overly simplistic, because the wiring alone does not account for the physiology of neural interactions, for the rich repertoire of spontaneous and task-dependent neural responses, or for their temporal patterning. At the same time, dynamic patterns of neural interactions cannot be fully interpreted unless structural connectivity is taken into account. Both structural and functional networks (or their union in a suitable model of effective connectivity) are needed to fully explain the time evolution of spontaneous network activity or of neural responses to perturbation.

Nodes and Edges

The construction of structural and functional brain networks from empirical data proceeds along several main steps (see figure 3.2; Bullmore and Sporns, 2009). The first step is the definition of network nodes, followed by an estimation of a (usually continuous) measure of association between pairs of nodes. These estimates are then compiled into an association matrix, which is often made sparse by removing weak relationships ("thresholding") in order to examine the structure of the strongest pairwise associations.[8] The final step is the calculation of graph measures from the fully weighted or thresholded association (adjacency) matrix and the statistical comparison of these measures to populations of random networks (as in the example discussed in chapter 2). Each of these steps requires choices in the processing and partitioning of empirical data sets. It is important to remember that graphs (sets of nodes and edges) are *descriptions* of real systems and that the choices made in parsing the system into nodes and in estimating measures of their mutual association will influence the results obtained from network analysis (Butts, 2009; Zalesky et al., 2010).

One of the most fundamental problems of graph analysis in the brain is the definition of nodes and edges. In some areas of network science,

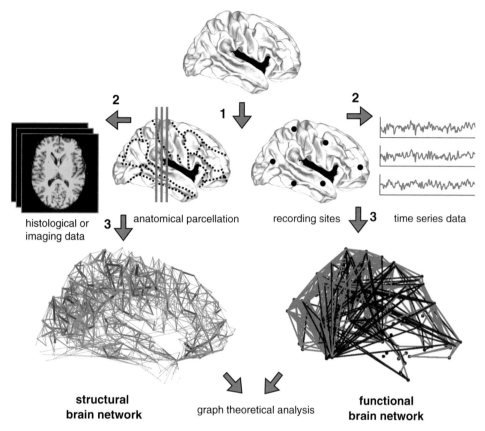

histological or   **3**   anatomical parcellation   recording sites **3**   time series data
imaging data

**structural   functional
brain network**   graph theoretical analysis   **brain network**

Figure 3.2
Constructing and measuring structural and functional brain networks. The diagram illustrates four major steps: definition of network nodes (step 1), estimation of association
measure (step 2), generation of an association matrix and a network composed of nodes
and edges (step 3), and graph theoretical analysis (step 4). Network representations are
from Hagmann et al. (2008) and Achard et al. (2006), modified and reproduced with permission. The diagram was redrawn and modified after Bullmore and Sporns (2009).

the definition of nodes and edges is quite straightforward. In social networks, nodes usually represent individuals that are part of a social group.
Studies of the World Wide Web typically identify nodes and edges as
hyperlinked web pages, and studies of citation or collaboration patterns
examine links between citing and cited documents or between groups of
researchers. In the case of the brain, nodes and edges are more difficult
to define. At first glance, the most natural partition is that of individual
neurons and their synaptic connections.[9] However, most neural recording techniques do not allow the direct observation of large numbers of

individual neurons. Techniques that resolve single neurons currently permit the observation of only a small number of cells embedded within a vast and mostly unobserved network. All noninvasive techniques, while covering a large part of the brain, record signals that originate from neuronal populations. Hence, virtually all studies of structural and functional brain networks require a parcellation of the recorded brain volume into distinct regions and connections. The rationale for the parcellation process imposes important constraints on the subsequent network analysis.

Node definition generally involves an anatomical parcellation into coherent regions on the basis of histological or imaging data. Objective parcellation, for example, of the cerebral cortex into a set of uniquely specified functionally coherent and nonoverlapping regions presents significant challenges that have still only been partially addressed (see chapter 4). Simple parcellation schemes based on anatomical landmarks are imprecise and insufficient to fully represent the true anatomical and functional diversity of the cortical architecture. More sophisticated approaches utilize information about structural and/or functional connectivity to define regions with a coherent connectivity profile, ideally obtained from individual brains (Johansen-Berg et al., 2004; Cohen et al., 2008). An alternative approach involves defining nodes as individual voxels in fMRI data or electrodes or sensors in electrophysiological or MEG experiments. This approach can be problematic due to shared variance among spatially contiguous recording sites, especially in EEG and MEG (Ioannides, 2007). Reconstruction of anatomical sources could conceivably map extracranially recorded electromagnetic potentials back into an anatomical partition, but source reconstruction algorithms still have limited coverage, accuracy, and resolution.

Edge definition involves the estimation of pairwise associations between nodes. Again, important choices have to be made, since there is a very wide range of potential measures of structural, functional, or effective association. Structural networks are constructed from measures of physical association—for example, the number of stained or reconstructed axonal fibers that link two nodes in an anatomical partition (see chapter 5). Functional networks are usually derived from symmetrical measures of statistical dependence such as cross-correlation, coherence, or mutual information. Effective networks can be defined on the basis of estimates for pairwise causal or directed interactions, obtained from time series analysis or from coefficients of models designed to infer causal patterns.

Connection, Correlation, Causation

The application of multiple recording techniques to the same neuronal preparation or the same individual brain can deliver multiple sets of associations within a single nodal partition. For example, noninvasive neuroimaging techniques allow researchers to simultaneously map structural and functional connections from recordings of dynamic time series data in the same individual. Can we use these data to deduce the complex chains of neural events causing other neural events in the course of perception and cognition? The inference of causality from a joint knowledge of anatomy and neural dynamics is a central question in theoretical neuroscience.

As defined earlier, functional connectivity records statistical dependencies between elements of a neural system or between neural recording sites. The relative ease with which measures of functional connectivity can be estimated has helped to promote their widespread use in the analysis of neuronal time series data. Bivariate statistical dependencies can be computed in the time domain as cross-correlation or mutual information, with the latter measure capturing both linear and nonlinear interactions. They can also be computed in the spectral domain as coherence, phase synchronization, or generalized nonlinear synchronization, for example, the synchronization likelihood (Stam, 2006). While these functional connectivity measures allow mapping of statistical patterns of dynamic coupling, they cannot reveal causal processes occurring among neurons or brain regions. For example, functional connectivity measures cannot detect whether dynamic coupling is due to direct and indirect interaction or due to a common external influence, such as shared input. Effective connectivity attempts to go beyond the fundamentally correlative construct of statistical dependence and aims to identify a network of causes or directed influences that explain the observed data. This endeavor faces a number of fundamental obstacles associated with the concept of "causality."[10]

The use of perturbations offers one approach for discerning causal patterns. Before the advent of sophisticated tracers for mapping neuroanatomical connections, neuronal stimulation was used to create localized perturbations and observe their effects on other parts of the brain. In a variant of this approach, called physiological neuronography, strychnine, which partially blocks inhibitory neurotransmission, was applied to a small patch of cortex, resulting in local disinhibition and propagation of excitatory activity away from the stimulation site. In anesthetized animals, it was found that strychnine-induced excitation did not spread across multiple synapses (Dusser de Barenne and McCulloch, 1939) and could thus reveal the extent of axonal connectivity emitted from the stimulated location. In an extensive series of studies, Dusser de Barenne and McCulloch (1938; Bailey et al., 1940) used strychnine neuronography to map directed functional relations mediated by interareal axons linking regions of the primate sensorimotor cortex. The diagrammatic summary of their results (see figure 3.3) essentially represents one of the earliest examples of a connection matrix of directed functional (and anatomical) relations between a set of brain regions. While neuronography was essentially abandoned half a century ago, other perturbational approaches for recording directed neural interactions continue today.[11]

One of the first formal definitions of effective connectivity originated in neurophysiology in the analysis of spike trains obtained from multielectrode recordings (Gerstein and Perkel, 1969; Aertsen et al., 1989; Aertsen and Preissl, 1991). Effective connectivity was defined as the minimal neuronal circuit model that could account for observed correlations between simultaneously recorded spike trains after stimulus-induced modulations of single neuron firing rates have been discounted. This circuit model was not intended to represent a unique solution to the "inverse problem" of inferring synaptic connections from spike trains. In fact, effective connectivity between individual neurons in cat visual cortex was found to exhibit rapid stimulus-locked modulations (Aertsen et al., 1989). In neuroimaging and cognitive neuroscience, effective connectivity, as originally defined by Karl Friston, attempts to reconstruct or "explain" recorded time-varying activity patterns in terms of underlying causal influences of one brain region over another (Friston, 1994; Büchel and Friston, 2000; Friston, 2009a). While there are conceptual similarities between effective connectivity in neurophysiology and in neuroimaging, there are also significant differences, primarily in temporal/spatial resolution and the nature of the recorded neural signal.

One approach to effective connectivity estimates directed interactions from observed neural data without making any assumptions about an underlying structural model or measuring the effects of perturbations. These methods utilize neural time series data to extract information about directed (or causal) interactions by exploiting the fundamental fact that causes must precede effects in time. One of the most widely used methods, Granger causality, was originally developed for social and economic systems (Granger, 1969). Based on time-lagged linear regression analysis, Granger causality captures the amount of information

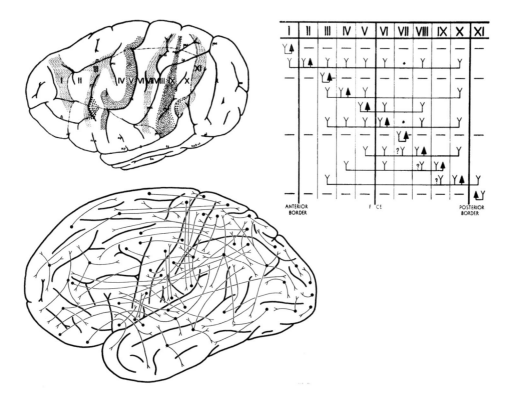

Figure 3.3
Mapping of connectivity with strychnine neuronography. The image on the top left shows the surface of the chimpanzee cortex, indicating the extent and location of functional subdivisions of the sensory cortex of the arm, numbered as bands II through X, and adjacent bands I and XI. The diagram on the top right shows a summary of the functional (and anatomical) relations detected with strychnine neuronography between cortical bands I through XI. "Anterior border" and "posterior border" mark the limits of sensory cortex, and "F CE" marks the fissura centralis (also called the Rolandic fissure). Black triangles schematically represent cell bodies, with excitatory axons and synapses ("Y") extending into other areas. Suppressive effects after the application of strychnine to bands I, III, VII, and XI are indicated by "–." The diagram represents an early example of a cortical connection matrix. The image on the bottom is a summary of directed functional (anatomical) relationships revealed by strychnine neuronography of chimpanzee cortex from Bailey and von Bonin (1951), reproduced with permission. Top illustrations are reproduced from Bailey et al. (1940) with permission.

about the future state of one variable that is gained by taking into account the past states of another variable. Granger causality has been widely applied in neuroscience (Kaminski et al., 2001; Ding et al., 2006)—for example, to EEG data sets obtained from large-scale sensorimotor networks (Brovelli et al., 2004) as well as fMRI time series (Goebel et al., 2003; Roebroeck et al., 2005; Bressler et al., 2008). A related measure based on information theory, called transfer entropy, is also based on temporal precedence cues and takes into account linear as well as non-linear interactions (Schreiber, 2000). Transfer entropy detects directed interactions between two variables by considering the effects of the state of one variable on the state transition probabilities of another variable.[12]

It is important to note that approaches to effective connectivity based on temporal precedence rely on several key assumptions (Friston, 2009a). Since these methods operate in discrete time, the parsing of the naturally continuous system dynamics into sequences of discrete states should conform to the time scale at which these states cause each other. Most importantly, the recorded variables must accurately preserve the temporal dependencies present within the system. This last assumption is violated if there are delays in the responses of these variables due to perturbations, as may be the case for fMRI signals due to regional variations in the hemodynamic response function (David et al., 2009). Such delays can disrupt the sequence of observed time series, possibly reversing the temporal order of cause and effect. Finally, Granger causality and related methods rely on statistical patterns of observed responses[13] but do not infer the hidden neural causes that underlie these observations.

In contrast to methods based on temporal precedence, there are several approaches for extracting effective connectivity under constraints imposed by a structural model of synaptic connectivity or interregional pathways. One of the earliest techniques is called covariance structural equation modeling (CSEM) and assigns effective connection strengths to anatomical pathways that best match observed covariance patterns, often recorded during performance of a specific cognitive task (McIntosh and Gonzalez-Lima, 1994; Horwitz et al., 1999). This technique has been applied in different cognitive domains, allowing the identification of time- and task-dependent differences in connectivity between a fixed set of brain regions. For example, McIntosh et al. (1994) used PET data to show that object or spatial vision tasks were associated with different effective connections among occipital, temporal, and parietal regions of visual cortex (see chapter 9, figure 9.5). In another example, an fMRI study of repetition suppression revealed that learning-related decreases in the activation of specialized cortical areas were accompanied by increases in effective connectivity extracted by path analysis (Büchel et al., 1999). One of the drawbacks of CSEM is that it does not explicitly model neural time series or temporal changes in experimental context (Stephan, 2004).

More recently, Karl Friston and colleagues have formulated a theoretical framework called dynamic causal modeling (DCM; Friston et al., 2003; Stephan and Friston, 2007). DCM uses statistical inference to estimate parameters for directed influences between neural elements, explicitly in the context of experimental perturbations (see figure 3.4). This inference is carried out by a comparison of neuronal models that include structural and biophysical parameters describing neural populations and their interactions, as well as a hemodynamic mechanism for the generation of fMRI signals. DCM identifies distributions of parameters that can account for observed fMRI data, and DCM also selects the model that describes the data most accurately and most parsimoniously by quantifying the model evidence. Unlike methods based on temporal precedence, DCM makes an inference on brain dynamics modeled as a system of coupled differential equations governing temporally continuous processes and derives estimates for parameters that relate directly to neuronal structure and biophysics. Hence, it explicitly tests hypotheses about how data are generated by inferring the form and coefficients of the neural system's equations of motion. Applications of DCM are discussed further in chapter 9.

The estimation of effective connectivity still presents a number of difficult technical and interpretational challenges. Structural equation modeling and dynamic causal modeling are sensitive to choices made about the underlying structural and/or dynamic model, while measures based on temporal precedence are sensitive to the rate and temporal resolution at which data are acquired. These difficulties notwithstanding, applications of effective connectivity are likely to grow in the future as they promise to reveal how brain responses are generated through temporally ordered dynamic processes unfolding in structural networks. Because computational models are a central component of effective connectivity and play an increasingly important role in studies of brain connectivity, we need to briefly review how such models are configured and tested against empirical data.

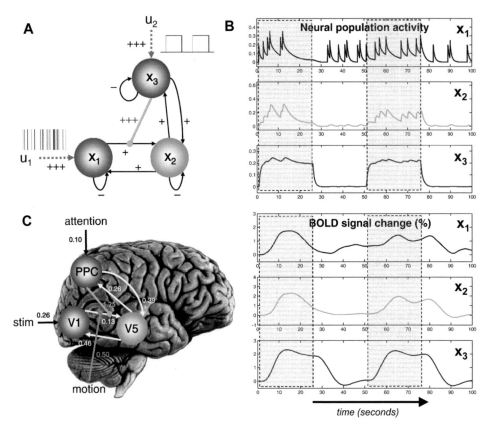

Figure 3.4
Effective connectivity. (A) A representation of a nonlinear neural model involving three neural regions (x_1–x_3) and their interconnections. Regions x_1 and x_3 receive external inputs (u_1 and u_2, respectively), and the output of region x_3 modulates the efficacy of the connection from x_1 to x_2. Plots in (B) show the time courses of modeled neural population activity (top) and synthetic blood-oxygen-level-dependent (BOLD) signal change (bottom). Note that activation of x_3 enables transmission of signals from x_1 to x_2. The model was used in dynamic causal modeling to estimate parameters in a neuroimaging study of attentional modulation of motion signals (C). Activity in the posterior parietal cortex (PPC = x_3) was found to modulate the efficacy of the connection from visual area V1 (x_1) to V5 (x_2) and thus the effect of sensory stimulation (stim). Adapted from Stephan et al. (2008); reproduced with permission.

Models of Brain Connectivity

Neither "armchair theorizing" nor formal mathematical analysis is sufficient to deal with the rich spatiotemporal structure of complex systems. Instead, computer simulations of such systems are necessary to form and test hypotheses and to gain mechanistic insight. Without the use of computer simulations, it would be impossible to explore complex physical processes such as the formation of planets from spinning circumstellar disks of gas and dust, the impact of human activity on climate change, or the folding of proteins.

Computational approaches to complex systems now pervade many scientific disciplines, and neuroscience is no exception. The extraordinary variety and complexity of neural activity patterns requires computational modeling of empirical data to achieve an understanding of the system that is both explanatory and predictive. Models are the basis of most, perhaps all, empirical investigation in neuroscience.[14] No hypothesis is formulated, no empirical measure is selected, and no experimental manipulation is devised without recourse to some sort of model or representation of the essential components and interactions and their expected behavior. Charts of cellular signaling pathways, box-and-arrow diagrams of cognitive processes, and circuit maps of neurons are models that inform and motivate empirical research. These models are often defined only implicitly and nonquantitatively. Increasingly, however, empirical researchers make use of models that are explicitly defined in a computational framework. The design of a computational model requires the choice of model components and the quantitative formulation of their unit and aggregate behavior. Thus, one important implication of computational modeling is the necessity to explicitly parameterize potentially ill-defined and qualitative concepts. Comprehensive surveys of computational neuroscience testify to the broad range of modeling approaches and the increasing integration of computational models and empirical investigation (e.g., Dayan and Abbott, 2001). In studies of brain networks and connectivity, models occupy an important role (Breakspear and Jirsa, 2007). Dynamic connectivity-based models are indispensable for understanding how the local activity of neural units is coordinated and integrated to achieve global patterns, and we will encounter such models frequently in the course of this book (see chapters 8–13).

The basis of all computational models is a set of state equations that govern the temporal evolution of the dynamic variables. These equations can take different forms. Often they are differential equations that describe the rate of change of a system variable. In brain models, such variables may stand for electrical membrane potentials, and the state equations describe how these potentials change as a result of changes in membrane conductances or synaptic inputs. The integration of these equations, usually carried out numerically by a computer, generates time series data that can be embedded in a geometric phase space. If the state equations describe two variables, a suitable phase space is the two-dimensional plane, and successive states of the system can be represented as a trajectory within this space. Given a set of initial conditions, the trajectory of the system will flow toward a bounded set of points that constitute an attractor. If the state equations are sufficiently complex, multiple attractors can coexist, and different initial conditions may end up on the same or different attractors. An attractor may be as simple as a single "fixed point" or have a more elaborate geometric shape such as limit cycles (in the case of periodic dynamics) or strange attractors (in the case of chaotic dynamics). An attractor is stable if the dynamic system returns to it after a small deflection. The set of points from which the system flows to a given attractor is its basin of attraction. As the parameters of a dynamic system are varied, the system trajectories may describe very different paths and approach qualitatively different attractors.

There are several systems of differential equations for describing the activity of individual neurons or of neuronal populations. Perhaps the most famous among these is the system of conductance-based coupled ordinary differential equations formulated by Hodgkin and Huxley (1952). The Hodgkin–Huxley model describes the generation of action potentials as a function of current flows through sodium, potassium, and chloride ion channels. Different models describe neural processes at different levels of scale. There are systems for modeling neural dynamics at the microscale of individual neurons (as in the case of the Hodgkin–Huxley equations), at the mesoscale of local populations of neurons such as columns, or at the macroscale of entire brain regions (Deco et al., 2008).

Synaptic interactions between neural elements are implemented by a coupling or connectivity matrix. Connectivity between neural masses creates large-scale neural models that aim to describe spatiotemporal dynamics of a large neural system based on realistic biophysical mechanisms. The connectivity structure is provided by a structural adjacency matrix (see chapter 2) that incorporates spatial (topological) parameters and, in many cases, also temporal (conduction delays) parameters. The temporal dynamics and attractors of coupled large-scale neural models can be analyzed with the tools of dynamical systems theory. Some models allow the mapping of simulated neural states to observables such as electromagnetic surface potentials or BOLD responses and thus enable direct comparison of model data to empirical data. Importantly, models can be manipulated in ways that are difficult or impossible in real neural systems. This allows systematic variations in biophysical parameters or in the space–time structure of the coupling matrix to be related to different dynamic regimes and global states attained by the large-scale system.

The prediction of the large-scale behavior of a complex system requires more than a description of the dynamic behavior of its components or a wiring diagram of its interactions. Model-based numerical simulations are often the only means by which such predictions can be generated— this is true for the complex spatiotemporal dynamics of molecules inside a cell, for the time evolution of social and economic systems, and for models of the global environment.[15] For example, computational models that attempt to predict future climate change are based on simulations of the entire "earth system," including the distribution of landmasses and oceans, solar energy input and dissipation, atmospheric and oceanic chemistry and flow patterns, as well as biological processes (McGuffie and Henderson-Sellers, 2001). These simulations are implemented as coupled differential equations on a three-dimensional grid covering the earth surface. Predictions of the long-term effects of perturbations or driving forces due to human activity are made on the basis of numerical simulations that are calibrated using data about the past of the earth's climate.

There are some parallels between these computational studies of the earth system and those of the brain. Perhaps, a "global brain simulator" will soon be on the horizon.[16] A feasible near-term goal of such a simulator would be the implementation of a realistic model of the large-scale dynamics of the human brain at a level of scale commensurate with that used in noninvasive neuroimaging and electrophysiology. Comprehensive data on brain connectivity (the "connectome"; see chapter 5) is essential to constrain such a model. If appropriately configured, a detailed "forward model" of the human brain would allow predictions about patterns of endogenous brain dynamics, about the responsiveness of the "brain system" to various exogenous stimuli, and about pathological changes in brain dynamics following damage or disease.

From Components to Patterns

There is great diversity in the way brain connectivity can be measured, computed, and represented, reflecting the many neural recording techniques that allow the direct or indirect observation of neural activity on different time and spatial scales. The distinct nature of neural signals obtained by techniques as disparate as cellular neurophysiology and functional neuroimaging can obscure the fact that underneath electrodes, sensors, and magnetic coils there is a single biological system, whose true structure and function is the object of the investigation. There is an urgent need for empirical data and computational models that provide insight into the relationship of neural signals from different recording modalities (hemodynamic responses, cellular or electromagnetic surface potentials) and, by extension, the ways in which brain connectivity estimated from these signals can be combined. The relationship between neural events in macroscopic brain systems, within millimeter-scale brain voxels, or among individual cells and synapses will be illuminated by more accurate models of connectivity at these different scales (Honey et al., 2010).

Connectivity translates unitary events at the cellular scale into large-scale patterns. Once the cellular machinery for generating impulses and for transmitting them rapidly between cells had evolved, connectivity became a way by which neurons could generate diverse patterns of response and mutual statistical dependence. Connectivity allows neurons to act both independently *and* collectively, thus providing the substrate for the "unitary action of the nervous system" that was so important to Camillo Golgi. The neuron doctrine has remained an important foundation of modern neuroscience, and yet its emphasis on the neuron as an autonomous anatomical and physiological unit of the nervous system should not be mistaken for the notion that the functioning of the brain can be reduced to that of its cellular substrate. Brain function is fundamentally integrative—it requires that components and elementary processes work together in complex patterns (Kelso, 1995). Connectivity is essential for integrating the actions of individual neurons and thus for enabling cognitive processes such as perception, attention, and memory.

The neuron doctrine, with its insistence on the functional autonomy of cellular elements of the brain, very much reflects the mechanistic leanings of the nineteenth century. A different and related mechanistic idea, functional localization, also originated during that time. It turns out that an analysis of brain connectivity can illuminate how function is localized and represented among nerve cells and brain regions.

4 A Network Perspective on Neuroanatomy

> Although I believe in the principle of localization, I have asked myself and still ask myself within what limits this principle can be applied. [...] There are in the human mind a group of faculties, and in the brain groups of convolutions, and the facts assembled by science so far allow to state, as I said before, that the great regions of the mind correspond to the great regions of the brain. It is in this sense that the principle of localization appears to be, if not rigorously demonstrated, so at least probable. But to know whether each particular faculty has its seat in a particular convolution, is a question which seems completely insoluble at the present state of science.[1]
> —Paul Broca, 1861

Few theoretical concepts have had a deeper, more confounding influence in the history of neuroscience than the concept of functional localization (Phillips et al., 1984; Young, 1990; Finger, 1994). The debate surrounding functional localization has raged for at least two centuries, pitching those who view brain function as resulting from the action of specialized centers against others who conceptualize brain function as fundamentally nonlocal and distributed. The battle plays out on the grand stage of whole-brain anatomy and in cellular physiology where highly specific responses of single neurons are usually interpreted as localized substrates of complex perceptual and cognitive functions.[2] This chapter explores how a more complete understanding of structure–function relationships in the brain can be achieved by taking a network perspective. I will argue that the problem of functional localization, or more generally the relationship between anatomical locations and mental processes, is productively addressed when the system is conceptualized as a complex network.

One of the goals of neuroanatomy is the identification of anatomical units (cells, cell groups, or brain regions) and the mapping of their interconnections to reveal brain architecture (Swanson, 2003; 2007). Once the brain's elements and connections have been determined, they collectively form a structural network that can be explored with the tools and methods of network science. For example, the organization and topology of structural brain networks provides quantitative information about the differential contributions of individual network elements to the overall architecture (see chapter 2). This information is useful when considering regional functional specialization in the brain. In most biological systems the elements of a given network display some level of functional specialization; that is, they participate in different system processes to a varying degree. Specialization among network elements can arise in two ways. It can be the result of differences that are intrinsic to each of the elements—for example, their intrinsic capacity to process information. Alternatively, or additionally, it can be the result of differences in their extrinsic connections, which determine the way the elements exchange information between each other. In other words, the functional specialization of each local element is determined in part by the intrinsic properties of the element and in part by its extrinsic network interactions. Thus, mapping the anatomy of brain networks offers important clues as to the functional specialization of each of the network elements.

An example from another domain of network biology may help to clarify this point. Modern molecular biology generates a wealth of genomic sequence data that poses significant challenges for identifying the functional roles of individual proteins. Classical methodologies for predicting protein function examine structural characteristics of individual proteins and infer function on the basis of structural similarities to other proteins with known functional roles. In contrast, network approaches to protein function prediction utilize information about interactions among proteins during specific cellular processes. Proteins often carry out functions by associating with other proteins to form protein complexes. These complexes are defined by protein–protein interactions, and a complete map of all such interactions (an interactome) thus provides important information about functional roles of individual proteins (Cusick et al., 2005). Unknown functions of proteins can be deduced from this map of interactions in several different ways (Vazquez et al., 2003; Sharan et al., 2007). Simple methods examine neighborhood relations and assign functions on the basis of a majority rule. More sophisticated methods attempt to identify modules consisting of proteins that participate in a common biological function. Proteins of unknown function that occur within such modules can then be given a predicted functional role. What all network-based protein function prediction methods have in common is that they exploit local and global features of the network structure to determine functional roles rather than viewing function exclusively as an intrinsic feature of isolated network nodes.

Thus, it appears that connectivity carries information about the functionality of elements in different kinds of biological networks. In this chapter, I will briefly examine the historical origins of the debate surrounding functional localization in the brain and consider how modern approaches to the analysis of the brain's microstructure and connectivity can create new bridges from structure to function. I will outline an emerging set of ideas where patterns of structural connectivity define functional specialization in the brain.

From Phrenology to Modern Cytoarchitecture

Phrenology, the identification of psychological and personality traits on the basis of protrusions or bumps on a person's skull, has been thoroughly debunked as a pseudoscience that lacks any plausible physiological basis and has no explanatory or predictive power. Despite the inadequacy of the correlational methods employed in phrenology, its originator, Franz Joseph Gall, has made a lasting contribution to psychological science by helping to establish its biological foundation. Gall promoted the idea that the brain forms the material basis for all mental function,[3] and his studies focused the interest of nineteenth-century anatomists and physiologists on the cerebral cortex as the seat of complex cognition. Gall's conception of the brain as composed of numerous and independent cerebral "organs of mind," each devoted to a specific and innately specified mental faculty, represented an extreme version of cerebral localization. Gall's ideas came under almost immediate attack from opponents like Pierre Flourens, whose lesion studies were suggestive of a much more diffuse organization of higher brain functions within the cerebrum. Ever since Gall, phrenology or "neophrenology" have been invoked, usually with negative connotations, in the discussion of historical or contemporary attempts to localize cognitive functions in discrete parts of the cerebral cortex.[4]

Clinical studies of the effects of lesions in the human brain—for example, those of Paul Broca—strongly supported the view that the integrity of specific mental functions depended on the integrity of specific brain centers (see chapter 10). These clinical observations were soon reinforced by histological evidence for structural differentiation of the brain that lent further support to localizationism. The anatomical studies of Korbinian Brodmann, Alfred Campbell, and others provided detailed and comprehensive maps of regional differences in the cytoarchitecture of the human cerebral cortex (see figure 4.1). One basis for these investigations was a histological stain discovered in the late nineteeenth century by Franz Nissl that allowed the selective visualization of cell bodies, in particular those of neurons. Campbell and Brodmann systematically charted the often subtle boundaries separating regions that differed in their staining pattern, marking variations in cell density, size, and layering. Remarkably, Brodmann's cortical maps and his regional classification scheme remain an important reference system for cortical localization even today.

Brodmann's observations on the regional differentiation of brain tissue offered a potential structural basis for functional localization and specialization. And yet, Brodmann rejected the notion that cytoarchitectonic regions of the brain operate in isolation from one another. Regarding complex brain functions, he wrote that "one cannot think of their taking place in any other way than through an infinitely complex and involved interaction and cooperation of numerous elementary activities [...] we are dealing with a physiological process extending widely over the whole cortical surface and not a localised function within a specific region" (Brodmann, 1909; quoted after Garey, 1994, p. 255).[5] However, Brodmann did not clearly articulate the role of connectivity in this process of coordination—in fact, he explicitly excluded fiber architecture from his cytoarchitectonic work. Alfred Campbell, on the other hand, viewed cytoarchitectonic specialization in the context of the patterning of cortical fiber bundles (Campbell, 1905). Campbell was among the first neuroanatomists to consider the role of regionally specific connectivity patterns in functional descriptions of the cortical system (ffytche and Catani, 2005). He is therefore regarded as one of the earliest advocates of the integrated study of structure–function relations in the human brain.

Despite the nuanced views and theories of some of its proponents, Brodmann and Campbell among them, descriptions of the highly

Figure 4.1
Anatomical parcellation of the human cerebral cortex. Maps show the left hemisphere as rendered by Alfred Campbell (1905), Korbinian Brodmann (1909), and Constantin von Economo (von Economo and Koskinas, 1925). Campbell distinguished 14 cortical fields, while Brodmann and von Economo divided the cortex into 44 and 54 regions, respectively.

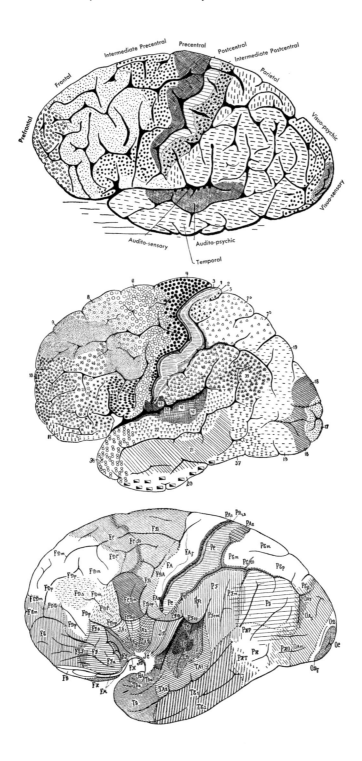

differentiated microarchitecture of the cortex fueled the simplistic notion that the diversity of mental and cognitive functions supported by the human brain came about by the actions of specialized brain regions that operated as independent "organs of the mind." However, this extreme variant of functional specialization was soon to be challenged. Karl Lashley's studies of the behavioral effects of ablations and white matter cuts in the rat brain and of the cortical localization of memory traces following learning led him to reject localization of function altogether. Instead, he formulated a set of opposing ideas such as cortical "equipotentiality" and "mass action" (Lashley, 1929) that emphasized the distributed nature of brain function. Later, Lashley's influential critique of the cytoarchitectonic approach (Lashley and Clark, 1946) cast doubt on the reliability and accuracy of cytoarchitectonic boundaries between cortical regions found in histological material. Lashley and Clark noted that the criteria for determining regional boundaries in cytoarchitectonic studies differed considerably between investigators, resulting in maps that were inconsistent and included a variable amount of detail.

Despite these criticisms, the study of cortical microstructure continues to provide important data on the structural differentiation and heterogeneity of cortical regions. A number of methodological innovations now allow the use of sophisticated statistical tools for the mapping of the brain's cytoarchitecture (Schleicher et al., 1999; Amunts and Zilles, 2001). These modern tools have confirmed some of the "classical" structural differentiations reported in earlier cytoarchitectonic studies. In addition, they have revealed numerous anatomical subdivisions that were missed previously. Automated analyses of cortical microanatomy utilize image processing and statistical techniques—for example, by examining the continuity of histological patterns across the cortical surface (see figure 4.2). One type of analysis proceeds by extracting linear density profiles quantifying cortical laminar patterns in histological sections. The statistical comparison of such patterns along the cortical surface allows the detection of sharp transitions, corresponding to putative boundaries between anatomically segregated cortical regions (Schleicher et al., 2005). Recent mapping studies of the auditory cortex have revealed additional regional subdivisions that were not contained in the classical Brodmann map (Morosan et al., 2001). More detailed and highly resolved cytoarchitectonic maps have also been constructed for human inferior parietal cortex (Caspers et al., 2006) and superior parietal cortex (Scheperjans et al., 2008). In addition to techniques based on histological stains, Karl Zilles and colleagues conducted systematic quantitative

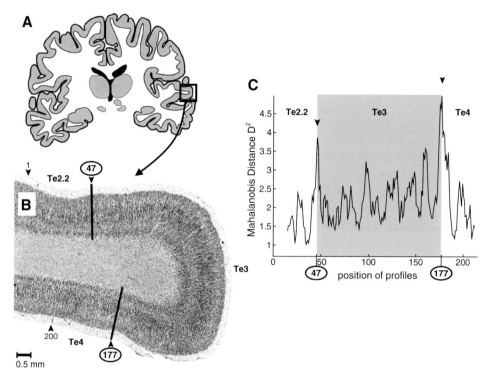

Figure 4.2
Objective identification of cytoarchitectonic boundaries. (A) Schematic drawing of a coronal section through the human brain. A portion of the superior temporal gyrus is marked, and a corresponding tissue section stained for cell bodies is displayed in panel (B). To extract borders between cytoarchitectonic areas, the cross-section of the cortex is covered by equidistant radial profiles that record the gray level index, an estimate of the volume fraction of cell bodies. Changes in the shape of these profiles are recorded by a distance measure, plotted in panel (C). Significant discontinuities in these profiles indicate an abrupt change of the pattern, corresponding to an areal boundary, in this case between temporal cortical regions Te2.2, Te3, and Te4. Images from Morosan et al. (2005), modified and reproduced with permission.

receptor autoradiography revealing regional and laminar densities of several neurotransmitter receptors (Zilles et al., 2004). These biochemical labeling approaches allow the parcellation of the cortex into physiologically and presumably functionally distinct regions. Most of these modern investigations have revealed additional regions that were not captured during the classic era of cytoarchitectural analysis, suggesting that these early attempts at subdividing the cortex underestimated the regional diversity of cerebral microstructure. Notably, virtually all modern cytoarchitectonic and receptor-labeling studies report significant intersubject and interhemispheric variability (Uylings et al., 2005). This variability requires probabilistic mapping techniques to construct reliable anatomical reference maps (Amunts and Zilles, 2006a).

The development of objective computational methods for determining areal boundaries in histological material is an important step toward a more complete characterization of the brain's cellular architecture. Recent studies have clearly confirmed the architectural heterogeneity of human cerebral cortex, and the impending arrival of comprehensive gene expression maps for the human brain will add an important new dimension.[6] Comprehensive cytoarchitectonic, receptor density, and gene expression brain maps will yield multivariate data on cell densities, laminar patterning, receptor types, and protein levels. The conjunction of these different measures allows inferences about functional differentiation that are more precise than those relying on a single structural attribute. A quantitative framework for combining multimodal data on the structure and physiology of brain regions (Kötter et al., 2001) relies on multivariate data analysis tools such as hierarchical cluster analysis and multidimensional scaling. These methods combine the assessment of "intrinsic" areal measures such as microstructural and receptor binding data together with "extrinsic" connectional information. These and other approaches contribute to achieving one of the basic premises of cytoarchitectonics, indeed of cerebral cartography in general (Zeki, 2005), that is, establishing links between local variations in microstructure and variations in function. Thus, modern cytoarchitectonic studies provide more than descriptive maps of cortical anatomy. They contribute to the identification of functional relationships among areas within the highly interconnected architecture of the cortex. In addition, modern cytoarchitectonic techniques are important tools for defining network nodes in the brain at the scale of macroanatomy.

Connectivity-Based Parcellation

The early focus on cyto- and myeloarchitecture as the main criterion for mapping anatomically segregated brain regions has yielded brain maps (such as Brodmann's) that continue to be in use today. Yet, cytoarchitecture alone, even when pursued with modern quantitative techniques, may still be insufficient for reliably detecting all anatomical boundaries between brain regions. While there is some evidence suggesting that similarities in cytoarchitecture may be indicative of functional relations (or at least interconnectivity), there are cases where regions currently viewed as microstructurally coherent are known to be functionally sub-divided (e.g., Brodmann's area 18). Furthermore, high-resolution cytoar-chitectonic studies currently require the use of postmortem brains, as they are difficult to conduct noninvasively in live tissue.[7]

Additional information about regional specialization can be derived from their interconnections. Numerous lines of evidence suggest that regional microanatomy and interregional connectivity of the cortex are mutually related. For example, Barbas and colleagues analyzed the laminar organization of areas in the monkey prefrontal cortex and found that the local cytoarchitecture could predict laminar termination patterns of connections between these areas with high accuracy (Barbas and Rempel-Clower, 1997; Barbas and Hilgetag, 2002). The origin of this relationship is not yet well understood but may involve developmental processes that lead to coregulated regional and connectional differentiation. Thus, the developmental linkage of cytoarchitecture and connectivity further clarifies the functional relationships between segregated cortical areas.

The topological pattern of corticocortical connections provides information that can aid in the definition of regional boundaries (Johansen-Berg and Rushworth, 2009).[8] The basic postulate is that projection neurons within a coherent brain region should share extrinsic (interregional) projection sources and targets, while projection neurons in different regions should have dissimilar connection patterns. If the connection profiles of neurons across the cortical surface can be measured, one can then use a clustering approach to extract homogeneous groupings that correspond to segregated brain regions. Such an approach would naturally result in a definition of network nodes (see chapter 3) that maximizes the information gained about internode connectivity, as additional subdivision of these nodes does not resolve the connection topology any further.

Node definition by clustering of connectivity can in principle be carried out on structural or functional connections. Behrens et al. (2003) used data on thalamocortical structural connectivity obtained by diffusion tensor imaging (DTI) to segment gray matter nuclei in the thalamus, with results that were reproducible between individual brains and consistent with neuroanatomical patterns previously described in nonhuman primates. Johansen-Berg et al. (2004) extended this approach toward identifying correlated structural and functional subdivisions within the cerebral cortex (see figure 4.3, plate 1). Diffusion magnetic resonance imaging (MRI) was used to determine the connectivity profile between

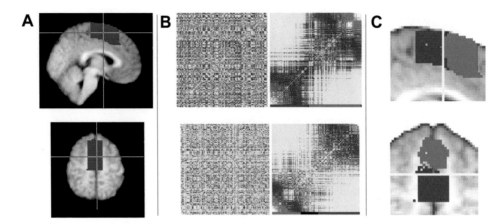

Figure 4.3 (plate 1)
Connectivity-based parcellation of cortical regions. (A) Voxel mask in medial frontal cortex shown in a sagittal (top) and axial view (bottom). (B) The matrix of cross-correlations between connectivity profiles of single voxels from the sagittal (top) and axial (bottom) sections of the medial frontal cortex shown in (A). High correlation implies similarity in the connection profile (hot colors), while low correlation implies dissimilarity (cool colors). In the plots on the right the voxels have been arranged using a spectral reordering algorithm to identify distinct clusters, labeled in blue and red along the axis at the bottom (black denotes voxels that remained unclassified). (C) Positions of the two clusters in anatomical space. Clusters are spatially contiguous, and they largely correspond to segregated functional volumes determined by functional magnetic resonance imaging. Plots reproduced from Johansen-Berg et al. (2004) with permission.

a set of seed voxels in medial frontal cortex and all other voxels across the whole brain. These connectivity profiles were then cross-correlated, and the resulting cross-correlation matrix served as the input to a spectral reordering algorithm that identified clusters of voxels with shared connectivity patterns. This structural imaging approach allowed the identification of connectivity-defined regions in medial frontal cortex.[9] In parallel, functional imaging experiments were performed on the same group of participants, probing for regionally specific activations within the same area of the brain. Comparison of structurally defined regions with regions defined by patterns of neural activation in fMRI revealed a high degree of overlap, which turned out to be significant even at the level of individual participants.

Johansen-Berg's connectivity-based parcellation of medial frontal cortex was replicated in a subsequent analysis (Anwander et al., 2007). These authors then used connectivity profiles obtained from diffusion MRI to partition a portion of the inferior frontal cortex corresponding to Broca's area. Previous cytoarchitectonic and receptor mapping work

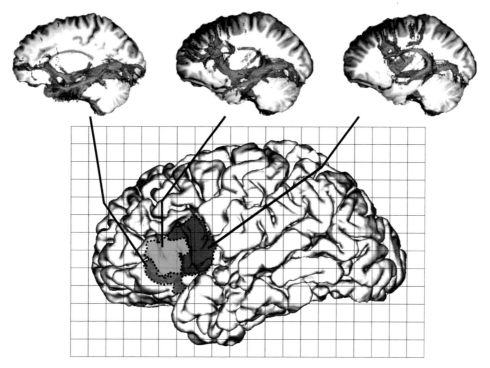

Figure 4.4
Parcellation of Broca's area in the left inferior frontal cortex. Broca's area appears segregated into three distinct subregions, derived on the basis of the similarities and dissimilarities of their long-range structural connections estimated from diffusion imaging followed by computational tractography. The tractographic signatures of the three subregions are shown at the top. The image at the bottom shows their anatomical location on the surface of the brain. Data are from a single subject reported in Anwander et al. (2007), converted to gray scale and reproduced with permission.

(Amunts and Zilles, 2006b) had shown several microstructurally defined subregions within Broca's area. Anwander and colleagues extended this work by showing that similar parcellations could be revealed in vivo in individual brains on the basis of patterns in connectional architecture. Examining data from six individual participants, a cluster analysis revealed three subdivisions of Broca's area, roughly corresponding to Brodmann's area 44, 45 and the deep frontal operculum (see figure 4.4). A comparison with a probabilistic map obtained on the basis of cytoarchitecture showed good agreement between the two parcellation methods. Broad agreement was also reported between the proposed anatomical parcellation and functional activation studies. As is the case for virtually all brain connectivity studies that examine individual participants, there were significant variations in area shape and size, sulcal pattern, and relation to cortical surface landmarks.

Cytoarchitectonic studies have not yet achieved whole-brain coverage, and connectivity-based segmentation approaches have not yet been applied to the entire cortex or more widely across the brain. Given the limitations of both histological and imaging methods, it may be difficult to achieve such whole-brain maps with uniform reliability and resolution. Nevertheless, connectivity-based parcellation, in conjunction with probabilistic maps of cellular microanatomy, has great promise for relating brain structure to function at the macroscopic scale. Additional criteria for defining boundaries of cortical regions may be derived from functional activation studies or from functional correlation patterns found in spontaneous or task-evoked fMRI time series data (Cohen et al., 2008; see chapter 8). The resulting maps will be more than mere descriptive tools—they will allow new ways to quantitatively analyze the functional contributions of individual brain regions and pathways within the global cortical network—for example, through connectional fingerprints.

Connectional Fingerprints

Once cortical regions have been defined on the basis of cytoarchitecture, receptor mapping, or connectivity-based parcellation, their mutual connections can be represented as a structural network. In such a network, each region is represented as a single node maintaining a specific pattern of internode (corticocortical) connections. Passingham et al. (2002) examined the relationship between cytoarchitecture and connectivity and concluded that both local structural differentiation and extrinsic connections contribute to define the functional specialization of each cortical area. Differences in cytoarchitecture between brain regions reflect differences in their intrinsic connectivity—for example, the definition of cell layers and relative proportions of cell types. As discussed earlier, these differences likely contribute to a given region's specific physiology or functionality. However, functional differences cannot be explained on the basis of cortical microstructure alone. Passingham and colleagues focused on the contribution of extrinsic or interregional connections and proposed the concept of the "connectional fingerprint," the idea "that each cytoarchitectonic area also has a unique set of extrinsic inputs and outputs, and this is crucial in determining the functions that the area can perform" (Passingham et al., 2002, p. 607).[10]

The hypothesis that connectional fingerprints are unique for each cortical area was tested by applying multivariate statistical techniques to anatomical data sets from primate prefrontal cortex (Stephan et al., 2001; see figure 4.5). The analysis showed that each area exhibited a unique set of extrinsic connections, and that areas could be grouped on the basis of the similarity of their connectional pattern. Passingham and colleagues suggested the term "connectional families" for clusters of regions that share similar patterns of connections. While it is difficult to objectively define cluster boundaries (due to the graded nature of the connectional similarity measure), the distance between two areas in this structurally defined connectional space may be predictive of their degree of functional relatedness. Support for this idea comes from earlier studies of Malcolm Young, who noted a high degree of similarity in connectional patterns among regions that are known to be functionally related (Young, 1992). Thus, clustering methods applied to connectional fingerprints may reveal not only structural but also functional similarities and relationships among segregated brain regions.

The concept of connectional fingerprints can be extended further—for example, by examining the hierarchical organization of connections around each node. Hierarchical fingerprints are constructed by taking into account connections not only within local neighborhoods but also within neighborhoods that are more than one step removed from the central node. In the primate visual system, such hierarchical fingerprints differ between areas belonging to the dorsal and ventral streams (Costa and Sporns, 2005). It is also possible to define "motif fingerprints," which describe the proportions of structural motifs of different classes that each node participates in (Sporns and Kötter, 2004; Sporns et al., 2007). Motif fingerprints are useful additional means for classifying nodes according to the way they are embedded in the network.

Classification of Nodes and Edges

Once a brain network has been defined, it is possible to quantify the contributions made by individual network nodes to the overall architecture (see chapter 2). Examples are so-called network participation indices (Kötter and Stephan, 2003), which measure relatively simple statistics of individual nodes such as the density, convergence/divergence, and symmetry of a node's afferent and efferent connections. Respectively, these indices have identified regions that are more or less densely

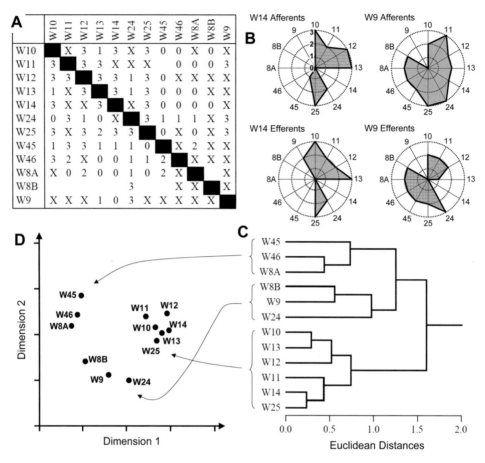

Figure 4.5
Connectivity fingerprints of macaque prefrontal cortex. (A) Matrix of anatomical pathways between prefrontal areas according to Walker (1940), graded in strength from 0 (absent) to 3 (strong)—X marks an existing connection of unknown strength (set to 2 in the other plots). (B) Connectional fingerprints of areas W14 and W9. (C) Hierarchical clustering analysis of Spearman correlations between areal connectivity vectors. (D) Multidimensional scaling of Spearman correlations, showing groupings of areas by similarity in the two principal dimensions. Panels (A) and (C) reproduced from Stephan et al. (2001) with permission. Panels (B) and (D) were generated from data shown in panel (A).

connected, that engage in widespread or more restricted interactions, and that predominantly receive or emit connections. Kötter and Stephan proposed that network participation indices could be related to modes of information transfer and thus be useful for defining nodes as either "senders," "receivers," or "relays."

Other network measures that are computed for single nodes provide additional information about the node's functional specialization. For example, important information can be gleaned from a comparison of a node's clustering coefficient and its average path length to other partners in the network. In mammalian cortex nodes that reside in highly clustered neighborhoods often tend to have long path lengths since they are relatively remote from nodes in other clusters. On the other hand, nodes that connect clusters to each other often have low clustering coefficients, since many of their neighbors belong to different communities, but a short path length, since they facilitate intercluster communication (Sporns and Zwi, 2004; see figure 4.6). Numerous other nodal graph measures are available, including centrality and efficiency (see chapter 2), and concepts from game theory can be applied to further assess the contributions of individual nodes to the global network (Kötter et al., 2007). Participation measures can also be constructed for individual network edges or for sets of edges that comprise coherent anatomical pathways.

Because they are mathematically interrelated, many nodal participation indices and network measures are partially redundant. For example, in most cases highly central nodes also have high degree (see chapter 2). However, this is not always the case, and therefore considering both node degree and centrality can provide additional information when it comes to classifying nodes on the basis of their contribution to the network. For example, as we will see in chapter 6, one major functional class is composed of nodes that are highly connected and highly central, so-called hubs. Hubs can be objectively identified on the basis of several network measures although a classification threshold must be applied since they normally do not form a class with sharply defined boundaries—all highly connected and highly central nodes are hubs, but to a varying extent. Current anatomical studies suggest that most hub nodes correspond to brain regions that were previously described on the basis of anatomical or physiological studies as multimodal, transmodal, or association areas. Hubs have been identified in several different regions of the brain, and it remains to be seen if all hubs display common functional properties, regardless of which brain areas they connect.

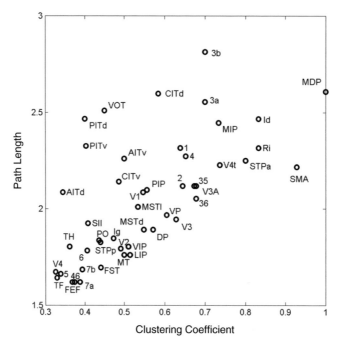

Figure 4.6
Relation of clustering coefficient and path length. The figure shows a scatter plot of areal clustering coefficients and path lengths for a matrix of 47 regions of macaque cortex (see figure 2.6). Note that regions that have high centrality (see figure 2.9) are found near the lower left corner of the plot, that is, they have low clustering and a short path length. Data were replotted from Sporns et al. (2007). For abbreviations of cortical areas see figure 2.6.

Variability in Brain Connectivity

Most anatomical mapping methods reveal not only species-specific and invariant patterns but also significant variability in corresponding structures across individuals. This variability is not surprising given the multitude of genetic and experiential factors that shape the morphology of the nervous system at all levels of organization. Should a network approach to neuroscience exclusively focus on population averages, or should it also take into account individual differences in connectional anatomy? There are many reasons to consider variability a significant factor in the organization of brain networks. Variability is an essential feature of many biological systems, and it is one of the major driving forces of evolution. According to the evolutionary biologist Ernst Mayr, a consideration of individual variability is what sets biology apart from other natural sciences. Biological variation is central to "population thinking," which stresses that "all organisms and organic phenomena are composed of unique features and can be described collectively only in statistical terms" (Mayr, 1959, p. 2).

Repeatedly in this chapter, we encountered evidence for individual variability in the structural composition and connectivity of brain networks, particularly those of the mammalian cerebral cortex. Individual variations are observed in all complex brains, whether they come from mammals, birds, or insects—no two brains from individual organisms are completely alike. This is true for cells within specific structures and for macroscopic brain regions and fiber tracts. Variability is encountered in vertebrate and invertebrate nervous systems. A functionally specialized interneuron in the locust, the descending contralateral movement detector, was found to be highly variable from animal to animal (Pearson and Goodman, 1979) with large variations in its branching structure as well as synaptic connectivity. The sizes of different brain regions in *Drosophila* display great variability, which likely reflects continual structural plasticity and reorganization (Heisenberg et al., 1995). In the human brain, there is significant intersubject variability at the macroscopic scale, which poses major challenges to brain mapping (see figure 4.7). Van Essen and Dierker (2007) proposed to distinguish four different types of variability, the variability of the macroscopic cortical folding pattern, the positioning of areas relative to these folds, as well as variability in areal size and connection patterns. In their terminology, the last two types of variability together constitute "variability in macro-circuitry" (p. 1050), and they note that this form of variability may be a structural basis for individual variations in cognition and behavior.[11] Individual variation in macroanatomy and connectivity is partly the result of genetic factors (Toga and Thompson, 2005; Chiang et al., 2009) and is reduced but not completely absent in monozygotic twins. A significant proportion of variable neuronal morphology and network structure is likely the result of experience- and activity-dependent processes, particularly at the scale of individual neurons and synapses (Butz et al., 2009).

Despite enormous differences in morphology and connectivity, human brain networks support behavioral and cognitive functions that are, for the most part, shared among all individuals. At the same time, specific variations in brain regions or fiber pathways alter network topology in ways that can be linked to individual differences in behavioral or cognitive performance (see chapter 9). Thus, brain networks combine a strong tendency toward functional homeostasis, the maintenance of function despite persistent variations in structure, with the capacity to express

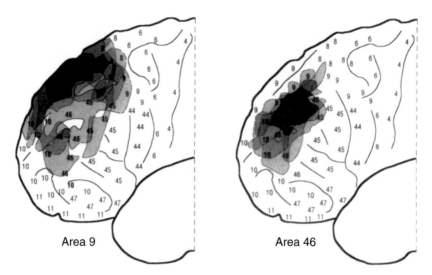

Figure 4.7
Intersubject variability in boundaries of cortical areas. The plots show five superimposed left-hemisphere reconstructions of cortical areas 9 and 46 based on their cytoarchitectonic profile. The outlines of the two areas in individual brains are marked by lines, and their overlap is indicated by the level of shading. Cortical territory occupied by area 9 or area 46 in all five individual brains is filled in black. Images from Rajkowska and Goldman-Rakic (1995), reproduced with permission.

variations in behavior. Functional homeostasis limits the phenotypic expression of variable neuroanatomy and is likely the result of coordinative network processes (Maffei and Fontanini, 2009). Functional homeostasis is found even in very simple networks. Prinz et al. (2004; Marder and Prinz, 2002) performed a modeling study of a three-cell model of the pyloric network of the crustacean stomatogastric ganglion, a circuit involved in the generation of rhythmic movements. The analysis examined many millions of circuit variants that differed in a number of biophysical parameters. Different parametric realizations of the circuit produced virtually indistinguishable dynamic behavior, suggesting that a given target network performance could be achieved with highly variable circuit designs. Prinz et al. suggested that networks may be regulated in terms of global functionality rather than by adjusting local settings of biophysical or morphological parameters. Such homeostatic mechanisms are essential for the long-term stability of the brain given the continual remodeling and structural turnover of its cellular and molecular components (Marder and Goaillard, 2006; Minerbi et al., 2009).[12]

Structurally variable but functionally equivalent networks are an example of degeneracy, defined as the capacity of systems to perform similar functions despite differences in the way they are configured and connected (Tononi et al., 1999; Edelman and Gally, 2001). Degeneracy is widespread among biological systems and can be found in molecular, cellular, and large-scale networks. Price and Friston have noted that human brain networks display degeneracy since different sets of brain regions can support a given cognitive function (Price and Friston, 2002). Cortical activation maps obtained from functional neuroimaging studies of individuals often show only partial overlap for a given cognitive task, suggesting that different individuals utilize different (degenerate) networks. The loss of a subset of all regions that are reliably activated in a given task may not disrupt task performance, indicating that individual regions may not be necessary or that recovery processes following brain injury can configure structurally different but functionally equivalent networks (see chapter 10). These examples of degeneracy in cognitive networks are suggestive of the idea that mechanisms promoting functional homeostasis may also operate at the scale of the whole brain to ensure that structural variations or disturbances do not lead to uncontrolled divergence of functional outcomes.

In addition to variability among neurons of the same type, nervous systems also exhibit striking diversity of neuronal cell types, distinguished by their characteristic cellular morphology. This morphological diversity is likely matched by an unknown degree of variability in the expression of cellular proteins involved in metabolism and interneuronal communication. Diversity and variability in cortical interneurons has been shown to affect network dynamics, with greater variability leading to less pronounced network synchrony (Soltesz, 2006). Diverse and variable cell morphology may thus help to regulate the excitability of nervous tissue, a potentially important factor in preventing pathological states such as epilepsy. The heterogeneity of interneurons has also been invoked as a source of greater "computational power" for cortical networks (Buzsáki et al., 2004).

Specificity and Randomness in Synaptic Connections

How specific or how random are synaptic connections between individual neurons? Early anatomical studies of neuronal circuits in the cerebral cortex as well as other structures such as the cerebellum suggested a degree of randomness of cellular connectivity (Sholl, 1953; Uttley, 1955). One of the prevailing ideas was that synaptic connectivity could be described by statistical distributions of synapses between cells of same or different types and that such descriptions were sufficient to explain the neural processing characteristics of a given circuit or structure. For example, Braitenberg and Schüz described the cortex as a "mixing device" whose corticocortical connections are "set up largely by chance and possibly refined by learning processes" (Braitenberg and Schüz, 1998, p. 64). Szentágothai acknowledged the existence of anatomically ordered long-range projections in the cortex, conveying specific axonal connections between different brain areas, but maintained that local synaptic connections between nearby cells appeared diffusely organized, with "cloud"-like arborization patterns (Szentágothai, 1977). In parallel with these neuroanatomical ideas, most early neural network models, dating as far back as the 1950s (e.g., Beurle, 1956), utilized random connectivity, an unorganized substrate that could be molded by learning and plasticity.[13]

Contrary to the idea of brain networks as "random nets," the development of new anatomical tracing and staining techniques that allow the visualization of the fine structure of morphologically and physiologically identified neurons in local circuits has provided abundant evidence that cells of different types form and maintain specific connection patterns. This structural specificity confers distinct biophysical and physiological properties to each cell type and is thus essential for neurons' normal operation. Computational studies suggest that specific neuronal morphologies—for example, dendritic branching patterns and synaptic distributions—support specific elementary computations (Stiefel and Sejnowski, 2007). Given that the cellular structure and the biophysics of neurons are intricately linked, it appears unlikely that any structural detail will ever be identified that is truly "without function." Much of the detail of cell structure and connectivity contributes to the cell's capacity to respond to and relay signals.

Are these ideas of randomness and specificity in cellular networks mutually incompatible with one another? Some confusion arises because of the way in which the terms "randomness" and "specificity" are applied to neuronal or synaptic structures. Many authors have used the term "randomness" to describe structural arrangements that are seemingly unorganized, presumed to be functionally insignificant, or just plain difficult to quantify and describe. Other authors have used the term "specificity" to emphasize that even the finest structural detail in the nervous system contributes to larger functional outcomes. What is considered random or specific may thus depend more on the amount of available information and less on the actual process by which a given structure has arisen. From a developmental perspective, randomness and specificity fulfill complementary roles as they jointly shape the generation and maintenance of synaptic connectivity. A developmental model for synapse formation (Jontes and Smith, 2000) involves a primarily undirected "exploratory" process of process extension, followed by selective consolidation or dissolution of contacts. The first process may be considered "random," while the second process conveys "specificity," since it is primarily driven by neural activity or biochemical interactions between participating cells.

As we probe the cellular architecture of the brain with ever more refined methods, we will undoubtedly discover more and more of its structural elaboration and detail. The structure of every neuron will reveal unique patterns of neuronal processes and intercellular junctions. "Randomness" then is reduced to that which is due to residual unobserved causes that are beyond current measurement—and given what we now know about cells as "molecular machines," it is likely that everything that appears random today will yield to a causal description in terms of molecular and cellular interactions at some later time. However, the fact that fine details of cellular anatomy are "specific" (causally determined) rather than truly "random" does not necessarily entail that a full description of the nervous system in structural terms must be framed at the level of the full-scale cellular, or even subcellular, anatomy. Homeostatic and coordinative processes within the nervous system ensure that variability at molecular or cellular scales generally does not perturb processes unfolding on larger scales. The modularity of the brain's architecture, a recurrent theme in this book (see chapters 6, 7, 8, 9, 12, and 13), effectively insulates functionally bound subsystems from spreading perturbations due to small fluctuations in structure or dynamics. Yet, while it is important to ensure that the loss of a single spine or the overexpression of a protein in a small number of synaptic sites does not result in alterations of global patterns of neuronal communication and connectivity, it is equally important that the neuronal architecture maintain variability and heterogeneity (Soltesz, 2006). Individual neurons, even those belonging to the same class, must remain different from one another to continually create dynamic variability as a substrate for adaptive change.

Neuroanatomy and Network Science

The failure of phrenology, and of subsequent localizationist accounts of brain function, resulted from an ill-conceived attempt to impose a classification of mental traits on the substrate of the brain. The main thrust of the effort was to search for the place where function was represented rather than ask how a given structural substrate can give rise to a broad set of functions.[14] The key question, however, is how cognitive function *emerges* from the specific anatomical and physiological substrates of the brain. Rather than begin with preformed notions of how cognition is carved up into distinct psychological functions or mental faculties, an alternative approach is to ask how brain networks can generate different classes of dynamic behavior and how these dynamics map onto cognition. Network neuroanatomy is essential for addressing this question and thus forms an indispensable conceptual basis for our understanding of complex brain networks.

Networks are a pervasive concept in neuroanatomy. The quantitative analysis of neuroanatomical networks can provide important clues for relating anatomical structure to physiological function. Network measures allow the objective characterization of how nodes (and edges, if desired) participate in the overall network. Nodes with shared attributes can be placed into a single structurally defined class—for example, "hub nodes" or "receivers." Regardless of whether they are spatially close or widely distributed across the brain, shared structural attributes can indicate that nodes are functionally related. Since structural connections shape functional interactions, these structural classes may be associated with different functional roles. Importantly, these functional roles are not assigned on the basis of the mental faculties of phrenology or "classical" domains of cognition but in terms of the functional specialization of nodes within the network.

Network approaches to neuroanatomy move us closer to resolving the long-standing debate between localizationist and distributionist accounts of brain function. The key step is to view local specialization as the result of patterned distributed interactions that confer different functional attributes to individual network elements. Since these interactions can be accessed with network mapping tools, they also allow a quantitative data-driven assessment of functionality and do not require assumptions about of how brain regions participate in various cognitive processes. Network approaches gain additional power because they can be applied to both structural and functional networks, thus allowing their direct comparison and interrelation. The relationship between structural and functional networks of the brain is beginning to bear results across multiple cognitive domains. These relationships strongly motivate the application of network approaches to neuroanatomy for providing mechanistic explanations of how, in Brodmann's words, cognition emerges from "a physiological process extending widely over the whole cortical surface."

Increasingly, modern neuroanatomical techniques require sophisticated tools for the acquisition, analysis, and representation of large data sets, developed by practitioners of neuroinformatics and computational neuroanatomy (Ascoli, 1999). A network perspective on neuroanatomy builds on the use of modern computational methods for analysis and representation of large data sets. To promote progress in computational and network neuroanatomy, we urgently need more extensive and comprehensive structural connectivity data sets than have previously been available. New methods will be needed to trace and map connections between neurons, cell populations, and brain regions. Several of these methods are poised to reveal structural connections in unprecedented detail, and they will greatly enrich our understanding of the principles that drive the anatomical and functional organization of the brain. We now turn to these new methods for mapping the brain's cells, circuits, and systems.

5   Mapping Cells, Circuits, and Systems

Instead of promising to satisfy your curiosity concerning the anatomy of the brain, I confess sincerely and publicly here that I know nothing about it. I wish, with all my heart, that I might be the only person to have to speak thus, for I would benefit, in time, from the knowledge of others and it would be a great blessing for the human race if this part of the body, which is the most delicate of all and which is liable to very frequent and very dangerous disorders, were as well understood as many philosophers and anatomists imagine it to be.[1]
—Nicolaus Steno, 1665

In 1665, the Danish-born naturalist Nicolaus Steno delivered a lecture to a select audience assembled at the house of the Parisian linguist and scholar Melchisédec Thévenot, entitled *Discours sur l'anatomie du cerveau* (Lecture on the Anatomy of the Brain). Later transcribed and published (Steno, 1965), this lecture became an important document in the early history of brain anatomy.[2] Steno's investigations into the structure of the human brain established him as one of the leading neuroanatomists of his time. He was among the first to pay close attention to the brain's white matter, composed of densely packed fibers whose neuronal origin and function would remain obscure for another two centuries. Steno believed that the organization of these fibers held the key for a deeper understanding of the human mind. However, then as now, the brain presented many challenges to neuroanatomy:

If, as I have just stated, the substance of the brain is little known to us, no more so do we know the correct way to dissect it. [...] For my part, I hold that the correct dissection would be one following the nerve filaments through the substance of the brain to see where they pass and where they come to an end. It is true that this method is so full of difficulty that I do not know whether one may hope ever to complete the task without very special preparations. The substance is so soft and the fibres so delicate that one scarcely knows how to touch them without breaking them. (Steno, 1965, pp. 124–125)

Steno viewed the brain's white matter as a set of specific pathways whose connectivity had functional importance:

[…] wherever fibres are found in the body, they maintain always a certain pattern among themselves, of greater or lesser complexity according to the functions for which they are intended. […] We admire the contrivance of the fibres in every muscle, how much more ought we to admire them in the brain, where these fibres, confined in such little space, carry out their individual functions without confusion and without disorder. (Steno, 1965, pp. 122–123)

Steno's view of the brain as a machine whose operations depend on the anatomical arrangement of fiber pathways is strikingly modern in spirit.[3] In fact, our understanding of the brain as an integrated functional system will be incomplete so long as we do not have a comprehensive description of its structural elements and interconnections. Descriptions of structural brain connectivity are sometimes referred to as the brain's "wiring diagram," a blueprint of sorts that charts the elements and connections of the brain in a way that is analogous to the layout of transistors and switches on a computer chip or in a complex electronic appliance. If obtained at high resolution, this blueprint would capture the entire cellular machinery of the brain and all its synaptic connections, encompassing approximately 10^{11} cells and 10^{15} connections in the case of the human brain.[4] Such a map is sometimes viewed as the "holy grail" of the study of intelligence, a road map to deciphering human cognition, or at least an essential milestone on our journey to a complete understanding of the brain.[5] Some authors have suggested that the wiring diagram is not only necessary but sufficient for understanding the brain and that there is no need for a global theory of how the brain operates. Rather, all that is required is to figure out how all its elements are connected and what mechanisms are involved in updating their individual states. However, the quest for the brain's wiring diagram cannot replace the search for theoretical principles that underlie brain network organization. Reliable and detailed maps of structural brain connectivity are necessary, but not sufficient, for formulating theoretical principles that capture the functioning of the brain as an *integrated system* with emergent and complex properties.

Even if the function of the brain cannot be reduced to its wiring diagram, there can be little doubt that structural brain networks shape patterns of spontaneous and evoked neural activity (see chapters 8 and 9). Simply put, in order to understand how brain networks function, one must first know how their elements are connected. In this chapter we will examine a range of empirical approaches to the mapping of structural brain networks at multiple scales of organization. Many of these approaches are currently undergoing rapid technological development and refinement, and several new methods for imaging and tracing neural connectivity are on the horizon. Given that most methods for mapping structural brain networks are still in the early stages of methodological development and application, it is premature to identify a single technique as the most promising or appropriate for capturing brain connectivity. In fact, it seems quite likely that a plurality of empirical approaches to brain mapping as well as new computational tools will be needed and that their integration into a common framework for capturing and recording structural brain connectivity will be essential for the ultimate success of the endeavor.

Defining the Brain's Connectome

In a 1993 commentary, Francis Crick and Ted Jones pointed to the lack of a connectional map of the human cortex, comparable to that compiled for the macaque monkey by David Van Essen and Dan Felleman (Felleman and Van Essen, 1991), and they challenged the field that such a map was essential for human neuroscience. In their words, "it is intolerable that we do not have this information for the human brain. Without it there is little hope of understanding how our brains work except in the crudest way" (Crick and Jones, 1993, p. 110). Indeed, a comprehensive description of the structural network of the human brain is of fundamental importance in cognitive neuroscience (Sporns et al., 2005). Together with Giulio Tononi and Rolf Kötter, I proposed the term "connectome" for such a data set. We stated as our central motivating hypothesis "that the pattern of elements and connections as captured in the connectome places specific constraints on brain dynamics, and thus shapes the operations and processes of human cognition" (Sporns et al., 2005, p. 249). Parallel to our proposal, Patric Hagmann suggested a similar approach to mapping structural connections in the human brain, which he termed "connectomics" (Hagmann, 2005). A principal goal of the connectome was the representation of structural brain networks in the form of graphs, collections of nodes and edges, which would allow the quantitative analysis of brain connectivity with the mathematical tools of network science. From the beginning we saw the connectome as a way to reveal structural principles of brain networks that would illuminate brain function, not merely as a database of "what connects to what."[6]

We chose the term "connectome" in deliberate analogy to the genome, the complete set of genetic information of an organism. We immediately recognized that, even when limiting the scope to the brain of a single species—for example, humans—there are significant challenges facing any effort to compile a comprehensive connectome data set. The human genome (Venter et al., 2001) consists of approximately 3×10^9 base pairs, linearly arranged in DNA molecules and perhaps containing little more than 20,000 protein-encoding genes (Pennisi, 2007). Despite the relatively straightforward composition of the genome, the assembly of a complete genome map has taken considerable time and resources and was eventually made possible by the adoption of innovative sequencing techniques that did not yet exist when the original goal of implementing a human genome program was formulated in 1986.[7] The connectome may require similar methodological innovation. The human brain's three-dimensional structure, its growth and development, individual variability, and the sheer number of components that it contains present challenges that far exceed those posed by the human genome (Insel et al., 2003).

Another fundamental challenge is the inherently multiscale architecture of human brain structural connectivity. When we first defined the human connectome (Sporns et al., 2005), we distinguished three relevant scales of organization, the microscale of single neurons and synapses, the mesoscale of anatomical cell groupings and their projections, and the macroscale of brain regions and pathways. We argued that the vast number, morphological variability, and structural dynamics of individual nerve cells and their processes render the microscopic scale an improbable target for an initial draft of the human connectome. The mesoscale offers much greater promise and may be feasible in the near term, especially in the case of smaller brains that can be studied with "classical" invasive anatomical techniques (described below). At the macroscale, techniques and approaches are currently available that allow the tracing of interregional pathways, including the noninvasive neuroimaging of white matter fiber tracts in the human brain. In the original proposal, we envisioned that a first draft of the human connectome would be assembled at the macroscale, and we proposed a strategy based on the combined use of diffusion and fMRI. We suggested the mapping of highly resolved structural and (resting-state and multistimulus/multitask) functional connectivity patterns, as well as their mutual comparison. We also emphasized the open-ended nature of any effort to compile a connectome, which ultimately may be extended to include information on neuronal and connectional subtypes, biophysical properties, metabolic signatures, and associated tissues like glial cells and brain vasculature.

Since our proposal was first published, others have suggested that the primary focus of connectomics should be on individual neurons and their synaptic connections (Lichtman and Sanes, 2008). To date, cellular techniques have not yet been applied to the comprehensive mapping of neural connectivity in large brains, and significant technical challenges regarding the reliability and sensitivity of these techniques remain to be addressed. Yet, even when applied to small volumes of tissue, these techniques will make an essential contribution—for example, by mapping local circuitry and interneurons which cannot be captured with neuroimaging methods. In the future, connectomics will most likely involve the mapping of brain connectivity at multiple scales and with multiple methodologies. Computational approaches may also play a role. Sebastian Seung suggested that it may not be necessary to acquire connectome data by "dense reconstruction" of a single brain specimen (Seung, 2009). Rather, connectomic data could be assembled via a (much simpler) "sparse reconstruction" approach—for example, by identifying and recording connected pairs of neurons.

A Simple Brain?

The microscopic roundworm *Caenorhabditis elegans* lives in the soil of temperate climates. Millions of individuals can be found underneath a single square meter of moist vegetated ground. The worm's tube-like body reaches a length of about 1 millimeter, and lacking vision or hearing, it is capable of sensing its environment through receptors responding to chemical, thermal, and tactile stimulation. Feeding mostly on bacteria in the ground, its behavioral repertoire ranges from relatively simple activities like locomotion or swimming to complex activities involving reproduction and even rudimentary forms of social interactions. Some of the worm's behaviors involve adaptation and learning—for example, the capacity to modify chemotaxic and thermotaxic behavior in response to changes in the environment.

For many years, *C. elegans* has been a favored model organism for developmental biologists, in part due to the ease with which it is grown in the laboratory and the relative simplicity of its body structure. *C. elegans* was also among the very first organisms whose genome was sequenced and mapped in its entirety, found to consist of ~100 million base pairs forming 17,000–20,000 genes.[8] Its body comprises ~1,000 cells, and the nervous system of the hermaphrodite adult worm consists of exactly 302 neurons arranged into a number of more or less distinct cell groupings or ganglia. These neurons are connected by several thousand chemical synapses and gap junctions. An important feature of the worm's nervous system is that the spatial position, number, and connectivity of its neurons are largely constant across individuals.

The nervous system of *C. elegans* has been mapped in exquisite detail. To this day, it remains the only nervous system of any organism whose connectivity structure is completely mapped at the level of individual cells and synapses. This remarkable feat was accomplished by painstaking reconstruction of the three-dimensional wiring pattern from electron micrographs (EMs) of a complete stack of serial sections, each about 50 nm thick (White et al., 1986).[9] The reconstruction work was performed largely by hand from a total of about 8,000 prints of EMs and took more than ten years to complete. The invariance of the structure of the nervous system across individuals, as well as the relatively simple morphology of many of its neurons—for example, the abundance of local connections and the relative lack of axonal or dendritic branches—aided in the reconstruction effort. Dmitri Chklovskii and colleagues recently performed a partial reanalysis as well as additional anatomical studies to generate a more complete reconstruction of the brain of *C. elegans* (Chen et al., 2006). The end result was a cellular connection matrix (see figure 5.1) comprised of a total of 279 nodes (neurons) linked by 6,393 chemical synapses, 890 electrical junctions, and 1,410 neuromuscular junctions.[10] A unique feature of the data set is that the spatial position of each neuron and hence the length of all synaptic connections are known. These data on the spatial layout of the worm's nervous system allowed a detailed analysis of wiring length (see chapter 7), providing important insights into spatial embedding and wiring minimization as possible constraints on neuronal placement and connectivity.

Since we possess the complete map of all cells and connections in the nervous system of *C. elegans*, do we now also have complete knowledge of how this brain functions and controls behavior? Indeed, the availability of the complete wiring diagram for *C. elegans* stimulated several projects aimed at creating a computational model of functional patterns of neural activity and behavior (e.g., Achacoso and Yamamoto, 1992). However, these efforts have not yet led to a full-scale computational model of the worm's nervous system, nor have they provided a complete description of its functional behaviors. There are several reasons for this

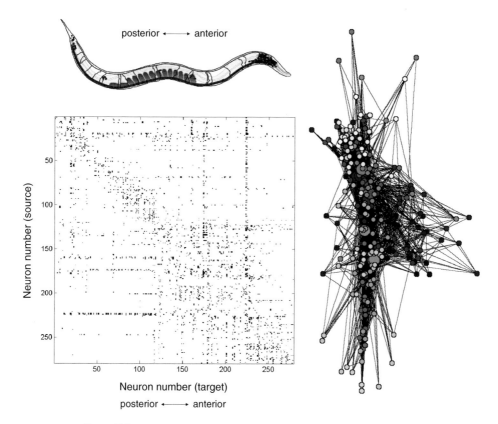

Figure 5.1
Connection matrix of *C. elegans*. The connection matrix shows (directed) chemical synapses
in black and (undirected) electrical synapses in gray. Neurons are arranged in order of
position along the main axis of the worm. Note that many connections are found near the
main diagonal, a first indication that wiring length is conserved (see chapter 7, figure 7.2).
Note also that some neurons are more highly connected than others—these neurons have
high centrality. The plot on the right is a visualization of the connectivity using the
Fruchterman–Reingold force-directed layout algorithm in Pajek (Bagatelj and Mrvar,
1998). Nodes (cells) are shaded according to their position along the main axis (light gray
= anterior, dark gray = posterior), and highly central nodes are displayed as large circles.
The sketch of *C. elegans* at the top is courtesy of Michael Nonet (Washington University),
and the connection matrix was constructed from data made available by Dmitri Chklovskii
and colleagues (http://www.wormatlas.org/neuronalwiring.html).

failure. Because of formidable technical challenges, we still lack essential information on the physiological properties of many of the neuronal cell types of *C. elegans* (Goodman et al., 1998). Further obstacles are that we know very little about the nature of the worm's sensory inputs or the way in which the worm's neural circuits control its motions and behavior. This situation reminds us that the complete wiring diagram is insufficient for reconstructing functional dynamics of a neural system in the absence of complementary information about the biophysical properties of neurons and synapses. These biophysical properties have a large role in determining the dynamic characteristics of neuronal activations, neural transmission, and synaptic plasticity. Most of the techniques surveyed in this chapter are limited to visualizing cellular or connectional morphology and cannot deliver these biophysical parameters.

Mapping Connections at Cellular and Subcellular Resolution

C. elegans is currently the only organism for which we have a (nearly) complete wiring diagram of its neuronal networks. The highly stereotypical nature and the small size of the brain of this species have helped significantly in creating and interpreting this important data set. Other brains have been partially mapped, revealing complex cell morphologies and wiring patterns. The mushroom bodies located in the protocerebrum of insects are believed to be the structures most closely associated with complex sensorimotor integration, learning, and social behaviors, and they comprise approximately 1 million neurons in the brain of the honey bee. The complex cellular and connectional anatomy of the bee mushroom body has been investigated with classical cell staining techniques (Mobbs, 1982). However, the sheer number and density of cellular processes in this structure will likely require techniques that allow the reconstruction of three-dimensional volumes of tissue at subcellular resolution. The complete mapping of the cellular anatomy of an insect brain is being pursued as one of the next research goals in this area (Adee, 2008).

New imaging tools, automated serial sectioning, and reconstruction techniques (Smith, 2007; Helmstaedter et al., 2008; Arenkiel and Ehlers, 2009) are crucial to the success of such an effort. These technological advances now make it possible to reconstruct the cellular anatomy of a block of neural tissue at submicrometer resolution. One promising approach, serial block-face scanning EM, allows the three-dimensional reconstruction of cellular processes and even organelles within large tissue blocks hundreds of micrometers on each side (Denk and

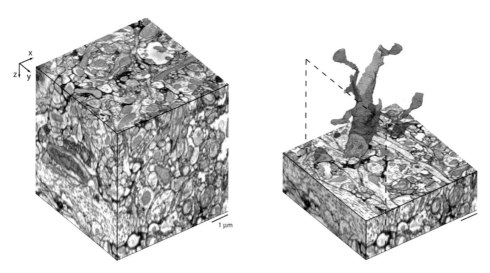

Figure 5.2 (plate 2)
Neuronal reconstruction with serial block-face scanning electron microscopy. The image on the left shows a 350 μm³ volume of adult rat cortex composed of 253 sections, each 30 nm thick. On the right is a volume reconstruction of a single manually traced spiny dendrite. Images are from Briggman and Denk (2006), reproduced with permission.

Horstmann, 2004; see figure 5.2, plate 2). Denk and colleagues argue that EM approaches are needed because the small diameters of many axonal processes as well as dendritic spines preclude the use of optical imaging methods (Briggman and Denk, 2006). Improved sectioning and imaging techniques will have to be complemented with improved reconstruction algorithms that allow the automated tracing of neurites. Complete ultrastructural mapping of neural connectivity of entire nervous systems will require the development of a comprehensive methodological framework that parallelizes serial section EM imaging, volume assembly, and data analysis to allow large-scale high-throughput collection and testing of connectivity information (Anderson et al., 2009). Future work will likely attempt the reconstruction of a single mouse cortical column (Helmstaedter et al., 2007), a task that will require the accurate mapping of synaptic connectivity on a scale that exceeds that of *C. elegans* by more than a million-fold. A unique feature of serial EM reconstruction is that it provides exquisite detail about the three-dimensional structure of neuronal and nonneuronal cells, which is important for understanding the biophysical properties of neural processes, spines, and synapses, as well as for neuron–glia interactions and models of brain tissue that take into account the spatial relations between cells.

Optical staining and circuit reconstruction tools have undergone significant technological improvements in recent years. One approach, called array tomography, combines optical fluorescence microscopy and scanning EM of ultrathin cryosections of immunolabeled neural tissue (Micheva and Smith, 2007; see figure 5.3). The method allows for a high-resolution three-dimensional map of the distribution of specific antigens in relation to cellular and subcellular structure. Imaging of synaptic markers and wide-field coverage might allow the construction of connectivity maps from tomographic volume images. Another approach involves the application of newly developed fluorescent intracellular or membrane dyes in transgenic mice. Lichtman and colleagues have developed a technique that labels individual neurons with distinctly colored immunofluorescent markers (Livet et al., 2007; see figure 5.4, plate 3). The distinct colors result from combinatorial expression of a small number of differently colored fluorescent proteins in transgenic animals ("Brainbow" mice). In these animals, labeled neurons can be traced by creating stacks of confocal microscopy images, each essentially a cross-section of the imaged tissue block, followed by the creation of a three-dimensional montage. The technique has produced breathtaking images

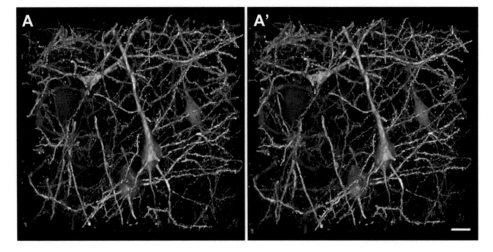

Figure 5.3
Array tomography. The images are a stereo pair of a volume rendering from an array tomograph of a block of mouse cerebral cortex, showing cell bodies and processes of several cortical neurons, studded with dendritic spines, as well as additional processes that intersect the imaged volume. Readers can see these images in three dimensions by crossing their eyes or viewing them through a stereoscope. Images from Micheva and Smith (2007), reproduced with permission.

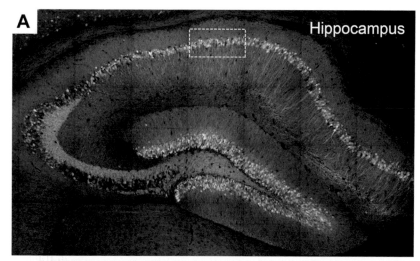

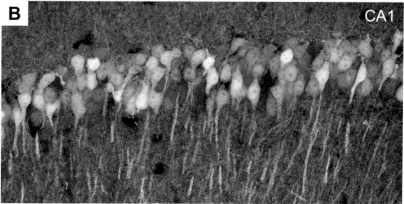

Figure 5.4 (plate 3)
Imaging of neural connectivity with combinatorial expression of fluorescent markers. Composite image of the mouse hippocampus (A) and magnified portion of the CA1 cell layer (B), from Livet et al. (2007), reproduced with permission.

of cellular neuronal architecture—for example, in the mammalian hippocampus—and it has been successfully applied to a portion of the mouse neuromuscular circuitry (Lu et al., 2009). A number of technical problems remain to be addressed (Lichtman et al., 2008), including limitations of optical resolution, uniformity of expression and stability of Brainbow markers, and the number of distinct colors expressed in a single animal, as well as extraordinary challenges for data collection and compression.[11] The technique currently requires the generation of transgenic animals that express fluorescent marker molecules and is therefore limited to animal species for which such transgenics can be successfully generated, effectively ruling out all primate species including humans.

It is too early to tell which technique will ultimately provide the most feasible and reliable approach to mapping neural circuits at the cellular or subcellular level. Perhaps a combination of serial EM, single-cell, and Brainbow labeling will be needed to acquire useful data sets in ways that are both fast and accurate. As more and more sophisticated data sets will become available in coming years, what will we learn about the structure of brain networks? Will microscale subcellular approaches, singly or in combination, soon deliver the complete wiring diagram of a brain that is significantly more complex than that of *C. elegans*? Several methodological and technological hurdles must be cleared before the cellular connectome of a complex brain can become a reality. While subcellular methods have provided tantalizing glimpses of neural wiring patterns, the complete mapping of, say, the full three-dimensional architecture of the approximately 80 million projection neurons in the mouse cortex still poses significant challenges in terms of resolution, tracing accuracy, and computational reconstruction. These challenges, while formidable, may well be overcome in the foreseeable future.

The cellular architecture of any complex nervous system exhibits tremendous heterogeneity and variability (see chapter 4). Several lines of evidence indicate that the cellular microanatomy of the brain is in constant flux, with spines and synapses, axonal and dendritic branches, and entire cells changing their morphology and connectivity, spontaneously and as a result of neural activity (Alvarez and Sabatini, 2007; Minerbi et al., 2009). At cellular or subcellular resolution, the connectome is therefore a "moving target," where each successful reconstruction of a block of neural tissue represents a snapshot of a dynamic architecture frozen in time. A collection of such snapshots would be invaluable for a systematic account of dynamic structural variability in neurons and circuits and for discovering what morphological or topological characteristics of connectivity remain invariant over time. An important goal for the connectome is to deliver a *description*, that is, a compressed representation of the *invariants* of neural connectivity, the structural regularities of brain networks that are characteristic for a given neuronal cell type, circuit, or brain region in a given species. For example, the reconstruction of individual mushroom bodies in the *Drosophila* brain or of individual columns in the mammalian neocortex should lead to the formulation of quantitative connectivity rules that capture statistical regularities in the patterning of cells and synapses, ideally in relation to genotype or environmental factors. Hence, for subcellular maps of brain connectivity to achieve their full potential, sophisticated neuroinformatics tools and statistical approaches to neuroanatomy are essential. Once an integration of empirical circuit mapping and computational analysis is accomplished, it will provide us with an unprecedented view of cellular networks that will inform more realistic physiological and neurocomputational models.

Tracing Long-Range Neural Connections

While comprehensive maps of the cellular connectivity of a complex brain may still be years away, there are several established and proven empirical approaches for the construction of connectome data sets at the level of mesoscopic and macroscopic projections between cell groups and brain regions (Kötter, 2007). These techniques usually involve the injection of a tracer into the living brain at a specific location which is then taken up by neurons in the proximity of the injection, transported along their projections, and ultimately visualized in histological sections or by optical imaging approaches. Tracers differ in the way they are transported, as well as in their sensitivity and persistence within the cell. The tracing of neuronal projections is usually carried out in vivo—for example, by injecting the plant lectin *Phaseolus vulgaris* leucoagglutinin, which labels the cell via binding to the cell membrane and allows detailed mapping of neuronal processes. Some tracing studies can be carried out in postmortem tissue—for example, through the use of lipophilic carbocyanine dyes (e.g., DiI and DiO). Neuroanatomical tracers are best suited to the mapping of long-range projection pathways, while local circuitry or processes of interneurons are often less well captured. Other approaches to the tracing of long-range projections involve myelin staining as well as a new class of optical imaging approaches using polarization microscopy. The latter technique allows insights into the three-dimensional arrangement of fiber bundles which can then be used to build three-dimensional trajectories of fiber pathways (Axer et al., 2002; Palm et al., 2010).

Axonal tracing methods have been widely applied in studies of the connectional anatomy of several mammalian species, including the mouse, rat, cat, and macaque monkey. For several of these species, systematic collation of individual tract tracing studies in the anatomical literature has led to the creation of consolidated and well-documented

neuroinformatics data sets. A landmark paper in 1991 combined anatomical information on hundreds of long-range projections in the cerebrum of the macaque monkey and provided the first large-scale structural
connection matrix (Felleman and Van Essen, 1991; see figure 5.5). The
matrix summarized information on 305 connections between 32 anatomically segregated visual and visual-association areas. The network
was found to be composed of multiple interconnected subdivisions
forming a distributed hierarchy (Van Essen et al., 1992), a result that was
confirmed on the basis of cluster analyses of the connectivity performed
by Malcolm Young (e.g., Young, 1992; 1993). Young and colleagues later
provided the first comprehensive connection matrix for the thalamocortical system of the cat (Scannell et al., 1995; 1999). This data set comprised a total of around 850 connections linking 53 cortical areas and 650
connections linking cortical areas to 42 thalamic nuclei.

These anatomical data sets have provided unique insights into the
connectional organization of cortex, including graph-theoretical analyses
which are reviewed in detail in the following chapter. They have also
spurred the development of dedicated neuroinformatics tools (Bota and
Swanson, 2007), most of which are openly accessible to the scientific
community.[12] For example, the online macaque cortex connectivity database CoCoMac provides a continually updated collection of anatomical
reports on structural connectivity among regions of the cortex and some
subcortical structures in the brains of adult primates of the genus *macaca*
(Kötter, 2004). Another such tool, the Brain Area Management System
(BAMS), records connections between anatomically distinct cell groups
and nuclei in the brain of the rat (Bota et al., 2005). As of 2007 (Bota
and Swanson, 2007), the matrix of axonal projections interconnecting 486
anatomically defined regions of the rat central nervous system contained
data on 22,178 distinct connections collected in the BAMS database for
a total coverage of 9.4 percent.

Weaknesses of the tract tracing approach are its invasiveness and the
need to combine a large number of studies involving many individual
brains of a given species in order to create a complete connection map.
Tract tracing is ill suited for studies in humans, for obvious reasons, and
the often gradual and patchy distribution of tracer across the brain is still
only incompletely captured in the often fairly qualitative, if not subjective, ways in which the data are reported. Nevertheless, its undeniable
success in tracing long-range pathways may make it a complementary
partner for optical or EM studies of cellular connectivity whose strengths
are in capturing local circuits and connections of interneurons.

Figure 5.5

Connectivity matrix for interconnections of macaque visual cortex. This figure summarizes observations from numerous anatomical studies, recording the confirmed presence ("+") or confirmed absence ("·") of interregional pathways, with untested connections corresponding to empty cells in the figure. Self-connections along the main diagonal are not recorded. From Felleman and Van Essen (1991), reproduced with permission. For abbreviations of cortical areas see figure 2.6.

A group of researchers, mostly from neuroanatomy and neuroinformatics, recently proposed a systematic plan for compiling neuroanatomical connectivity data at a mesoscopic scale (Bohland et al., 2009), utilizing "classical" anatomical tracers. The plan aims at whole-brain coverage and the development of standardized and automated techniques for mapping and validating connection patterns, as well as open access and interoperability with existing neuroinformatics tools. A specific target is the mapping of the mesoscopic connectivity of the mouse brain, with possible extension to primate species in the near future. Bohland and colleagues argue for a focus on the mesoscopic scale of local populations of neurons that share functional properties and connectional patterns and that can generate information about species-specific invariant patterns of anatomical connectivity, rather than an effort to map all microscale synaptic connections, citing technological obstacles as well as an unknown degree of interindividual variability. This effort, if carried out, could provide a fairly fine-grained connectivity matrix for an entire mammalian brain within a reasonably short time frame.[13]

Noninvasive Mapping of Human Brain Connectivity

Invasive anatomical techniques such as tract tracing cannot be used in humans. The structural connectivity of the human brain is accessible by postmortem examination of dissected brain tissue (see figure 5.6) or by utilizing in vivo noninvasive brain imaging (see figure 5.7, plate 4). However, postmortem neuroanatomy faces numerous obstacles, not the least of which is the rapid deterioration of neural tissue after death,[14] and there is a lack of suitable postmortem tracing techniques. More promising, at least in the short term, are noninvasive neuroimaging approaches such as structural MRI and diffusion MRI.

Structural MRI utilizes differences in magnetic resonance (MR) signals produced by different types of brain tissue to visualize and quantify the three-dimensional arrangement of structural subdivisions of the brain—for example, cell nuclei and cortical gray matter. Structural MRI measures not only reveal variations in the volume or surface area of specific brain structures but also allow the inference of structural connectivity. Correlations in the thickness or volume of gray matter between two cortical areas, usually measured across brain data sets from multiple participants, have been shown to be associated with the presence of a fiber tract linking these areas. The mechanism that leads to these correlations is currently unknown but possibly involves correlated metabolic or

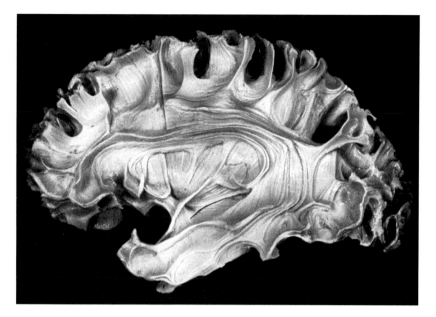

Figure 5.6
Dissection of the human brain to reveal fiber architecture. The image is from an atlas of the human cortex by Ludwig and Klingler (1956), prepared from postmortem tissue by carefully freezing the specimen followed by gradual removal of tissue around major fiber pathways. The largest pathway shown here is the superior longitudinal fasciculus, which connects frontal, occipital, and temporal cortex. Image reproduced with permission.

trophic processes, genetic factors, or experience-related factors. Cortical thickness correlations have been used to assemble some of the very first whole-brain connection matrices (He et al., 2007c) and are discussed further below.

The diffusion of water molecules in biological tissue is the primary signal measured by diffusion imaging (Johansen-Berg and Behrens, 2009). In the gray matter of the brain, changes in the direction of MR gradients do not result in large changes in the diffusion pattern of water molecules since diffusion is largely isotropic. Diffusion anisotropy, however, is often observed in the brain's white matter, with a maximum that generally coincides with the spatial orientation of nerve fibers within each voxel. Hence, the signal generated by diffusion imaging can provide information about the direction of fiber tracts within individual voxels of the brain. The spatial resolution of the signal is limited by the voxel size and could be improved by imaging at higher field strength. A more fundamental limitation encountered in DTI is that the diffusion tensor

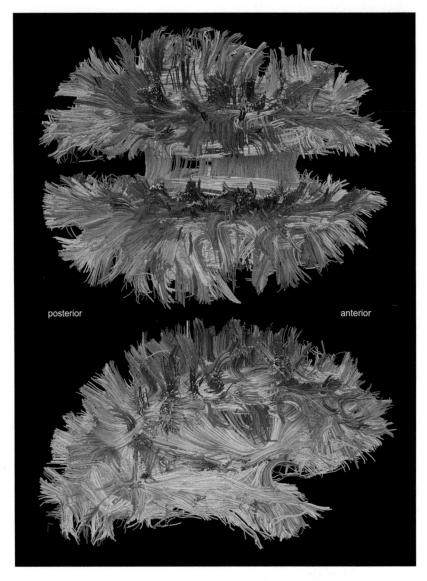

posterior   anterior

Figure 5.7 (plate 4)
Diffusion spectrum imaging and tractography of cortical connectivity. Images show dorsal
and lateral views of the brain of a single human participant. Images courtesy of Patric
Hagmann (Ecole Polytechnique Fédérale Lausanne).

captures only a single diffusion direction per voxel, which does not account for crossing fibers. Heterogeneous fiber directions within single voxels can be revealed with imaging techniques that utilize multiple diffusion directions, for example, high angular resolution diffusion imaging (Tuch et al., 2002), q-ball (Tuch et al., 2003), and diffusion spectrum imaging (DSI; Wedeen et al., 2005; see figure 5.7, plate 4). The nature of the diffusion weighted signal requires the application of computational algorithms for probabilistic estimation or fiber reconstruction from the set of diffusion profiles of individual voxels. These tractography algorithms are fundamentally inferential in nature, that is, they attempt to construct fibers that are consistent with the observed distribution of diffusion anisotropy. The development of tractography algorithms is an active field of research in its own right. Deterministic approaches to tractography rely on finding optimal streamlines within the tensor field, while probabilistic approaches aim to provide statistical estimates for the existence of fiber pathways.

Diffusion MRI and tractography data are often difficult to validate against more "classical" anatomical techniques, such as tract tracing. In the case of the human brain, tract tracing is unavailable, although further technology development might produce viable tracers for postmortem connectivity studies. To date, only a handful of studies have acquired diffusion imaging data in species for which anatomical tract tracing data are also available. In validation studies of macaque cortex, Dauguet et al. (2007) performed tract tracing as well as DTI in the same animal. While DTI appeared to reconstruct major white matter pathways correctly, some differences were seen in fine anatomical detail. Schmahmann et al. (2007) first used DSI to identify a number of long-range association tracts in the macaque brain and then compared these tracts to a large set of previously assembled histological tract tracing data (Schmahmann and Pandya, 2006). The study revealed considerable agreement between these two different anatomical approaches, thus providing indirect support for the validity of diffusion imaging data obtained from the human brain, where tract tracing data are not available. Hagmann et al. (2008) compared a connection matrix of a single macaque hemisphere obtained with DSI to tract tracing data in the CoCoMac database. Only about 6 percent of all cortical fibers derived from DSI were in places where pathways had been reported absent in previous anatomical studies. Taken together, the comparison of structural connectivity obtained with diffusion weighted imaging and with "classical" tract tracing anatomy reveals a high degree of overlap.

Complete agreement between tract tracing and diffusion imaging may never be achieved since both techniques probe structural connectivity only at specific spatial scales and with limited resolution. With regard to whole-brain connectivity data, diffusion imaging has certain advantages over tract tracing techniques. Unlike tract tracing, diffusion MRI allows the acquisition of large volumes of data under conditions of relative homogeneity in terms of resolution and sensitivity from a single brain. The compilation of tract tracing data for the brain of a given species requires numerous injections and histological reconstructions across the brains of many individuals, thus rendering the result a "mosaic" of connectivity. Another advantage of the noninvasive neuroimaging approach is that it offers the potential for parallel recording of structural (DTI/ DSI) and functional (fMRI) data in the same individual brain, which allows unique insights into structure–function relationships (see chapters 8 and 9). A major disadvantage of diffusion imaging is that it does not currently allow the determination of the direction of a fiber pathway.

Noninvasive imaging techniques have been in use for a number of years and have delivered profound insights into the spatial arrangement of fiber tracts of the human cerebrum. Recently, investigators have begun with the acquisition and analysis of whole-brain data sets for mapping human structural connectivity. One of the first such data sets exploited cross-correlations in cortical thickness obtained from a database of 124 human brains (He et al., 2007c). The resulting connection matrix was analyzed using a broad array of graph theory methods (Chen et al., 2008). Whole-brain structural connection matrices of the human brain have also been obtained by Bassett et al. (2008) from a cohort of healthy participants as well as participants with a clinical condition.

Several studies have constructed whole-brain structural connection matrices derived from diffusion MRI. Iturria-Medina and colleagues (2007; 2008) derived connection probabilities for between 70 and 90 cortical and basal brain regions on the basis of DTI data. Gong et al. (2009) also used DTI and a similar parcellation scheme of 78 cortical regions to create an average structural network for a cohort of 80 young adult participants. DSI was used in two studies by Hagmann et al. (2007; 2008). Hagmann's group first partitioned the cortical surface into anatomical regions defined by a standard landmark-based template and then subdivided these regions further into between 500 and 4,000 equally sized regions of interest (ROIs). Fiber densities were then derived for each pair of ROIs, resulting in a more highly resolved connection matrix. For a partition into approximately 1,000 ROIs (500 per cerebral hemisphere) this procedure yielded between 13,000 and 15,000 distinct connections. An example of a structural connection matrix rendered within a standard landmark-based cortical parcellation is shown in figure 5.8 (Hagmann et al., 2008). The corresponding connectivity backbone of the full resolution connection matrix displayed in spatial coordinates gives a first visual impression of the contributions of both short- and long-distance projections between regions of the cerebral cortex (see figure 5.9, plate 5). I will discuss the network architectures of these data sets in the following chapter.

A direct comparison of connection matrices obtained in these studies is made difficult because of the adoption of different parcellation schemes (which define the network nodes and hence their connections as well) and acquisition methods. Further complications arise because different authors use different ways to measure the "strength" or "density" of individual fiber pathways. The strengths of pathways are reported as fiber counts or densities in some studies and as connection probabilities in others. Diffusion imaging methods deliver weighted (symmetrical) connection matrices, which are then in some cases thresholded and reported as a binary pattern. The field is in great need of improved standardization of cortical parcellation and a more rigorous definition of the strengths or densities of reported fiber pathways. Particularly promising is the use of structural connections (see chapter 4) or functional mapping criteria (see chapters 8 and 9) for defining the anatomical boundaries of brain regions. These methods may ultimately allow the parcellation of an individual brain into internally coherent regions that constitute well-defined network nodes.

Noninvasive brain imaging, including high-resolution diffusion imaging, currently represents the most promising avenue for mapping comprehensive structural connectivity data sets at the macroscale. In the near future, we will see more comprehensive coverage of subcortical regions and pathways as well as improved spatial resolution for mapping smaller fiber bundles and anatomical subdivisions. Diffusion imaging techniques are undergoing rapid technological development, which makes it likely that this chapter's summary of diffusion MRI approaches to the connectome will soon be in need of revision.

The Future of the Connectome

Which of the methodological approaches to structural brain connectivity surveyed in this chapter will yield the most detailed, most accurate, and

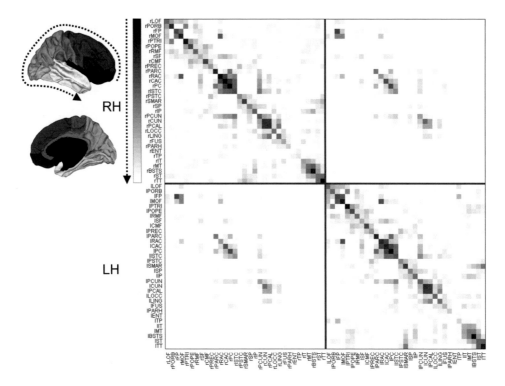

Figure 5.8
Regional connection matrix of human cerebral cortex. Cortical regions in the right and left cerebral hemispheres (RH and LH, respectively) are ordered along a frontotemporal gradient (see insets on left), thus largely preserving their spatial proximity. Note the high incidence of connections along the main diagonal of the matrix, indicative of the high proportion of short connections linking neighboring areas. Replotted from data reported in Hagmann et al. (2008). Abbreviations of anatomical areas are as follows (prefix "r" denotes right hemisphere, and "l" denotes left hemisphere): BSTS, bank of the superior temporal sulcus; CAC, caudal anterior cingulate cortex; CMF, caudal middle frontal cortex; CUN, cuneus; ENT, entorhinal cortex; FP, frontal pole; FUS, fusiform gyrus; IP, inferior parietal cortex; IT, inferior temporal cortex; ISTC, isthmus of the cingulate cortex; LOCC, lateral occipital cortex; LOF, lateral orbitofrontal cortex; LING, lingual gyrus; MOF, medial orbitofrontal cortex; MT, middle temporal cortex; PARC, paracentral lobule; PARH, para-hippocampal cortex; POPE, pars opercularis; PORB, pars orbitalis; PTRI, pars triangularis; PCAL, pericalcarine cortex; PSTS, postcentral gyrus; PC, posterior cingulate cortex; PREC, precentral gyrus; PCUN, precuneus; RAC, rostral anterior cingulate cortex; RMF, rostral middle frontal cortex; SF, superior frontal cortex; SP, superior parietal cortex; ST, superior temporal cortex; SMAR, supramarginal gyrus; TP, temporal pole; TT, transverse temporal cortex.

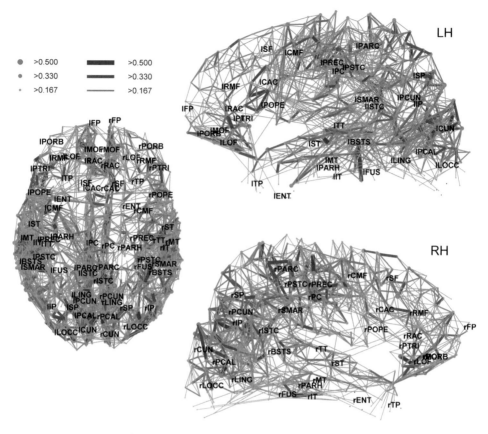

Figure 5.9 (plate 5)
Backbone of the structural connectivity of human cerebral cortex. Nodes (998 regions of interest) are coded in red according to the node strength, and edges (approximately 4,000 shown in this plot) are coded according to the connection strength (fiber density). LH, left hemisphere; RH, right hemisphere. For abbreviations of anatomical areas see figure 5.8. Replotted from data reported in Hagmann et al. (2008).

most reproducible brain network? The answer to this question is far from obvious. There are many different empirical approaches to how structural connectivity of the brain is recorded and processed, each with some considerable strengths as well as weaknesses. Each approach provides data that illuminate different aspects of structural connections, often at different levels of scale. A major future challenge will be to merge information across these different scales, to yield structural networks that can inform a broad range of physiological experiments and models, from single cells to systems. Challenges are also posed by the numerous methodological and computational hurdles that must be cleared in order to reveal the important invariants of structural connectivity. The essence of such a description is that it is a meaningful compression of the full-scale pattern, capturing its essential topology.

Cellular and subcellular reconstruction methods can deliver connectivity data on neural circuits with unparalleled spatial resolution, and they are poised for significant technological advances in the near future (Eisenstein, 2009). Cellular mapping techniques are also the only methods currently available to map the anatomy of neural tissue in its entirety, including all other cell types and structures within which nerve cells are embedded (glial cells, cerebral vasculature, etc.). All serial sectioning and reconstruction methods face significant methodological obstacles—for example, establishing reliability in tracing long processes over millimeters or even centimeters of tissue. Because of these obstacles, these methods may have greater probability of success, at least initially, when applied to small nervous systems or to small blocks of tissue containing local circuitry. With regard to the complete mapping of larger and more complex brains, these techniques still face significant challenges, not only in terms of data acquisition and processing, but also in terms of the dimensionality, variability and stability of cellular structural connectivity (Lichtman and Sanes, 2008). Other, complementary methodologies might be of use in addressing these challenges.

Particularly promising are combinations of techniques that aim to reconstruct connectional architecture with those that probe for functional coupling. As we discussed earlier, the physical wiring diagram usually only contains the morphological aspect of structural connectivity, but the presence of a physical connection does not reveal its strength or physiological efficacy. The efficacy of synapses in the cerebral cortex varies over a wide range, with a large number of synapses that are weak or "silent." Dhawale and Bhalla (2008) have proposed combining structural labeling and tracing of cells (e.g., using the "Brainbow" method) and functional circuit mapping, by presynaptic stimulation and measurement of postsynaptic responses in large numbers of neurons using optical imaging. Such a dual approach could distinguish between "silent" and active synapses and assign synaptic efficacy to structurally identified sites of intercellular contact. In functional neuroimaging, the combined analysis of structural and functional connectivity has already begun (see chapter 8), and relationships have begun to emerge between the presence and strengths of structural pathways and the magnitude and consistency of functional coupling.

Several "connectome projects" are on the horizon. In the United States, the National Institutes of Health are embarking on a "Human Connectome Project," whose major goals parallel those originally suggested in Sporns et al. (2005). This project will use existing MR methodologies to map human brain connectivity in a large population of healthy adults. Other approaches are being pursued in parallel. Serial EM seems poised to deliver the complete subcellular structure of a cortical column within the next few years, and cellular labeling techniques such as "Brainbow" may soon be applied in an attempt to map all cells and connections within a significant portion of a mammalian brain. Classical neuroanatomical tracing techniques will be used in a systematic attempt to obtain the first complete connectome at the mesoscale, possibly of the mouse brain. Researchers in human neuroimaging have already utilized diffusion MRI and fMRI techniques to reconstruct whole-brain networks, and these approaches are increasingly being deployed in developmental and clinical studies (see chapters 10 and 11). There is little doubt that these different methodologies will continue to become more refined and reliable, and entirely new techniques may soon appear on the horizon. As techniques mature, it would be fruitful to explore avenues for mutual cross-validation or for combining multiple technologies to map structural connectivity in ways that harness the often complementary strengths of each approach.

"To extend our understanding of neural function to the most complex human physiological and psychological activities, [...] it is essential that we first generate a clear and accurate view of the structure of relevant neural centers, and of the human brain itself, so that the basic plan—the overview—can be grasped" (Cajal, 1995, p. 39). Cajal's dream is about to be fulfilled. The next few years will likely see a rapid proliferation of data on structural connectivity in human and animal brains. Network analysis techniques will then be needed to extract their statistical patterns and regularities. The next chapter surveys what we know to-date about the topology of structural brain networks.

All the neurons in the central nervous system are reciprocally connected by numerous pathways, some having great and others lesser degrees of complexity. This wealth of connections is due not only to the high number of neurons and pathways, but also to the branching of the axons and their collaterals and to the overlapping of the fields of distribution of the branches of the different axons. The number and complexity of central pathways are best described by saying that, with but few exceptions, at least one pathway can be found connecting any two central neurons [...]. Obviously many of these complicated paths are physiologically impassable, because the impulses sooner or later fail to reach the threshold of an intervening neuron, but others actually do play an important role in the physiology of the central nervous system.[1]
—Lorente de Nó, 1938

Lorente de Nó sought to identify functional principles of the cerebral cortex from the action of neurons organized into elementary circuits.[2] These circuits were defined by the patterning of axonal ramifications and synaptic connections, and they could be represented in diagrams not unlike those found in present-day graph theoretical descriptions of structural brain connectivity. Lorente de Nó realized the important role of recurrent connections in the central nervous system,[3] an idea that proved to be highly influential in later physiological accounts of reverberant neural activity. He also realized that elementary circuits did not operate in isolation but were anatomically and functionally linked, with central neurons arranged into complex "synaptic chains." The resulting networks were amenable to theoretical analysis: "Recent advances in the knowledge of the physiology of the synapse [...] make it possible to analyze in greater detail the physiological significance of the arrangement of the neurons in synaptic chains. The interest of the analysis consists in that it is possible to reduce the actual anatomical complexity of the nerve centers to simple diagrams suitable for theoretical arguments" (Lorente de Nó, 1938, p. 207). Lorente de Nó advanced his own "theoretical

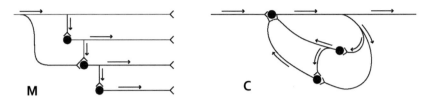

Figure 6.1
Two fundamental types of neural circuits, after Lorente de Nó (1938). These two arrangements of neurons, the multiple (M) and closed chain (C), reflect the two principles of plurality and reciprocity. These arrangements resemble network motifs. Redrawn after Lorente de Nó (1938).

arguments" suggesting that cortical circuitry can be characterized by a combination of "plurality" and "reciprocity" (see figure 6.1). Importantly, neurons in the central nervous system were linked by an "exceedingly large number of interlacing pathways" (Lorente de Nó, 1938, p. 241) that shaped the conduction and circulation of central nerve impulses. He recognized that such interlacing pathways provided numerous opportunities for neurons to influence each other, either directly or indirectly, resulting in network interactions that are essential for integration in the central nervous system.

Since then, the bewildering complexity of structural brain connectivity, its abundant variability and dynamic change, has posed many challenges for neuroanatomists and physiologists. As we discussed in the previous chapter, neuroanatomical data continue to be difficult to collect and analyze, and complete circuit diagrams for most neural structures of most species, notably humans, are still incomplete or lacking altogether. Can we, at this early stage, discern overarching network principles that govern the structure and function of cellular or large-scale neural systems? Graph theoretical analyses have allowed us to make some first steps toward elucidating important architectural features of structural brain networks. As a result of these studies, simple notions of "randomness" in brain connectivity have given way to a renewed emphasis on specific network attributes, such as highly nonrandom distributions of motifs, small-world organization, and the existence of modules and hubs. How pervasive and common are these attributes, and what does their occurrence imply for the function of the brain?

The Nonrandomness of Brain Networks

Data sets recording large-scale connectivity within the mammalian thalamocortical system have been available since the early 1990s. It was immediately noted that these networks exhibited attributes characteristic of an organization that was neither entirely random nor entirely regular. The first connection matrix of the macaque visual cortex (Felleman and Van Essen, 1991; see figure 5.5) was sparse (only about 30 percent of all possible connections had been confirmed as present), and the majority of pathways between cortical regions were found to be reciprocal.[4] Closer inspection revealed the existence of multiple parallel processing streams whose constituent brain areas were organized into a cortical hierarchy (Van Essen et al., 1992). This anatomical organization provided a structural substrate for functional specialization in the visual cortex documented by physiological recordings and lesion studies (Ungerleider and Mishkin, 1982; Van Essen and Maunsell, 1983).

Malcolm Young's quantitative analyses of macaque cortical connectivity revealed additional nonrandom structural features (Young, 1992; 1993). Utilizing a multivariate statistical technique (nonlinear multidimensional scaling) to visualize the topology of connection patterns (figure 6.2), he demonstrated specific connectional relationships between

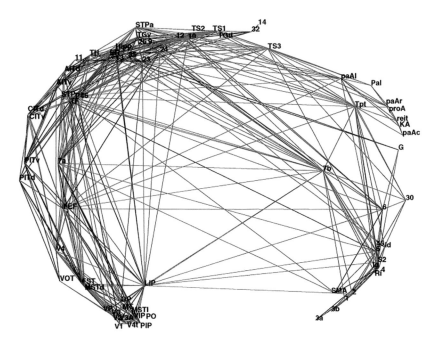

Figure 6.2
Multidimensional scaling of macaque cortical connectivity. Positions of cortical areas are determined on the basis of similarity in their connectivity patterns, with areas that have similar connection patterns placed close to one another. Reproduced from Young (1993) with permission.

brain regions, including the existence of largely segregated and hierarchically organized dorsal and ventral processing streams in primate visual cortex and their convergence onto regions of temporal and frontal association cortex. This organization was inferred on the basis of structural connection data, and it could explain a wide range of physiological and cognitive findings. Young noted that the existence of areas of reconvergence of the two functional streams such as polysensory regions of the superior temporal lobe and prefrontal cortex was suggestive of their functional role in visual integration.

Young also noted that neighboring brain regions on the cortical surface are more likely to be connected than pairs of regions that are separated by greater distances. This overabundance of short-range corticocortical pathways cannot be explained on the basis of a random model of cortical connectivity. At the same time, not all corticocortical pathways conform to a lattice-like regular pattern because a significant proportion of pathways extend over long distances. Connections that link nearby regions contribute to one of the most conspicuous nonrandom features of large-scale cortical connectivity, the existence of clusters or modules (see below). These clusters, for the most part, form compact groupings that occupy contiguous regions on the cortical surface. In order to test whether spatial proximity could explain all or at least a large fraction of the topology of interregional pathways, Young and colleagues attempted to predict cat cortical connectivity on the basis of simple nearest-neighbor and next-door-but-one models (Scannell et al., 1995). It turned out that these models could only account for a fraction of the existing connections, thus indicating that the cat cortex was neither random nor entirely regular, or lattice-like, but instead combined features of both random and regular connectivity.

As noted in chapter 2, random networks have degree distributions that are fairly homogeneous, indicating a single characteristic scale of network connectivity, while the degree distribution of other network architectures is much more heterogeneous, possibly even scale-free. Are structural brain networks single-scale or scale-free? Given the small size of most currently available connection data sets (in many cases comprising less than 100 nodes), the question is difficult to settle and may require the arrival of more highly resolved structural data sets. Because of the cost of adding connections in the brain, it seems unlikely that structural brain networks, including those at the large scale, can exhibit scale-free degree distributions across a wide range of degrees (Amaral et al., 2000). Since all brain nodes, regardless of how they are defined, are spatially embedded, there must be strict upper limits on the number and density of connections that can be sustained at any given node, due to basic spatial and metabolic constraints. Other networks that are spatially embedded and where similar constraints on node degree apply, such as transportation networks, have been shown to exhibit exponential or exponentially truncated scale-free degree distributions (Amaral et al., 2000; Guimerà et al., 2005). Even if structural brain networks will not turn out to be scale-free, the degree distributions analyzed so far all exhibit deviations from a simple Gaussian or exponential profile that is characteristic of random networks. For example, brain regions that maintain a large number of connections are generally more abundant than would be expected based on the assumption of random degree distributions.

While there is convergent evidence for the nonrandom and nonregular organization of brain networks at the large scale, the degree to which cellular networks are either random or regular is much less well understood. A primary reason for this gap in our knowledge is the relative lack of cellular connectivity data sets acquired in a format that allows graph analysis. At the time of writing, most such data sets consist of very small numbers of neurons and do not comprise entire networks, or they report connection probabilities between cells and cell types rather than actual wiring patterns. In the few available cellular connectivity data sets—for example, the nervous system of the worm *C. elegans* (see chapter 5)—nonrandom features abound. As was already noted by White (1985), the connection pattern of *C. elegans* is highly nonrandom, in that connections between neurons predominantly occur within local neighborhoods, resulting in conservation of axonal lengths (see chapter 7). Spatial proximity of connected neurons is likely to be just one among several factors that account for the nonrandomness of the overall topology. Given that a nervous system as compact as that of *C. elegans* needs to support a wide range of behavioral capacities, it is likely that functional considerations provide an additional set of tight constraints on connectivity.

In the case of pyramidal cells in the mammalian neocortex, one of the most robust observations on cellular interconnectivity is that the probability that two cells are synaptically connected falls off with their mutual distance (Braitenberg and Schüz, 1998). The relationship has a bell-shaped profile and drops to near zero as distances grow to several millimeters (Hellwig, 2000). At longer distances, connections are often patchy and locally clustered, possibly linking cell groups that have similar response properties. Such connection patterns can be described by distance-dependent probabilistic distributions that govern cellular and synaptic densities. Inferences of synaptic connectivity from observed functional interactions have provided some additional insights into various nonrandom properties of cellular cortical networks. For example, when synaptic connections in rat visual cortex were probed (Song et al., 2005), synaptic strengths were found to observe a lognormal distribution with a "heavy tail," indicative of a greater than expected abundance of strong synaptic connections embedded "in a sea of weaker ones" (see figure 6.3). Stronger connections also showed a tendency to be more highly clustered, which favors more densely connected structural motifs. Different sets of experiments demonstrated the existence of independent subnetworks of highly coupled excitatory neurons that are intermingled within single cortical columns (Yoshimura et al., 2005) and of a high degree of cellular precision in functional maps of orientation selec-

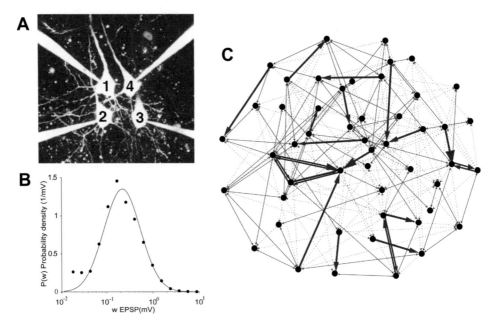

Figure 6.3
Nonrandom features of synaptic connectivity in rat cortex. (A) Fluorescent image of four rat cortical neurons taken during a quadruple whole-cell recording. The recording setup allows the estimation of connection strengths between these cells. (B) Across many recordings, the distribution of connection strengths has a lognormal profile, exhibiting a normal (Gaussian) appearance in this semilog plot. Most connections are weak, while strong connections are more abundant than would be expected if their strengths were exponentially or normally distributed. wEPSP, synaptic connection strength, measured as the amplitude of the excitatory postsynaptic potential. (C) A statistical reconstruction of the synaptic network, depicting the "skeleton of strong connections in a sea of weaker ones" (Song et al., 2005). Reproduced from Song et al. (2005).

tivity (Ohki et al., 2005), which allows cells to express distinct functional properties even in close spatial proximity, thus enabling functionally independent communities to coexist within a single volume of space. Developmental studies (Yu et al., 2009) suggest that these observations may have an anatomical basis. Taken together, these empirical findings indicate that probabilistic rules based on spatial proximity alone are insufficient to describe cellular cortical connections and that cellular circuits form precise patterns with currently unknown topology. Critical information on the nature of these patterns will become available once volumes of cortical tissue have been comprehensively mapped with ultrastructural or cellular labeling techniques (see chapter 5).

Act Locally: Motifs and Motif Distributions

The pronounced tendency for synapses to connect cells within local neighborhoods results not only in high clustering but also in an over-abundance, relative to random architectures, of particular classes of structural motifs. The occurrence of a large number of densely connected three-node motifs ("triangular sub-circuits") in the brain of *C. elegans* was already noted by White (1985, p. 281), a feature he attributed to the prevalence of local connectivity in the worm's nervous system.[5] Detailed quantitative studies (Milo et al., 2002; 2004a; Reigl et al., 2004; Chen et al., 2006) have confirmed an overabundance of a subset of motif classes in the nervous system of *C. elegans*. The relative abundance of each motif class was determined on the basis of a comparison of the actual network to a null model, constructed as a population of random networks with identical sequences of node degree. However, it is likely that the existence of some highly enriched motif classes is at least partly due to the predominance of short connections that link neurons in local communities (Artzy-Randrup et al., 2004; Milo et al., 2004b). Comparison of motif classes across networks of different origin (e.g., neuronal, cell transcription, and ecology; Milo et al., 2004a) may require the construction of domain-specific random models. The issue has implications for arguments about the evolutionary origin of network topology in general and the functional importance of specific enriched motif classes in particular (see below).

While only very few motif analyses of cellular networks are currently available, indications are that they show characteristic nonrandom distributions. Recording from multiple neurons in the mammalian cortex, Song et al. (2005) have demonstrated a much greater than expected likelihood for reciprocal connectivity (a motif involving only two nodes), as well as for a specific set of triadic motifs of cells, particularly those that involve highly clustered connections. Whether this observation is due to spatial biases in the recordings, preferentially local connectivity, or specific computational roles of these motifs that provide an adaptive advantage to the organism is currently unknown.

As will be discussed in the following chapter, the spatial proximity of segregated regions on the cortical surface is thought to contribute to the patterning of corticocortical connections at the large scale. When investigating the abundance of motif classes in large-scale cortical networks—for example, those of the cat and macaque monkey cortex—it is therefore important to compare the actual networks against at least two null models that capture effects of randomness and spatial regularity. When this dual comparison was performed, cat and macaque cortex were found to contain an overabundance of a single three-node motif (Sporns and Kötter, 2004). The motif was comprised of two sets of reciprocal connections (a "dyad") joined at a single node (motif class 9 in figure 6.4). When the contributions made by individual nodes to the overall motif distribution ("motif fingerprints"; see chapter 4) were examined, this "dual dyad" motif was found to be enriched at putative hub nodes that are characterized by relatively low clustering, short path lengths, and high centrality (Sporns et al., 2007). Because hub nodes maintain connections linking different network communities or modules, a greater than expected proportion of their neighbors will not be mutually connected, thus leading to an aggregation of dual dyad motifs at these nodes.

Why are motifs of potential interest in brain networks? Motifs represent different topological patterns of structural connections that link small subsets of nodes within a "local" neighborhood (defined topologically, and not necessarily implying small metric distances between nodes). In principle, different motif classes could support different modes of information processing, and their distribution within a larger network could therefore be considered of adaptive value. Modeling studies have shown that the way in which small groups of units are structurally interconnected constrains their dynamic interactions. Different structural motifs facilitate specific classes of dynamic behavior—for example, periodic or chaotic behavior (Zhigulin, 2004)—or promote dynamic stability (Prill et al., 2005). Another way in which structural motifs contribute to neural function derives from the idea that more densely connected motifs contain a larger number of potential subcircuits ("functional motifs"; see Sporns and Kötter, 2004).[6] A greater number of potential

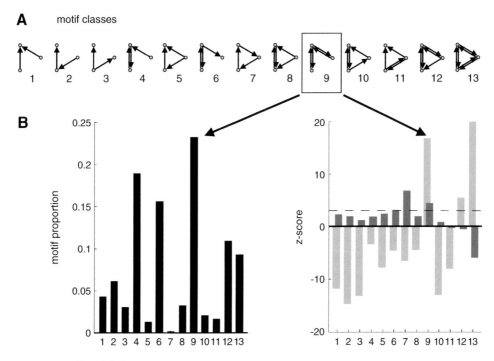

Figure 6.4

Motifs in macaque cortex. (A) All 13 possible motif classes for three nodes linked by directed edges. (B) Motif frequency distribution for a structural connection matrix of macaque cortex containing 47 nodes and 505 directed edges (see figure 2.6). Motif counts are compared (right panel) against populations of random (light gray) and lattice networks (dark gray). Only one motif class (motif class 9, referred to as the "dual dyad" motif) is found in significantly increased proportion relative to both random and lattice controls. Data were redrawn from Sporns et al. (2007).

subcircuits allows greater diversity in the topology of functional and effective interactions that are expressed in the brain at any given time. Yet another functional aspect of motifs relates to synchronization. Different motif classes exhibit different capacities for synchronization in networks with conduction delays (D'Huys et al., 2008). The high proportion of dual dyad motifs in large-scale connectivity data sets has been linked to the capacity of such motifs to promote zero phase-lag synchrony across great spatial distances and hence long conduction delays in cortex (Vicente et al., 2008). Taken together, these studies suggest that specific classes of neural motifs contribute to specific network functionalities.[7]

These studies appear to support the argument that certain motif classes may have been selected for in evolution because they confer adaptive value to the organism. However, nonrandom motif distributions may also have arisen as a result of selection pressure on other network components or processes—for example, the need to accommodate developmental constraints or to conserve wiring and metabolic energy (see the next chapter). In that sense, nonrandom motif distributions may be secondary features of network architectures, reflecting their rules of construction rather than their adaptive value. A recent re-examination of motifs in cellular networks cast doubt on their interpretation within an adaptive framework and traced their emergence to network construction rules such as duplication mechanisms (Solé and Valverde, 2006). Viewed from this perspective, motifs may be phenotypic characteristics that are by-products of true adaptations, or "spandrels" of complex network design.[8] Because of their mutual dependence and partial redundancy, it is probably premature to attribute adaptive advantages to each and every nonrandom network attribute. The fundamentally intertwined nature of many of the network attributes discussed in this chapter (motifs, modules, hubs) makes it difficult to disentangle selective contributions made by one but not another attribute. The detection of a statistically significant network feature does not automatically imply that the feature has adaptive value (see chapter 7). Simple random models, often employed in graph theoretical studies of networks, provide statistical validation but often make little biological sense as they fail to take into account biological rules of growth, spatial embedding, or metabolism.

Small Worlds Everywhere!

The seminal paper by Watts and Strogatz (1998) first presented evidence for the small-world organization of neural systems (see chapter 2). The paper reported that the clustering of the neural network of *C. elegans* was significantly increased relative to equivalent random networks, while its path length remained approximately the same. Only very few additional examples of structural cellular networks have since been examined for small-world attributes. A study of the medial reticular formation by Humphries and colleagues (Humphries et al., 2006) provided an example of small-world connectivity in the vertebrate brain at the cellular scale. Humphries et al. did not find evidence for a scale-free organization of the network's degree distribution. In general, the high density of local or short-range connections in many nervous system structures, together with a small admixture of long-range connections, should favor a small-world topology. Synthetic connectivity matrices that combine these two types of connection profiles exhibit high clustering and short path lengths (Sporns and Zwi, 2004). Some early quantitative studies of cellular circuits of mammalian neocortex show the presence of small-world features and suggest an important role for inhibitory connections in maintaining dynamic balance (Binzegger et al., 2009). Networks constructed from physiological recordings have begun to reveal clusters and hub nodes within functional cellular networks of cerebral cortex (Yu et al., 2008) and "superconnected hub neurons" in hippocampus (Bonifazi et al., 2009).

Soon after the paper by Watts and Strogatz was published, small-world attributes were also described in cat and macaque cortex (Sporns et al., 2000a; Hilgetag et al., 2000), and their existence has since been confirmed in all studies, without exception, of the large-scale anatomy of the mammalian cortex (Bassett and Bullmore, 2006).[9] An interesting question concerns the cross-species comparison of network attributes—for example, those indicating the presence of a small-world network. Has the "small-worldness" of the mammalian cortex increased over evolutionary time, or does it covary with brain size? Cross-species comparisons of small-world attributes are made difficult by the use of incompatible anatomical partitioning schemes and by a general lack of structural data for many species. A possible experimental avenue is the acquisition of connectivity data sets from brains of different organisms using a consistent methodology, for example, high-resolution diffusion MRI of post-mortem whole brains (Wedeen et al., 2009). Network analysis might then address the question of whether small-world features have undergone any kind of evolutionary trend (see chapter 7).

Mapping studies of the human brain have provided additional support for the ubiquity of small-world architectures. A connection matrix of the human brain derived from cortical thickness correlations revealed short path lengths and high clustering of cortical regions (He et al., 2007c). These clusters were later shown to be related to known functional subdivisions (Chen et al., 2008), supporting the idea that extrinsic connection patterns partly determine the intrinsic functionality of brain regions. Other studies used DTI to create cortical connectivity maps. A series of studies investigated networks of 70–90 cortical and basal brain gray matter regions derived from diffusion imaging of 20 participants using graph methods that preserve connection weights (Iturria-Medina et al., 2007; 2008). These networks were shown to exhibit robust small-world properties, and they contained an abundance of motifs in classes similar to the ones identified in tract tracing data from nonhuman mammalian cortex. Iturria-Medina and colleagues were the first to report individual variations in small-world attributes, which may be the result of macro-scale variability in the structural connectivity of individual brains (see chapter 4). The study also reported high betweenness centrality for a small set of brain regions, including the precuneus, the insula, the superior parietal cortex, and the superior frontal cortex. Several of these findings were confirmed in an independent study reporting graph analyses of DTI-derived connection matrices of 78 cortical regions (Gong et al., 2009). Once again, cortical networks were found to exhibit small-world attributes, and several regions of high centrality were identified, including the precuneus and the superior frontal gyrus.

Small-world attributes were also found for connection matrices created from DSI data sets of individual human participants. The nodes of the network were obtained from a random partition of the cortical surface into equally sized ROIs, numbering between 500 and 4,000 (Hagmann et al., 2007). High clustering and short path lengths were found at all partitions, indicating that small-world attributes persist across multiple scales and that their detection is somewhat independent of the cortical parcellation scheme used to define the network. These results were confirmed in a more extensive analysis of 998 ROI cortical networks obtained from five participants (Hagmann et al., 2008) using graph methods that preserved the experimentally obtained fiber densities for individual pathways. This study found evidence for not only high clustering at most nodes but also positive assortativity for the network as a whole. Positive assortativity, the tendency for highly connected nodes to be connected to one another, is rarely seen for other types of biological networks such as those formed by interacting proteins or signaling pathways (Newman, 2002) and is more common in social systems such as coauthorship networks. Positive assortativity is inconsistent with an organization where hubs are dispersed and disconnected but is found in network architectures that contain highly and densely connected core regions with interlinked hubs. Small-world measures are not independent of the network size or of the resolution at which brain network data are acquired (Humphries and Gurney, 2008; Wang et al., 2009a). As the spatial resolution of the network partitioning scheme is increased, a greater proportion of all connections are revealed as local or short-range, thus increasing the clustering coefficient of the network as well as the small-world index and the assortativity. Thus, the presence of network characteristics such as small-world attributes or assortativity is robust across scales, but numerical estimates for these measures depend on the prior definition of nodes and connections.

Most recent analyses of small-world structural brain networks have gone beyond merely reporting global statistics of clustering and path length. Several studies have identified clusters of brain regions or nodes, as well as critical hub nodes that link them with one another, an architecture that is highly characteristic of mammalian cortical connectivity at the large scale. This particular type of small-world architecture plays a significant role in shaping functional and effective connectivity (see chapters 8 and 9). Presently, it is much less clear whether cellular circuitry exhibits similar or different topological characteristics. As we noted in chapter 2, there are multiple ways in which a small-world network can be constructed, not all of them involving structural modules and hubs. Future studies are needed to more fully reveal the nature of the small world in cells and circuits.

Structural Modules in Mammalian Neocortex

The term "modularity" has many meanings and connotations within brain and cognitive sciences. Some of the more cognitive or psychological formulations of "modularity of mind" have attracted considerable attention, and their potential relationship with structural and functional network modules will require a separate discussion later in the book (see chapter 9). Here, I refer to modules strictly in a graph theoretical sense, defined as communities of nodes that share greater numbers of mutual connections within each community and fewer connections between them. Community detection in graphs generally involves the application of well-described clustering algorithms that are either agglomerative (starting from small groupings and constructing progressively larger ones) or divisive (subdividing larger units into smaller ones). Mark Newman and colleagues (Newman and Girvan, 2004; Newman, 2006) developed several community detection algorithms that are particularly well suited for detecting communities of arbitrary number and size based on a simple measure of modularity (see chapter 2).[10] These algorithms have been widely applied in the analysis of complex networks in transportation, social, ecological, and metabolic systems. In all these applications, modularity is the result of an objective analysis of network connectivity and not based on intuitive or subjective classification criteria for network elements or on their intrinsic characteristics. These and other related clustering methods are being increasingly applied to structural as well as functional brain networks, and they have begun to reveal the brain as a set of interconnected communities of structurally and functionally related elements, arranged on multiple scales from cells to systems.

Predating the graph-based community detection algorithms of Newman and colleagues, Young and colleagues applied multidimensional scaling to connection data sets and retrieved clusters of cortical areas that resembled known functional subdivisions in macaque and cat brain (Young, 1992; 1993; Scannell et al., 1995). Connections between nodes were translated into spatial relationships, and dimension reduction allowed the visualization of the set of spatial distances in two dimensions, thus revealing clusters of nodes that shared connectional patterns. Claus Hilgetag developed a different method termed "optimal set analysis," a stochastic optimization technique that arranged nodes into clusters such that a global cost function based on the distribution of intra- and inter-cluster connections is minimized. Implemented as an evolutionary algorithm, the method was applied to large-scale mammalian connection matrices (Hilgetag et al., 2000). In the case of the matrix of areas and connections of the macaque visual cortex, the method revealed two main clusters that closely corresponded to the dorsal and ventral streams of the primate visual cortex. For cat cortex, clusters corresponded to predominantly visual, auditory, somatomotor, and frontolimbic areas (see figure 6.5). It was noted that the cluster structure, once identified, may aid in the prediction and discovery of previously unknown connections. Hilgetag and Kaiser (2004) commented on the relationship between clusters in anatomical connectivity and the spatial proximity of many cluster members. Their proposal for a spatial growth model that can reproduce some features of the cluster structure observed in large-scale brain networks will be discussed in chapter 11.

Various structural connection matrices obtained from human brain data sets have been subjected to graph-based community detection methods. Chen et al. (2008) performed a modularity analysis with Newman's modularity measure on a connection matrix of human cortex previously derived from intersubject correlations in cortical thickness (He et al., 2007c). Several densely connected modules were identified whose members corresponded to functionally distinct groups of areas related to vision, movement, or language (see figure 6.6). Interlinking hub regions tended to be areas of multimodal or association cortex. Based on data sets derived from DSI, Hagmann et al. (2008) identified

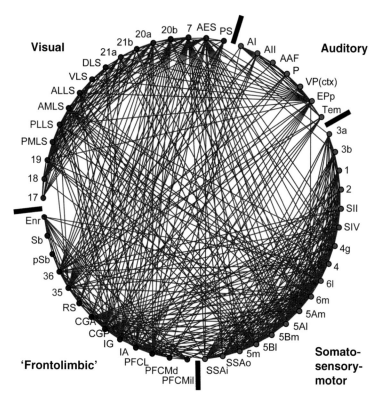

Figure 6.5
Clustered organization of cat cortex. Regions of cat cortex are arranged on a circle such that regions with similar connectivity patterns are placed near each other. Note the appearance of clustered communities corresponding to known functional subdivisions. The ordering is based on Hilgetag et al. (2000), and the image is from Hilgetag and Kaiser (2004), reproduced with permission.

modules in networks of 998 cortical regions of interest. Six structurally distinct modules were identified consisting of frontal, temporoparietal, and medial cortical regions (see figure 6.7). Modules consisted of spatially contiguous brain regions reflecting the large number of short connection pathways linking adjacent areas. Connector hubs linking multiple modules were located along the anterior–posterior medial axis of the brain and included highly connected regions such as the rostral and caudal anterior cingulate cortex, the paracentral lobule, and the precuneus. More fine-grained modularity analyses carried out on restricted subsets of ROIs revealed additional, hierarchically nested, modular arrangements. For example, clustering of ROIs within the visual cortex

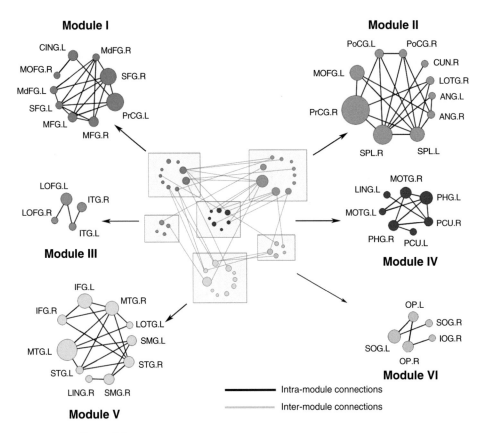

Figure 6.6
Structural modules of human cerebral cortex, identified from correlations of cortical gray matter thickness. Modularity analysis based on the modularity measure by Newman (2006) revealed 6 modules, consisting of between 4 and 10 cortical regions. Modified and reproduced from Chen et al. (2008).

yielded segregated dorsal and ventral clusters, corresponding to separate functional processing streams.

These initial studies indicated that modules mostly consist of regions that are spatially close, functionally related, and connected through hub nodes. Additional data on functional modules derived from physiological recordings (see chapters 8 and 9) confirm these patterns although the degree to which structural and functional modules can be mutually aligned is still unknown. It should also be stressed that, in many cases, reported patterns of modularity represent optimal configurations, selected for lowest cost under a cost function based on attraction/repulsion or for highest modularity score in graph-based methods.

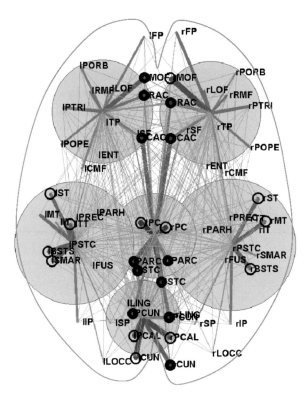

Figure 6.7
Structural modules of human cerebral cortex, identified with diffusion imaging and tractography. The plot shows a dorsal view of the brain, with the anterior–posterior axis running vertically from top to bottom. Brain regions form 6 modules whose position and size are indicated by the gray disks. Connector hubs are shown as solid black circles, and provincial hubs as open black circles. Modified and redrawn after Hagmann et al. (2008). For abbreviations of anatomical areas see figure 5.8.

However, quite often other, less optimal configurations (with greater or fewer numbers of modules) coexist within the network. The full pattern of modularity in any real-world neuroanatomical network likely involves a nested hierarchy, ranging from coarse clusterings, for example, the two cerebral hemispheres, to much more fine-grained groupings, such as functional brain systems (e.g., visual, auditory, somatomotor cortices), individual anatomically segregated areas, gray matter nuclei, or columnar arrangements of cells. This concept of hierarchical modularity stands in marked contrast to the more widely used notion of serial hierarchy based on patterned feedforward and feedback connections (see chapter 9).

Modularity involves a decomposition of a larger network into smaller units, and it has important functional connotations. It has been noted repeatedly that nodes that form a module often appear to be functionally related. For example, several of the modular groupings detected on the basis of structural connectivity in mammalian cortex involve areas with similar functionality, for example, areas within the dorsal stream of the visual cortex or within somatomotor cortex. As discussed earlier (see chapter 4), the functionality of a network node results in part from its afferent and efferent connections. Areas within structural modules are functionally related because they share many of their inputs and outputs, including connections to many other members of the same community. This pattern of preferential interconnectivity ensures that processing occurs primarily within the module, thus preserving the informational specialization of each region. However, specialized modules are not sufficient to explain cognition—the operations of individual modules must be coordinated in order to ensure system-wide coherence and information integration. We need specialized nodes that interlink modules: network hubs.

Hubs in the Brain

Hub nodes are among the most intriguing structural features of brain networks. Hubs have attracted much attention in network science since they often correspond to nodes that have special integrative or control functions. For example, hubs in protein interaction networks correspond to proteins whose deletion is often lethal to the organism (Jeong et al., 2001). In social networks, hub nodes are individuals who are highly connected and often occupy positions of leadership and power. Not surprisingly, in a social context, centrality is generally conceptualized as an influence measure. While the mechanisms of information flow in the brain are rather different from those in social systems, it is likely that neuronal hubs have a privileged role in organizing network dynamics and exert strong influence on the state of more peripheral nodes. By virtue of their structural connections, hub nodes integrate a highly diverse set of signals and are in a position to control the flow of information between otherwise relatively segregated parts of the brain. Since much of the "between-modules" information flow travels through hubs, the rate at which they relay signals would have a large impact on system-wide communication. Because of their position on many of the network's short paths, any perturbation of the state of a hub node would be able to spread quickly across the network. Hubs also contribute to brain economy. The existence of hubs as specialized "integrators" helps to conserve wiring length and volume since most regions can access information from most other regions through a few long-distance connections that access a small set of hub nodes. Taken together, there are numerous ways by which hub nodes can exert special influence on other parts of the brain—we will return to a more complete discussion of the integrative processes taking place at hub nodes in chapters 8 and 9.

Criteria for hub identification vary across different studies. In some cases, hubs are identified as "highly connected nodes," that is, primarily on the basis of node degree or strength. In scale-free networks that have heavy-tailed degree distributions, hubs are identified as nodes that are highly connected, for example, highly linked and frequently visited web sites in the case of the World Wide Web. In the case of structural brain networks, which may not exhibit scale-free degree distributions for reasons discussed earlier, the reliable identification of hub regions should take into account a combination of node degree, motif fingerprint, and centrality measures (Sporns et al., 2007). Hubs should be both highly connected and highly central, and in addition they can be identified on the basis of their low clustering coefficient and high aggregation of characteristic motifs—for example, the dual dyad (see figure 6.4). Based on these multiple criteria, a detailed analysis of the structural connectivity of macaque cortex revealed several putative hub regions, including prefrontal area 46, the frontal eye fields, and parietal areas 7a and 7b, as well as visual area V4 and somatosensory area SII, among others (Sporns et al., 2007).

Another useful distinction is that between a provincial hub and a connector hub, introduced by Guimerà and Amaral (2005) in studies of metabolic networks (see chapter 2). This classification is dependent on a previously determined partitioning of the network into modules. Provincial hubs are nodes that have high degree and centrality but whose connections are mostly contained within a single module of the network. Their position within the network allows them to facilitate the exchange and integration of information *within* a single segregated community. In contrast, connector hubs also have high degree and centrality, but their connections run mostly *between* two or more modules. Thus, they can promote information flow between otherwise segregated communities. In the study of the macaque cortex of Sporns et al. (2007), visual area V4 and somatosensory area SII were classified as provincial hubs. For example, area V4 maintains a large number of reciprocal pathways with other visual areas, and its structural embedding identifies it as a crucial link between dorsal and ventral visual streams (see figure 6.8). Most of its projections are short, underscoring its role as a hub within a single spatially coherent module. Lesions of V4 result in a variety of functional disruptions, including deficits in visual recognition and attention. In comparison, prefrontal area 46 also has high degree and centrality, but its connections link areas across multiple modules in macaque cortex, and it is therefore classified as a connector hub. Many of the projections of area 46 travel across long distances, for example, those connecting to parietal and temporal visual regions. Area 46 is known to be involved in

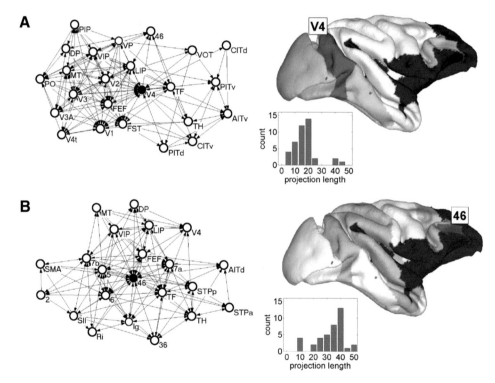

Figure 6.8
Provincial and connector hubs in macaque cortex. Network diagrams show area V4 (A) and area 46 (B) and their neighbors (left panels), as well as their spatial arrangement on the cortical surface (right panels; V4 and 46 shaded in dark gray, neighbors in medium gray). Both areas have high degree and high centrality (see figure 2.9). Area V4 connects almost exclusively to other visual areas via short projections (average length 17 mm), while area 46 maintains more widespread projections (average length 33 mm) with a mixture of visual, sensorimotor, and multimodal areas. V4 can be classified as a provincial hub, and area 46 as a connector hub. Modified and reproduced from Sporns et al. (2007). For abbreviations of anatomical areas and corresponding connection matrix see figure 2.6.

the integration of polysensory inputs, in relating external sensory inputs to internal goals, and in maintaining information in working memory. Lesions of area 46 have been shown to cause impairments in various complex cognitive tasks and to disturb internal drive and awareness.

While the special roles of areas like V4 or 46 have been previously noted in the context of physiological studies, their identification as hubs on the basis of their anatomical connectivity provides a structural basis for their involvement in diverse cortical functions. Following the idea that connectional fingerprints are associated with functional specialization (see chapter 4), the physiological characteristics and functional profiles of these hub regions are at least partly the result of their diverse and distributed pattern of structural connections. Further support for the close relationship of structure and function comes from the observation that many of the hubs identified in structural graph theoretical studies correspond to areas of the brain that had previously been classified as multimodal, transmodal, or high-level association regions.

Several authors have examined structural connectivity data sets obtained from the human cerebral cortex for highly connected or highly central regions. Gong et al. (2009) reported high centrality for the precuneus and medial frontal cortex (see figure 6.9, plate 6). Hagmann et al. (2008) identified several provincial and connector hubs on the basis of an optimal partitioning into six modules (see figure 6.7). Connector hubs were located along the anterior–posterior axis, including anterior and posterior cingulate cortex and the precuneus. Nodes with high degree and high centrality were found in areas of lateral prefrontal and parietal cortex, as well as along the cortical midline (see figure 6.10, plate 7). The most conspicuous aggregation of hubs was located in the posterior medial cortex, comprising portions on the precuneus, the posterior cingulate cortex, and parts of the retrosplenial cortex (see figure 6.11, plate 8). The structural prominence of this complex of brain regions derives from its high degree of connectedness as expressed in the graph measures of node degree and strength, as well as its high betweenness centrality, independently reported in several graph theoretical analyses of the structural connectivity of the human cerebral cortex (Iturria-Medina et al., 2008; Hagmann et al., 2008; Gong et al., 2009; Li et al., 2009).

As we will see in chapters 8 and 9, the precuneus/posterior cingulate cortex occupies an equally central position in functional networks of the human brain, in particular those engaged during cognitive rest (Greicius et al., 2003; Fransson and Marrelec, 2008), and it corresponds to an area of extremely high metabolic activity (Gusnard and Raichle, 2001). The

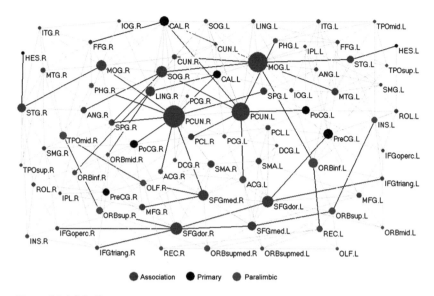

Figure 6.9 (plate 6)
Topological organization of human brain structural connectivity obtained with diffusion tensor imaging. Brain regions are arranged using a spring embedding algorithm, and symbol size indicates the magnitude of a region's betweenness centrality. Regions are classified as belonging to association, primary, or paralimbic cortex. Reproduced from Gong et al. (2009) with permission.

region is homologous to the macaque monkey posteromedial cortex, known to maintain extensive and widely distributed connections with numerous cortical and subcortical regions (Parvizi et al., 2006). In the past, the functional roles of the precuneus were not well understood,[11] in part because of the scarceness of neurophysiological recording data and the reported involvement of the precuneus in an extremely broad range of diverse cognitive phenomena. For example, activation of the precuneus has been reported in self-referential processing, imagery, and episodic memory (Cavanna and Trimble, 2006), and its level of activation is associated with the level of consciousness (Laureys et al., 2004). Administration of general anesthetics such as propofol induces large regional decreases in cerebral blood flow in the precuneus, cuneus, and posterior cingulate cortex (Fiset et al., 1999), and deactivation of posterior medial cortex is associated with loss of consciousness (Kaisti et al., 2002). Lesions of the posterior medial cortex, while rare because of its redundant arterial blood supply and protected location deep within the skull, result in severe disturbances of cognition and consciousness (Damasio, 1999).[12] Could this intriguing confluence of diverse functional

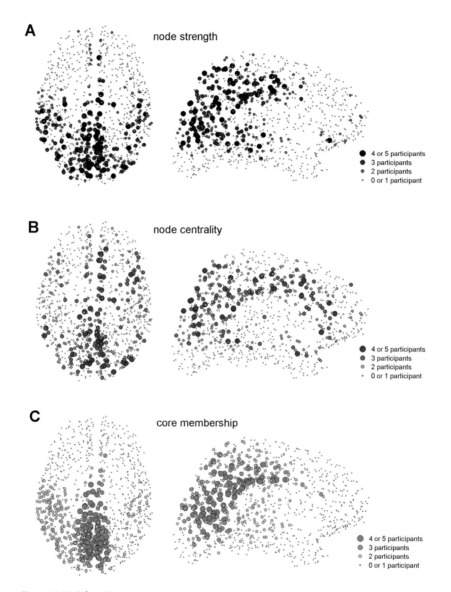

Figure 6.10 (plate 7)
Anatomical distribution of node strength, node centrality, and core membership. All plots show summary results obtained for brains of 5 participants. (A) Network nodes with high node strength. The plot shows how consistently region-of-interest (ROI) strength ranked in the top 20 percent across participants. (B) Network nodes with high centrality. The plot shows how consistently ROI centrality ranked in the top 20 percent across participants. (C) Average network core across participants. The plot shows how consistently ROIs were included in the core across participants. Data as shown in Hagmann et al. (2008).

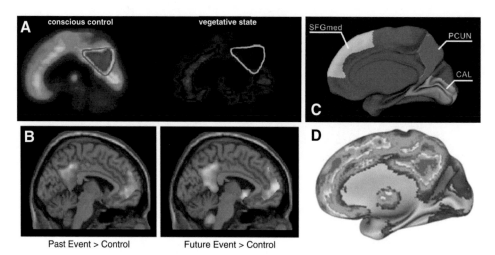

Figure 6.11 (plate 8)
The precuneus/posterior cingulate in brain imaging and network analysis. (A) Resting metabolism in a healthy participant and in a patient in the vegetative state. Images show glucose metabolism (high values in hot colors) shown in the sagittal plane, with the precuneus/posterior cingulate cortex outlined in red. The region exhibits the highest metabolic rate in the healthy participant and the lowest in the vegetative patient. Image is from Laureys et al. (2004), reproduced with permission. (B) Sagittal slice of functional magnetic resonance imaging activations obtained during the elaboration of past (left) and future (right) events, both relative to a control task. Image is from Addis et al. (2007), reproduced with permission. (C) Map of betweenness centrality obtained from structural connectivity of the cerebral cortex, indicating several structural hubs (PCUN, precuneus; SFGmed, medial superior frontal gyrus, CAL, calcarine cortex). Image is from Gong et al. (2009), reproduced with permission. (D) Cortical hubs estimated on the basis of node degree obtained from resting-state functional connectivity of the cerebral cortex. Image is from Buckner et al. (2009), reproduced with permission.

roles, from brain metabolism to consciousness, be the result of the area's high centrality within the cortical system?

The existence of hub nodes is essential to maintain network-wide information flow. Their loss or dysfunction has disproportionate effects on the integrity and functionality of the remaining system. Studies of social or technological systems have shown that hubs are points of vulnerability that may become subject to "targeted attack." I will further examine this aspect of structural hubs when I discuss the effects of lesions and disease states on brain networks. However, despite their highly central structural embedding and diverse functionality, hub nodes should not be mistaken for "master controllers" or "homunculus regions," capable of autonomous control or executive influence. Their influence derives from their capacity to connect across much of the brain and promote functional integration, not from special intrinsic processing power or capacity for "decision making." Hubs enable and facilitate integrative processes, but they do not represent their outcome, which instead is found in the distributed and global dynamics of the brain.

Small World—Big Deal?

A broad range of natural, social, and technological systems exhibits small-world connectivity (see chapter 2). The ubiquity of this architecture is suggestive of a universal functional role that transcends specific network implementations and mechanisms (Watts and Strogatz, 1998). As we have seen in this chapter, small-world architectures are abundant in structural networks of the brain, across a number of species and systems—but are small-world networks of functional importance? Small-world architectures in the brain are implemented as networks of modules and hubs, and these architectural features have clear relevance for the functional organization of the brain. As we will see in coming chapters, the dual hallmarks of the small world, high clustering and short path length, play crucial roles in shaping dynamic neuronal interactions at cellular and large scales. Not only do patterns of functional interactions themselves exhibit small-world features (see chapters 8 and 9), but there is mounting evidence that disruptions of small-world organization are associated with disturbances in cognition and behavior (see chapter 10). The next chapter will demonstrate that modular small-world architectures also promote the economy and efficiency of brain networks by allowing for structural connectivity to be built at low cost in terms of wiring volume and metabolic energy demand and by enabling efficient information flow across the entire network. Furthermore, economical and efficient small-world networks can generate functional dynamics that express highly diverse states (see chapter 12) and high complexity (see chapter 13).

Thus, the small-world architecture of neuronal networks, at the scale of cellular and large-scale systems, provides a structural substrate for several important aspects of the functional organization of the brain. The architecture promotes efficiency and economy, as well as diverse and complex network dynamics. Each of these functional aspects is of critical importance for the organism and its evolutionary survival, and it is important that small-world networks can promote all of them *simultaneously*. A brain network that is economically wired but not capable of rapid and flexible integration of information would be highly suboptimal, as would be an architecture that supports great computational power but utilizes an inordinate amount of space or energy.

These considerations naturally lead to the idea that the small-world architecture of brain networks has been selected for in biological evolution. Are small-world networks an adaptation, or can their ubiquitous appearance be explained in some other way? To begin to answer this question, we need to consider brain networks not only as topological patterns but also as physical objects that consume space, energy, and material.

7 Economy, Efficiency, and Evolution

After reviewing the many shapes assumed by neurons, we are now in a position to ask whether this diversity [...] has been left to chance and is insignificant, or whether it is tightly regulated and provides an advantage to the organism. [...] all of the morphological features displayed by neurons appear to obey precise rules that are accompanied by useful consequences. What are these rules and consequences? [...] all of the various conformations of the neuron and its various components are simply morphological adaptations governed by laws of conservation for time, space, and material.[1]
—Santiago Ramón y Cajal, 1899

Nervous systems are physical objects of staggering complexity. In the human brain, at least a million billion synapses and thousands of miles of neural wiring are compressed within a volume of around 1,400 cm^3, forming a dense web of cellular connections that is yet to be completely mapped. When examining the physical structure of the brain, one cannot help but be struck by its high economy and efficiency. Santiago Ramón y Cajal was among the first anatomists to clearly express the idea that the conservation of basic resources such as space and biological material has governed the evolution of neuronal morphology and connectivity (see figure 7.1). Recently, the availability of network data sets and computational modeling tools has allowed this idea to be more fully explored. There can be little doubt that space and energy constraints can have direct effects on the physical realizability of a nervous system. For the brain to function properly it must fit inside the head.[2] The brain's "wiring," its constituent neuronal and nonneuronal cells and all their processes, cannot occupy a volume greater than that afforded by the bony enclosure of the skull. Furthermore, the metabolic cost of operating the brain's neural elements should only be a fraction of the total energy budget of the body. The wiring and metabolic cost that result from the architecture and operation of the brain impose narrow limits on structural brain connectivity that cannot be circumvented. Detailed studies of neural

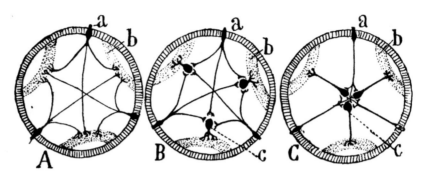

Figure 7.1
Cajal's example for wiring economy. The diagrams show cross-sections of idealized invertebrates, with three sensory neurons (a) each of which innervates three muscles (b). (A) Only sensory neurons are present and the total wiring cost is high (approximately 6 times the diameter of the cross-section). (B) The appearance of separate motor neurons (c) and the aggregation of their cell bodies in ganglia (C) lowers the wiring cost (to about 3 times the diameter of the cross-section). Reproduced from Cajal (1995, p. 14) with permission.

morphology and spatial layout of neural connectivity in brains of several species support the idea that neural elements are arranged and connected in ways that make economical use of limited resources of space and energy. The brain's connectivity pattern appears to have been shaped over evolutionary time to provide maximal computational power while minimizing the volume and cost of physical wiring.

Much of this chapter will examine this "wiring minimization" hypothesis. To what extent has brain connectivity been shaped by spatial and metabolic constraints? Are the elements and connections of brain networks optimally economical (in a spatial or metabolic sense), and is this optimality the direct result of natural selection? Are functional design constraints compatible with economical spatial embedding and low metabolic cost? As we will see, multiple lines of empirical and computational evidence suggest that brain architectures balance competing spatial, metabolic, and functional demands. Rather than being optimal for any single factor, brain connectivity jointly satisfies these multiple demands. The combination of these demands is likely to have shaped the neuronal morphology and connection topology of nervous systems ranging from *C. elegans* to humans.

The Cost of Neuronal Communication

The economy of neuronal architecture involves a combination of factors that come into play during growth and development of the nervous system, as well as during its operation in the adult organism (Laughlin and Sejnowski, 2003). Economy during development may imply that neural structures require only a small number of molecular cues for regulation of elementary processes such as cell proliferation, differentiation, migration, and axonal outgrowth and guidance. Economical design may also result from a combination of conserved wiring length or volume, short axonal conduction delays, fast signal propagation, and low metabolic cost of neural activity and spike propagation. All of these factors contribute to the overall cost of neuronal communication between spatially remote neurons and brain regions.

Mechanisms of neural development lead to the formation of specific long-range neural pathways that link neurons over great distances or within local volumes of space. Temporally regulated patterns and gradients of a small number of attractive or repulsive guidance molecules can shape growing axons into complex anatomical networks (Dickson, 2002; Williamson and Hiesinger, 2008). For example, molecular guidance cues are critically involved in the establishment of topographic maps (Sur and Rubenstein, 2005). Topography supports a number of important computational functions (Thivierge and Marcus, 2007) and is also compatible with an efficient arrangement of wiring between neural areas. The spatiotemporal control of molecules involved in axonal patterning of topographic projections thus supports economical wiring in structural brain networks. A further example includes the intra-areal connections in the cerebral cortex, which are mostly made within local volumes of space and tend to be reciprocal and patchy (Douglas and Martin, 2004). These synaptic patterns are shaped by distributions of morphogens that control axonal outgrowth as well as synapse formation and stabilization. Thus, molecular developmental mechanisms can account for the observed abundance of topographic and local connections and, consequently, for at least some aspects of wiring minimization in neural structures such as the cerebral cortex.

Given that developmental mechanisms play a major role in shaping connectivity and naturally promote short wiring, what is the role of development in theories of wiring minimization? Most proponents of conservation principles, including Cajal,[3] have suggested that economical features of cell morphology and connectivity arose as a result of selection for utility and adaptive advantage rather than as a result of developmental processes. An alternative view proposes that developmental processes may also directly contribute to conserved wiring patterns. Following the same general principles that govern the evolution of animal forms (Carroll, 2005), evolution may have favored developmental processes that give rise to economical brain connectivity, including short wiring and low metabolic cost. It is also worth pointing out that many developmental processes that unfold in a growing organism are not a direct consequence of natural selection. For example, the physical and chemical forces that shape spatial gradients of morphogens and the capacity of cells to respond to external cues in a concentration-dependent manner naturally favor topographic and clustered connectivity. Physical processes such as diffusion or adhesion do not arise as the result of natural selection but can nevertheless promote specific patterns of morphology and connectivity such as short wiring. Furthermore, morphology and function are closely intertwined. For example, the prevalence of short-range connections, particularly in cortical maps, has important functional and computational implications. Developmental mechanisms that favor short-range over long-range (or randomly arranged) connections not only are conserving cortical space and volume but also have direct consequences for the computational operations carried out in neural maps (Nelson and Bower, 1990; Thivierge and Marcus, 2007) and for the emergence of a modular neural architecture (Jacobs and Jordan, 1992).

The constraints imposed by wiring volume on axonal patterning have been recognized for some time. Mitchison (1991) demonstrated that minimizing the volume of axonal branching in intra-areal connectivity can account for observed arrangements of cells and connections in cortical maps—for example, interleaved stripes and blobs formed by distinct cell populations that occur in visual cortex. Segregation of cells that have distinct patterns of inputs favors economical wiring, and the same idea was invoked as an explanation for the existence of multiple segregated cortical areas whose inputs are distinct and whose physiological properties are functionally specialized (Mitchison, 1991; 1992). Cherniak (1992) applied a network optimization framework to identify the critical parameters that are optimized in the design of branching neuronal structures such as dendritic and axonal arbors. Results suggested a minimized wiring volume, rather than wiring length, signal propagation speed, or surface area. Cherniak concluded that local network volume minimization may be sufficient to account for observed neuroanatomy, "without introduction of, e.g. the ideas of optimization of subtle electrophysiological signal-processing roles for the junctions, or of the abstract flow of information through them" (p. 509). More recently, the idea of pure volume minimization has been supplemented by more detailed models that explain the topology of dendritic branching by using a combination of wiring constraints and graph theoretical measures, such as path length between synaptic inputs and the base of the dendritic tree (Cuntz et al., 2007). The model suggests that a conjunction of biophysical and topological factors is sufficient to account for the observed shapes and morphologies of neuronal processes.

Another aspect of the cost of neuronal communication involves the relationship between connection length and axonal conduction delays. Conduction delays have important effects on processing speed, dynamic coupling, and other integrative processes within populations of neurons. Recent studies have reaffirmed the importance of neuronal conduction delays in determining connectional features of structural brain networks (e.g., Chklovskii et al., 2002), despite earlier suggestions that delays may play only a minor role (e.g., Mitchison, 1991).

Finally, metabolic demand should be mentioned as another costly aspect of long connections. The generation of spikes by neurons and their propagation along axons requires considerable amounts of metabolic energy. In unmyelinated axons, the cost of neuronal communication increases with axonal length and has been estimated at around one third of the total metabolic cost for each single spike (Lennie, 2003), likely imposing tight constraints on the architecture of structural brain networks. In virtually all species, neural tissue operates at very high energetic cost, both during active processing and at rest. This cost is seen to have led to further selective pressure toward energy efficiency. Niven and Laughlin (2008) examined data on the energy consumption of neuronal structures in the visual system of a wide range of animal species. They concluded that energy efficiency may have played a key role in the evolution of the morphology and physiology of neural systems, including the way in which neurons encode and transmit information.

Neuronal Placement and Connection Length in *C. elegans*

The availability of the complete anatomical arrangement of neurons in the brain of the nematode *C. elegans* (see chapter 5), including their connectivity and spatial location, has provided a rare opportunity to investigate the role of resource constraints in determining wiring patterns. In the mid 1990s, Christopher Cherniak advanced a theory to explain the spatial layout of nervous systems and, specifically, that of *C. elegans*. He suggested that the physical positions of network components were arranged such that total connection cost was minimized, a principle he termed "component placement optimization" in analogy to principles used in the design of electronic microcircuits (Cherniak, 1994;

1995). Combining data on the physical location and connectivity of neurons in *C. elegans*, Cherniak showed that the spatial positions of ganglia or cell groupings are highly optimal, with the actual placement exhibiting minimal wiring cost among about 40 million alternatives. An examination of the spatial layout of individual neurons was not feasible at the time.

The central idea in Cherniak's theory was that neurons (or ganglia) are placed at spatial locations such that their total wiring length is minimized. The theory was framed in an evolutionary context, with the implication that optimal component placement conferred an advantage in natural selection. However, it was left unspecified how the spatial placement of neurons could be varied independently of connectivity in any real nervous system. Placement of neurons is not independent of the formation of connections since both events unfold within the same developmental process. Spatial distributions of morphogens guiding connectivity are regulated by other developmental factors such as cell migration and differentiation. These factors follow specific spatial and temporal rules that cannot be independently varied to produce "suboptimally" wired variants. Instead, if two neurons are spatially close within the developing organism, biochemical mechanisms (such as graded molecular cues) make it more likely that these neurons are also connected (Young and Scannell, 1996). Developmental processes thus produce a tendency for neurons to be "connected, because they are adjacent," not "adjacent, because they are connected" as suggested by component placement optimization.

Critics of the component-placement-optimization approach disputed the privileged role of wiring minimization by questioning whether the wiring of *C. elegans* is indeed minimal. Cherniak's original study only provided an analysis of the placement of 11 ganglia. More recent studies have been able to determine whether *C. elegans* is minimally wired at the level of individual neurons. Chen et al. (2006) performed a painstaking reanalysis of the wiring diagram of *C. elegans*, which led to an updated and more complete connection matrix (see chapter 5). Given the wiring diagram, Chen et al. compared the most economical layout of individual neurons and connections to the actual set of spatial positions recorded in the organism. Predicted neuronal positions were found to be close to actual ones for most neurons; however, some neurons showed significant deviations from their predicted optimal positions (see figure 7.2). Thus, it appears that wiring minimization can account for much of the neuronal layout, with some important exceptions that may relate to functional

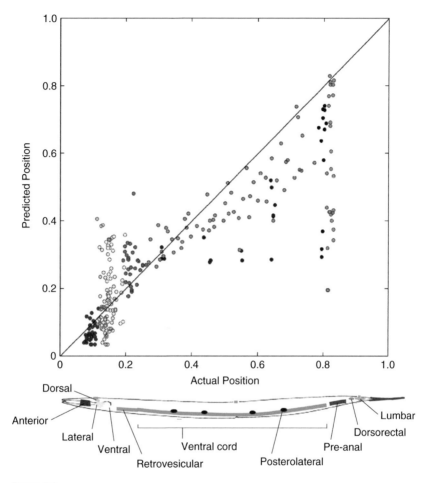

Figure 7.2
Wiring economy in *C. elegans*. Scatterplot of neuron positions along the main axis of the worm's body versus positions predicted by a wiring-minimization model. Dots along the main diagonal of the plot correspond to perfect predictions. Overall, the discrepancy between actual versus predicted positions is less than 10 percent. The sketch at the bottom shows the location of the main ganglia and cell groupings (cf. figure 5.1). Modified and reproduced from Chen et al. (2006) with permission.

demands which violate the minimization rule. Two other studies also indicate that the actual wiring of *C. elegans* does not embody a global minimum in wiring cost. Ahn et al. (2006) were able to generate a spatial layout for neurons in *C. elegans* that further reduced wiring cost by about 50 percent. Given the distribution of connection lengths, much of the "suboptimal" connection cost in the real worm appeared to be due to the existence of long connections spanning around 80 percent of the worm's body length. A similar reduction in wiring cost was obtained by Kaiser and Hilgetag (2006). Again, much of the excess in wiring cost was found to be due to long-distance connections.[4]

There is broad agreement that wiring minimization *alone* cannot account for the exact spatial layout of neurons in the nervous system of *C. elegans*. While the actual layout seen in the real organism does conserve space and material, other functional considerations are also likely to play a role. An examination of the efficiency and economy of neural wiring in the mammalian cerebral cortex offers additional clues to the nature of these functional constraints.

Neuronal Wiring in the Mammalian Brain

One of the most robust features of corticocortical connectivity is the prevalence of short-range connections. This pattern prevails among individual cortical neurons as well as between segregated brain regions. Anatomical studies have demonstrated an exponential decrease of connection probability with increasing spatial separation between cortical neurons (Braitenberg and Schüz, 1998; Hellwig, 2000; Liley and Wright, 1994). While these connection probabilities approach zero at distances of several millimeters, cortical cells can make horizontal connections that extend over greater distances, in addition to long-range projections to targets in other regions. Similar biases of connections toward spatial proximity are seen not only among individual cells but also at the large scale of brain regions and systems, ultimately shaping cortical topology into spatially coherent modules (see chapter 6). Among the segregated areas of the cerebral cortex, connections occur with high probability between adjacent or neighboring areas and with much lower probability between areas that are separated by greater distances (Felleman and Van Essen, 1991; Van Essen, 1997). However, not all adjacent cortical regions are mutually connected. Young's analysis of the wiring pattern in macaque cortex (Young, 1992; 1993) showed that only a fraction of interregional pathways could be explained on the basis of regional proximity on the cortical surface. Within more spatially confined sets of brain regions—for example, those of the primate prefrontal cortex—neighboring areas were found to be anatomically linked with a probability of 0.94, and these probabilities progressively decreased as distances between areas increased (Averbeck and Seo, 2008).

The macroscopic anatomical organization of the mammalian cortex is characterized by the segregation of cell bodies and axonal connections into gray matter and white matter, by an arrangement of gray matter into a sheet surrounding a white matter core, and by various degrees of folding of the cortical surface. Ruppin et al. (1993) noted that given the preponderance of short-range over long-range connections in cortical networks, the combination of these three characteristics supports volume minimization and results in a volume-efficient architecture (see also Murre and Sturdy, 1995). Wen and Chklovskii (2005) have argued that the segregation of much of the vertebrate brain into gray matter and white matter is a consequence of joint optimization for the competing requirements of high connectivity and minimal conduction delay. Based on measurements of the gray matter "wire fraction," defined as the proportion of volume occupied by axons and dendrites within gray matter, Chklovskii et al. (2002) suggested that cortical circuits are organized such that conduction delays are near-minimal and synapse numbers are near-maximal. In a similar vein, Klyachko and Stevens (2003) performed computational analyses of the spatial layout of macaque prefrontal cortex and concluded that the actual spatial arrangement of these cortical areas minimizes the total volume of the interconnecting axons. An extension of the component-placement-optimization framework to the positioning of brain regions within mammalian cerebral cortex (Cherniak et al., 2004) suggested that cortical regions are placed such that connection lengths between them are minimized.

Cortical folding contributes to conserving wiring length.[5] Van Essen (1997) suggested that the compactness of cortical wiring may be due to physical tension along developing axonal pathways and the consequent folding of the cortical surface (see figure 7.3). Such a process of tension-based morphogenesis would naturally promote short wiring lengths and small conduction delays. In cat and macaque cortex, local connections between brain areas are denser within gyri than across sulci (Scannell, 1997), a finding that is consistent with the tension-based folding model. Further support for a significant role of physical forces, such as tension exerted by corticocortical connections in the folding of the cortex, was provided by Hilgetag and Barbas (2005; 2006). Axonal tension should result in projections that are predominantly straight rather than curved, and a quantitative analysis of corticocortical pathways in macaque prefrontal cortex provides support for this hypothesis. Folding was found to have differential effects on the cellular architecture of cortex that is folded inward or outward, influencing cell density and the spatial layout of cortical columns. Hence, the effects of folding far exceed wiring optimization. Instead, it appears that mechanophysical forces operating

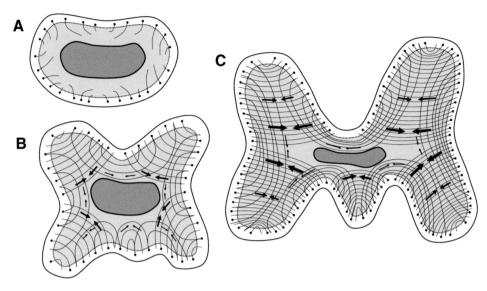

Figure 7.3
Tension-mediated folding of the cerebral cortex. (A) At early developmental stages, newly differentiated neurons emit axons. (B) Axons reach target structures, and the formation of axonal pathways results in the onset of tensile forces that pull strongly interconnected regions closer together. (C) Outward folds begin to appear, separating more strongly connected regions. Simplified and redrawn after Van Essen (1997).

within growing brain tissue can have profound effects on several key aspects of brain connectivity. The mechanics of cortical folding may introduce variations in the way cortical tissue responds to or processes information. As discussed earlier (see chapter 4), cortical folding patterns are variable across individuals, even between monozygotic twins. Among healthy adults, larger brains are more highly folded, possibly as a result of increased axonal tension during development (Im et al., 2008).[6] Disturbances of cortical folding may be associated with brain diseases such as schizophrenia and autism that exhibit disorganized structural and functional connectivity (see chapter 10). Brain shape and brain function are once again revealed to be interdependent.

Intuitively, if wiring volume or length were the only factor according to which neural connectivity is optimized, then the existence and, in many cases, evolutionary elaboration of long-range projections between distant cortical regions is hard to explain. An optimally short wiring pattern would look like a two-dimensional grid or lattice, with connections that link only neighboring nodes. This point was examined in more detail by Kaiser and Hilgetag (2006), who reanalyzed optimal spatial arrangements for several brain connectivity data sets including *C. elegans* (see above) and mammalian cortex by taking into account metric distances between neurons or areas. Remarkably, these networks could be spatially rearranged such that the total cost of wiring decreased by more than 30 percent, due to the existence of "nonoptimal" long-distance connections in the primate cerebrum (see figure 7.4). These long-distance connections are essential for keeping path lengths between pairs of cortical regions short and, thus, for enabling efficient information flow within the network. In fact, networks that minimize wiring cost but lack any long-distance connections showed significantly increased path lengths,

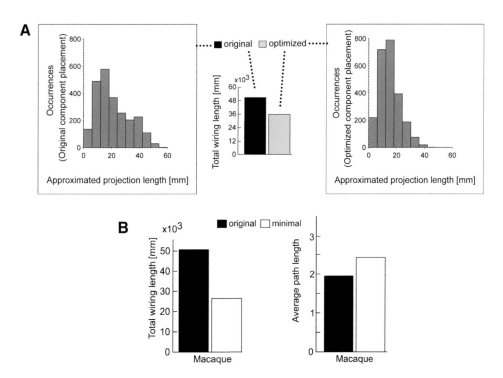

Figure 7.4
Wiring cost in macaque cortex. (A) Projection length before and after component placement optimization. The "original" distribution was derived by determining Euclidean distances between all pairs of connected regions. The "optimized" distribution was derived from an optimal "wire-saving" rearrangement of cortical regions determined by a simulated annealing optimization algorithm. Optimal placement of regions reduced wiring cost by an additional 32 percent over the original pattern, predominantly by eliminating long-distance pathways. (B) Wiring length and path length in minimally rewired macaque cortex. Rewiring was carried out by preferentially connecting neighboring regions without changing the overall density of connections. Minimizing wiring cost comes at the expense of an increase in path length. Modified and reproduced from Kaiser and Hilgetag (2006).

indicative of an increased number of processing steps. Kaiser and Hilgetag concluded that optimal wiring length alone cannot account for the observed wiring patterns—instead, the topology of structural brain connectivity appears to be shaped by several different factors, including wiring as well as path length.

Thus, a cortical architecture with short path length (or high efficiency; see below) may confer a selective advantage to the organism. A drive toward maintaining short path length may partly explain the appearance and expansion of long-range fiber pathways in evolution. One such pathway, the arcuate fasciculus, is a prominent fiber tract in the human brain and links cortical regions in the temporal and lateral frontal cortex involved in language (see figure 7.5). Rilling et al. (2008) compared the

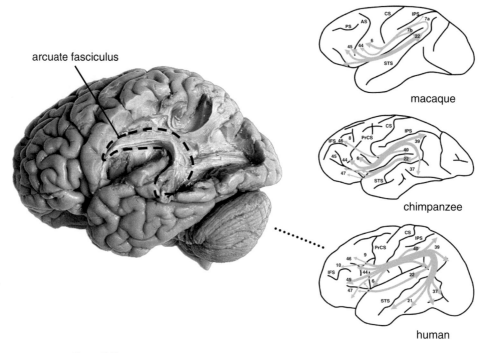

Figure 7.5
Evolution of a long-distance fiber pathway, the arcuate fasciculus. The image at the left shows an anatomical preparation exposing the arcuate fasciculus in the left cerebral hemisphere of the human brain (image courtesy of the Digital Anatomist Project, Department of Biological Structure, at the University of Washington). Sketches at right show a schematic summary of the connectivity of the arcuate fasciculus in three primate species, obtained by diffusion imaging and tractography. Note the expansion of the tract and the appearance of new links between the frontal and temporal cortices in humans. Modified and reproduced from Rilling et al., 2008, with permission.

anatomy of this tract in postmortem brains of several primate species, imaged with diffusion MRI. The tract is significantly smaller and differently organized in the cortex of nonhuman primates compared to the cortex of humans. Rilling et al. suggested that the elaboration and modification of the arcuate fasciculus, together with the increased differentiation of connected cortical regions, represents a structural substrate for the evolution of human language. The selective evolutionary expansion of the arcuate fasciculus is interpreted as evidence against the notion that language arose as an incidental by-product of brain-size enlargement. Viewed from the perspective of network topology, selective pressure on maintaining functional integration and efficient information flow in a larger brain may also have contributed to the evolutionary expansion of the arcuate fasciculus. This expansion led to the emergence of a new structural network that became available for functional recruitment by communication and language.

Efficient Information Flow

Network-wide communication and functional integration are facilitated by short path lengths (see chapter 2). This aspect of the topology of structural brain networks has been quantified as "brain efficiency." Efficiency as a network measure was first introduced by Latora and Marchiori (2001; see chapter 2) to express the capacity of networks to facilitate information exchange. The efficiency with which two nodes communicate was defined to be inversely proportional to the shortest distance between these nodes. The global efficiency of the network is the average of the efficiency over all pairs, including disconnected pairs (see chapter 2). Local efficiency is a nodal measure of the average efficiency within a local subgraph or neighborhood. While global efficiency is related to the path length, local efficiency is related to the clustering coefficient. Latora and Marchiori suggested that local and global efficiency characterize a network in terms of its ability to support parallel information transfer. Small-world topology is closely associated with high global and local efficiency, often achieved with sparse connectivity at low connection cost (Latora and Marchiori, 2003).

Latora and Marchiori (2001; 2003) provided a range of examples of real-world networks with high global and local efficiency. Among these were several neuronal networks, including those of *C. elegans*, cat cortex, and macaque monkey cortex. In all cases, the topology of structural brain networks exhibited high global and high local efficiency, consistent with their small-world architecture (see chapter 6). Latora and Marchiori noted that the coexistence of high local and high global efficiency allows the network to balance localized processing, fault tolerance, and large-scale functional integration. Human brain networks also enable highly efficient parallel information flow. Achard and Bullmore (2007) applied efficiency to functional brain networks acquired with fMRI during cognitive rest (see chapter 8) and showed that such networks exhibited small-world properties with globally and locally efficient information flow. This high efficiency could be achieved at relatively low cost, where cost was defined as the number of edges in the network. Other studies have since confirmed that small-world topology of brain networks is associated with high efficiency of information flow.

Neuronal synchrony is thought to play an important role in information flow and system-wide coordinative processes. The two main cellular components of mammalian cortex, excitatory principal cells and inhibitory interneurons, jointly account for much of the computational capacity of the network and its ability to form synchronized assemblies. György Buzsáki and colleagues have argued that this computational capacity is enhanced by the great morphological and physiological diversity of cortical interneurons (Buzsáki et al., 2004). This diversity of network elements counteracts opposing demands on the size and connection density of the network, thus achieving a compromise between computational needs and wiring economy. Computational models show that long-range connections are crucial for producing network-wide synchronization, but their addition to the network increases the wiring cost. An efficiency function that trades off increases in synchronization with increases in wiring defines an optimal range within which global synchrony can be achieved with the addition of a modest number of long-range connections. Within this optimal range, the network exhibits a small-world architecture characterized by high clustering and short path length.

Robustness and Evolvability

If the brain were a system composed of billions of independent variables, its very existence would be a mystery, since a system of such complexity could hardly have evolved through the slow and gradual accumulation of heritable variation. In a more general sense, the problem of how complex biological organization can evolve applies to all organisms, and it has puzzled evolutionary theorists since Darwin. More recently, the issue has been reframed as "evolvability" or evolutionary adaptability, the capacity to generate heritable, selectable phenotypic variation (Kirschner and Gerhart, 1998; 2005). This capacity is not simply accounted for by random mutations, because it matters how such mutations are translated into variable phenotypes. Evolvability is compromised if most mutations result in lethality or seriously disrupt the functioning of the organism. Thus, a degree of robustness is highly desirable, such that the phenotypic effects of most random mutations are neutralized or at least reduced. At first glance, robustness appears to limit the evolvability of a system by reducing the number of genetic variations that are phenotypically expressed and upon which natural selection can act. However, neutral mutations can also promote evolutionary innovation (Wagner, 2005) by creating a set of systems that vary in their genetic makeup yet function equally well. This pool of stable variants can become useful if novel external challenges are encountered that turn the hidden reservoir of genetic variability into adaptations. In summary, "robustness implies that many mutations are neutral and such neutrality fosters innovation" (Wagner, 2005, p. 1773).

Robustness and evolvability are supported by the modular organization of biological systems, found everywhere from gene and protein networks to complex processes of embryonic development (Raff, 1996; Wagner et al., 2007). Modularity promotes robustness by isolating the effects of local mutations or perturbations and thus allowing modules to evolve somewhat independently. Networks of dependencies between system elements reduce the dimensionality of the global phenotypic space and effectively uncouple clusters of highly interacting elements from each other. Modularity itself should therefore offer an evolutionary advantage and thus affect evolvability. The mechanisms by which the modularity of biological systems may have arisen are a matter of much debate (Wagner et al., 2007). Modularity may have evolved along two routes, by integration of smaller elements into larger clusters or by parcellation of larger systems into segregated smaller ones (Wagner and Altenberg, 1996).

The dissociability (or "near decomposability"; see chapter 13) of biological systems extends to the brain's small-world architecture. Whether the modular organization of the brain has supported its evolvability is unknown and would depend in part on whether phenotypic characteristics of individual modules, or regions within modules, are shown to be under the control of locally expressed genes. In support of this notion, a recent analysis of regional gene expression patterns during human brain development revealed a high percentage of genes that were expressed in a regionally specific pattern (Johnson et al., 2009). Individual brain regions were found to express partially segregated sets or modules of coregulated genes. An intriguing possibility is that modular gene transcription supports the independent evolution of regional phenotypes and thus forms a substrate for functional innovation. Structural brain connectivity may support this process by helping to coordinate gene expression patterns among remote locations in the brain through generating dynamic correlations.

Models of evolutionary processes suggest that modular processing emerges in the presence of a highly variable environment (Lipson et al., 2002). This modularization is also observed in more complex models of evolving networks exposed to an environment posing variable goals or challenges (Kashtan and Alon, 2005). If these varying goals contained common subgoals, networks evolved modular structure where the individual modules become specialized for these subgoals. However, if varying goals do not have common subgoals, networks fail to evolve modularity. These models suggest that network modules become specialized for recurrent task demands of the environment. In addition to allowing efficient processing and conferring a degree of robustness in evolution, brain network modularity has a deep impact on the relation of network structure to network dynamics, a topic we will more thoroughly explore in coming chapters (chapters 8, 9, 12, and 13). Among these dynamic effects of modularity is a tendency toward increased dynamic stability as shown by Variano et al. (2004). Networks optimized for dynamic stability (within a linear systems framework) were found to exhibit hierarchical modularity, a structural feature that rendered their dynamics both stable and robust against structural mutations. Other dynamic effects of modularity include limiting the spread of perturbations between modules and shaping the pattern of dynamic dependencies and synchronization (see chapter 12).

Brain Size and Scaling Laws

Size is of fundamental importance to the organization of all living organisms (Bonner, 2006). Size has a major impact on the shape and form of the organism's body and on the way in which the organism interacts with its environment. Size also plays a major role in the anatomical arrangement and connectivity of the brain (Striedter, 2005). Many of the variations in brain structure and connectivity that are observed across species can be explained on the basis of variations in size. The absolute size of a nervous system has straightforward effects on the total number of neurons and the fraction of brain volume the neurons occupy as well as on their regional density and patterns of connectivity. If a given brain is scaled up or down in size, the physical embedding of the brain requires corresponding changes in its anatomical connection patterns. It is impossible to change the physical dimensions of a nervous system without also changing its connection topology. Therefore, evolutionary changes that affect the size, as well as the general morphology, of an organism's body have inevitable consequences for the connectional organization of its nervous system.

Comparative analyses of morphological variables recorded across numerous extant species have revealed a number of stable and robust scaling relationships, relating the sizes and shapes of anatomical structures.[7] In most cases, these scaling relationships are not isometric but allometric. Isometry implies that a change in the size of an organism does not alter the proportional sizes of its components and hence does not change its shape and form. Allometry, instead, is found when a change in body size results in proportionally larger or smaller component structures. Many physiological and metabolic processes, as well as morphological features, scale allometrically with body size, and it has been known since the nineteenth century that the brain is no exception. The exact shape of the relationship of body–brain allometry depends on the taxonomic groups that are included in the analysis (e.g., Jerison, 1973; Gould, 1975), but an allometric (not isometric) relationship is obtained in virtually all cases.

Allometric scaling has a significant impact on the connectional organization of the brain. This is most readily seen when one considers the effect of an increase in the absolute size of a brain on its internal connectivity (see figure 7.6). Deacon (1990) contrasted two scenarios resulting from an increase in the number of neural elements, which we term "proportional" and "absolute" connectivity (following Striedter, 2005). Proportional connectivity ensures that all neural elements remain directly linked to one another, and the number of axons thus scales exponentially with the number of neurons. In the case of absolute connectivity, the same number of axons per neural element is maintained. It is immediately obvious that absolute connectivity is much more economical with regard to the number and lengths of axonal wires but that it poses some constraints on network topology if global coherence of the

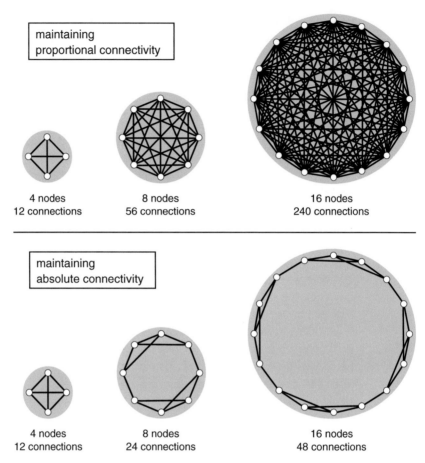

Figure 7.6
Network allometry and two models for scaling of connectivity. In both cases, network size increases from 4 to 8 to 16 nodes. If networks maintain "proportional connectivity" (top), the number of axons (and the wiring cost) rises exponentially. If networks maintain "absolute connectivity" (bottom), the number of axons increases linearly. Modified and redrawn after similar diagrams in Deacon (1990), Ringo (1991), and Striedter (2005).

network is to be maintained. Naturally, what emerges is a form of small-world connectivity, a combination of local clustering and interconnecting bridges and hubs.

Available data on scaling relations between neuron number and density, brain size, and relative proportions of gray and white matter support the notion that brains maintain absolute connectivity as their sizes change. As mammalian brain size increases over four orders of magnitude from mouse to elephant, neuronal density decreases by a factor of 10, which indicates that the increase in brain size is associated with an increase in the total number of neurons. Neocortical gray matter and white matter exhibit an allometric relationship but do not scale with an exponent close to 2 as would be expected if proportional connectivity were maintained. Instead, white matter only increases with an exponent of ≈4/3, much closer to the expected value for absolute connectivity. Zhang and Sejnowski (2000) have argued that this empirical power law can be explained as a necessary consequence of the basic uniformity of the neocortex and the need to conserve wiring volume (see figure 7.7).

Evolutionary changes in the absolute size of the brain, including the neocortex, thus result in progressively less dense connectivity and

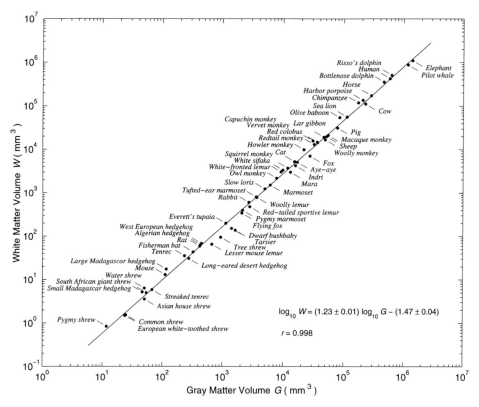

Figure 7.7
Scaling relationship between neocortical gray and white matter volume. Data from 59 mammalian species were assembled by Zhang and Sejnowski (2000). While white and gray matter volumes range over five orders of magnitude, the ratio of white to gray matter volumes varies over only one order of magnitude, resulting in a power law with an approximate exponent of 1.23, or 4/3 after a correction for cortical thickness is taken into account. Reproduced from Zhang and Sejnowski (2000) with permission.

increased modularity (Stevens, 1989). Stated differently, sparse connectivity and modularity are inevitable outcomes of increases in brain size. Brain architecture cannot sustain boundless increases in size, as long conduction delays soon begin to offset any computational gains achieved by greater numbers of neurons (Ringo, 1991). Larger brains are also naturally driven toward greater functional specialization as it becomes necessary to limit most connectivity to local communities while ensuring their global functional integration. One way in which evolution can create larger brains, or larger structures within brains, is by manipulating timing in neural development, with structures that develop over a more extended time and mature later becoming larger in size (Finlay and Darlington, 1995). Evolutionary changes of developmental mechanisms thus become a powerful force that shapes network topology. The tight limits imposed by allometric scaling laws on the density of axonal connections in large brains or large brain structures may put significant selectional pressure on additional features of connectivity that promote the brain's functional coherence. Hence, small-world architectures may thus be partly the result of the evolutionary emergence of larger organisms with larger brains.

What Drives the Evolution of Brain Connectivity?

This brief survey of the many factors that shape the evolution of brain morphology has raised more questions than it has been able to answer. Nevertheless, one conclusion is apparent: the intricacies and interdependencies of evolutionary and developmental mechanisms render it highly unlikely that brain connectivity has been "optimized" for any single structural or functional measure. The architecture of brain networks combines low wiring cost, high computational power, efficient information flow, and (as I will discuss in more detail in chapter 13) high neural complexity. Taken together, these factors reconcile the constraints of brain economy, eloquently expressed by Cajal, with the demands of efficiency in communication and information flow. It is likely that the optimization of any single factor would result in an undesirable decrement of one or more of the other factors. For example, minimization of wiring cost alone tends to eliminate long-range pathways that are vital for global information exchange, while optimization of information processing requires a prohibitive increase in the number of neural elements and interconnections. A corollary of this idea is that brain connectivity represents a viable compromise of economy and efficiency.

It is tempting to interpret the brain's economical wiring or efficient information flow as adaptations that have been selected for and optimized in the course of evolution.[8] For example, the notion of wiring optimization implies that low wiring cost represents an adaptive trait of brain anatomy and that phenotypic variants whose brains were suboptimal with regard to wiring cost have been selected against. However, wiring economy also partially correlates with dynamic and functional characteristics, as well as with scaling relationships between body size and gray and white matter volume. Furthermore, wiring patterns are partly controlled by physical forces such as axonal tension that leads to the prominent folding pattern of the cerebral cortex. This raises the question of whether some of what we see in the wiring patterns of structural brain networks is the result of physical forces rather than the outcome of natural selection. The realization that not every observable phenotypic trait is the result of adaptation has led to sharp disagreements among evolutionary theorists.[9] This ongoing controversy suggests that any characterization of complex brain networks as "optimally adapted" or "maximally efficient" should be viewed with an abundance of caution. Optimal design is incompatible with the fact that evolutionary mechanisms cannot anticipate functional outcomes before they are realized as part of a living form and then become subject to variation and selection. It is therefore problematic to argue that observations about the structural economy or functional efficiency of extant brain networks are the outcome of a process of optimal design. This mode of explaining brain network topology in terms of a final cause (efficiency, optimality) is reminiscent of teleology, an idea that has had a difficult time in the history of biology.

Brain structure, including the topology of brain networks, is part of an organism's phenotype. Currently existing animal forms occupy only part of a large phenotypic space of possible forms, most of which have not and will not be realized. Extending this argument, currently existing nervous systems only occupy a small subspace within the much larger space of all possible, physically realizable, phenotypic arrangements of cells and connections. Given the vast number of combinatorial possibilities, it seems likely that there are regions of phenotypic space with brain connectivity that is more economical and more efficient than the connectivity of all extant species, including humans. These regions may have been missed by historical accident, or they may be unreachable because these brains cannot be built with the available toolkit of developmental biology—we just cannot "get there from here." Developmental processes are crucial for determining which regions of phenotypic space can be accessed given the genetic makeup of an organism and its lineage. The brain's niche in this space is partly determined by the development and evolution of the rest of the body. The appearance or modification of new body structures has a profound impact on brain architecture and will often be accompanied by structural changes in brain networks. These linkages and cross-dependencies make it highly unlikely that we find ourselves on a path toward anything resembling optimality. This is not to say that brain networks do not make economical use of limited bodily resources or are not efficiently integrating information, but we have no way of knowing if they do so *optimally*. Fortunately, the fundamental demands of wiring economy and processing efficiency can be reconciled. Had they turned out to be incompatible, I would not be writing this sentence and you would not be reading it.

8 Dynamic Patterns in Spontaneous Neural Activity

A main function of the neural cell is of course to transmit excitations, and earlier ideas of anatomy and physiology made the central nervous system appear, in principle, a collection of routes, some longer, some shorter, leading without reversal from receptors to effectors—a mass of conductors that lies inactive until a sense organ is excited, and then conducts the excitation promptly to some muscle or gland. We know now that this is not so. [...] Electrophysiology of the central nervous system indicates in brief that the brain is continuously active, in all its parts, and an afferent excitation must be superimposed on an already existent excitation. It is therefore impossible that the consequence of a sensory event should often be uninfluenced by the existing activity.[1]
—Donald Hebb, 1949

At the outset of his seminal book *The Organization of Behavior*, Donald Hebb framed this discussion of "existing activity" in the central nervous system in terms of the psychological problems of attention and set, and he pointed to mounting neurophysiological evidence, gathered from EEG and cellular recordings, for spontaneous brain activity in the absence of afferent stimulation. Today, the existence of spontaneous or endogenous neural activity has been demonstrated in many systems and with a broad array of methodological tools, and yet its importance for the functioning of the brain is only beginning to be grasped (Buzsáki, 2006). One way to characterize brain function is to focus entirely on the brain's responses to well-defined environmental stimuli. This "reflexive mode" of brain function largely neglects or disregards the existence of endogenous patterns of activation that are not directly attributable to external stimulation. Instead, this theoretical framework treats the brain as a system in which the essential neural process is the transformation of inputs into outputs. Endogenous patterns of neural activity do not participate, except as a source of "noise" that must be overcome by purposeful activation. Until now, much of the interest in theoretical neuroscience has focused on stimulus-driven or task-related computation, and considerably less attention has been given to the brain as a dynamic, spontaneously active, and recurrently connected system (e.g., Vogels et al., 2005; Raichle, 2010).

The previous four chapters (chapters 4–7) have focused on structural brain networks, the physical wiring patterns traditionally described by neuroanatomy, particularly those found in the mammalian cerebrum. Even cursory examination of structural brain connectivity reveals that the basic plan is incompatible with a model based on predominantly feedforward processing within a uniquely specified serial hierarchy. Whether considering individual neurons or entire brain regions, one finds that the vast majority of the structural connections that are made and received among network elements cannot be definitively associated with either input or output. Rather, they connect nodes in complex and often recurrent patterns (Lorente de Nó's "synaptic chains"). Even in regions of the brain such as primary visual cortex that are classified as "sensory," most synapses received by pyramidal neurons arrive from other cortical neurons and only a small percentage (5 percent to 20 percent) can be attributed to sensory input (Douglas et al., 1995).[2] Cortical areas that are farther removed from direct sensory input are coupled to one another via numerous mono- and polysynaptic reciprocal pathways. This prevalence of recurrent anatomical connections suggests that models which focus exclusively on feedforward processing in a silent brain are likely to capture only one aspect of the anatomical and physiological reality.[3] As will be discussed in more detail in chapter 9, recurrent or reentrant processes make an important contribution to the shaping of brain responses and to the creation of coordinated global states. This coordination is essential for the efficient integration of multiple sources of information and the generation of coherent behavioral responses. In addition to recurrent processing induced by external perturbations, anatomical recurrence also facilitates the emergence of endogenous, spontaneous dynamics. These dynamics are more accurately captured as series of transitions between marginally stable attractors, as sequences of dynamic transients rather than stable states (see chapter 12).

The next four chapters address the patterns of dynamic network interactions that emerge from the brain's physical wiring, as a result of spontaneous activity (chapter 8) or in response to stimuli and perturbations (chapter 9), and how these interactions are affected by physical injury or disease (chapter 10) or shaped by growth and plasticity (chapter 11). Dynamic interactions between large populations of neurons are an essential ingredient for relating neural activity to cognition and behavior. These dynamic interactions can be estimated with a broad range of measures that capture the association between neural time series data or model its causal origins, resulting in functional or effective brain connectivity (see chapter 3). Analysis of functional connectivity measured during spontaneous activity reveals characteristic patterns at multiple spatial and temporal scales. Empirical and modeling studies demonstrate that the spatial and temporal patterning of endogenous brain activity reflects the structure of the underlying anatomical brain network and exhibits characteristic topology consisting of functional modules linked by hub regions. The existence of spontaneous patterns of neural activity raises the question of their relevance for task-oriented processing. We will explore the possibility that spontaneously generated network states form an internal functional repertoire. The observation and modeling of endogenous or spontaneous brain activity provide a unique window on patterns of self-organized brain dynamics—an intrinsic mode of neural processing that may have a central role in cognition.

Spontaneous Activity in Cellular Networks

Nervous systems do not depend on external input to provide representational content but instead rely on such inputs for context and modulation. This view of brain function, as articulated by Rodolfo Llinás, implies that "the significance of sensory cues is expressed mainly by their incorporation into larger, cognitive states or entities. In other words, sensory cues earn representation via their impact upon the pre-existing functional disposition of the brain" (Llinás, 2001, p. 8). In order for the brain to achieve this degree of autonomy, neurons must be capable of spontaneous discharge—for example, through intrinsic oscillatory electrical properties. Numerous types of central nerve cells are indeed capable of producing spontaneous rhythmic variations in their membrane potential across a wide range of frequencies (Llinás, 1988). Mutual coupling through synaptic connections promotes phase synchrony and coherence, resulting in synchronized groups of cells that are joined together to create large-scale functional connectivity. According to Llinás, intrinsic electrical properties and functional coupling are the two essential ingredients that enable spontaneous and stimulus-independent neural activity.[4]

In nearly all instances where it has been empirically observed, spontaneous neuronal firing exhibits characteristic spatiotemporal structure. Spontaneous neural activity therefore is not stochastic "noise" but rather is organized into precise patterns. For example, numerous studies have shown that populations of cortical neurons coordinate their spontaneous activity, presumably via their anatomical interconnections, and exhibit characteristic correlation patterns. Neurons in mouse visual cortex are found to be spontaneously active and show synchronization as well as repeating patterns of sequential activation within distinct cellular networks (Mao et al., 2001). Pharmacological blocking of excitatory neurotransmission abolishes network synchronization, while some neurons maintain their ability to engage in spontaneous firing. This suggests that spontaneous cortical activity is shaped by two components, the intrinsic electrical properties of "autonomous" neurons and the spreading and synchronization of neural activity via excitatory connections. The important role of recurrent connectivity in shaping spontaneous as well as evoked cortical responses has since been confirmed in additional studies. For example, MacLean et al. (2005) found that thalamic input triggered patterns of cortical response that were strikingly similar to those seen during spontaneous cortical activity, suggesting that the role of sensory input is to "awaken" cortex rather than impose specific firing patterns (see figure 8.1). This observation has far-reaching implications for models of cortical information processing to which we will return in later chapters.

One consequence of spontaneous dynamic interactions is the correlated transition of populations of cortical neurons between a more quiescent (DOWN) and a more depolarized (UP) state (Steriade et al., 1993; Sanchez-Vives and McCormick, 2000), characterized by two different levels of the subthreshold membrane potential. The responsiveness of the cortex to sensory stimuli is generally decreased during DOWN states and increased during UP states.[5] Synchronized UP states occur in populations of cortical neurons in virtually all regions of the cerebral cortex, and they represent spatially organized "preferred network states" that are dynamically stable and persist on a time scale far longer than that of feedforward sensory processing (Cossart et al., 2003). These self-maintained depolarized network states are likely constrained by recurrent intracortical structural connections. In vivo recordings of populations of cells in rat neocortex demonstrated that transitions of cortical neurons to coordinated UP states result in sequential firing patterns that are stereotypically organized (Luczak et al., 2007). Dynamic patterns triggered after transition to an UP state are shaped by cellular physiology and anatomical connections that link populations of neurons. Importantly, these sequential patterns can unfold in the absence of sensory

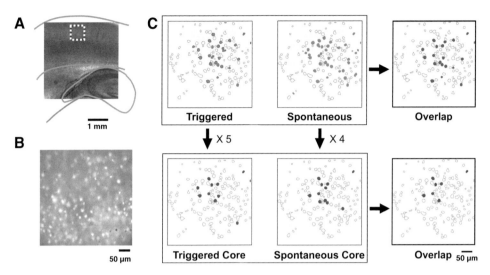

Figure 8.1
Overlap between spontaneous and evoked activity in mouse somatosensory cortex.
(A) Image of somatosensory cortex slice preparation indicating the location of recordings
shown in subsequent panels (square box), overlaying layer 4 of cortex. (B) Single frame
of layer 4 cortical neurons stained with a fluorescent voltage-sensitive calcium dye. Cell
bodies of neurons are brightly stained and are drawn as small circles in the following plots.
(C) Activity of imaged neurons illustrating network patterns that arise in response to
thalamic stimulation (left, "triggered") or spontaneously (middle, "spontaneous") and their
mutual overlap (right, "overlap"). Note that repeated activation, either through stimulation
or spontaneously, generates patterns that exhibit significant similarity (bottom), with a
number of "core neurons" that are consistently activated during both spontaneous and
evoked activity. Images are modified and reproduced from MacLean et al. (2005) with
permission.

input and on time scales of hundreds of milliseconds. Luczak et al. (2009)
suggested that population spike patterns form a constrained space, a
"vocabulary" or repertoire of dynamic states that is widely explored
during spontaneous activity and more narrowly subsampled by sensory
responses.

Several network models have attempted to shed light on the mechanisms by which coordinated UP states arise or terminate. For example,
Compte et al. (2003) created a detailed biophysical model of 1,024 pyramidal cells and 256 interneurons that reproduced slow oscillations
between episodes of sustained low-rate neural activity and periods of
silence (UP and DOWN states, respectively). The model suggested that
the synchronized UP state is sustained by local excitatory recurrent connections. A multilayer model of several interconnected cortical and thalamic regions consisting of 65,000 neurons linked by several million

synaptic connections also reproduced spontaneous slow oscillatory activity patterns that were synchronized through corticocortical connections (Hill and Tononi, 2005). Spontaneous activity patterns and responses to sensory stimuli resembled those seen in experimental studies and, through modeled effects of neuromodulators, the system was able to reproduce the transition of cortical dynamics from wakefulness to sleep.

Relationships between structural connections and patterns of dynamic network correlations are difficult to observe directly at the level of individual cells and synapses, in part because anatomical connections are not easily traced within most preparations. Nevertheless, the stereotypical nature of spontaneous cortical activity (MacLean et al., 2005) strongly suggests the idea that preferred network states are sculpted by a backbone of intracortical connections. Interestingly, MacLean et al. identified a set of "core neurons" that participated in many separate instances of spontaneous or stimulus-evoked activations (see figure 8.1). These core neurons may represent a separate functional class with distinctive physiological properties that is highly influential in shaping dynamics due to their structural embedding within the cellular network.[6]

Several studies of ongoing neuronal activity have attempted to relate spontaneous activity patterns to the known functional architecture of sensory cortex. In vivo spontaneous activity of cortical neurons has been investigated with a wide array of techniques, including EEG, optical imaging with voltage-sensitive dyes, and recording of single neuron or population activity. The spatiotemporal organization of spontaneous activity closely resembled firing patterns seen during stimulus-evoked or task-related activation. A series of studies by Amos Arieli and coworkers using voltage-sensitive dye imaging of cat primary visual cortex revealed that spontaneous activity consists of a series of dynamically switching cortical states that correspond to cortical representations of visual orientations (Arieli et al., 1995; 1996; Kenet et al., 2003; see figure 8.2). Patterns of spontaneous activity recorded with voltage-sensitive dyes are correlated with the ongoing discharge of simultaneously recorded single cortical neurons (Tsodyks et al., 1999). Their resemblance to stimulus-evoked orientation maps strongly suggests that spontaneous dynamic patterns are shaped by intracortical structural networks that define orientation columns. Arieli and coworkers put forward the idea that these intrinsic cortical states, constrained by the network architecture, serve as an internal context for sensory processing or reflect a set of expectations about probable patterns of sensory input from the environment.

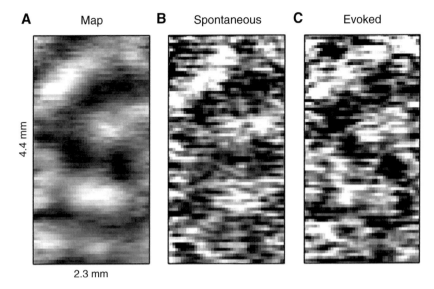

Figure 8.2
Spontaneous and evoked orientation-selective responses in visual cortex. The images are taken from optical recordings of neural activity in area 18 of the cat. (A) The panel shows a map of neural responses, acquired during the presentation of visual stimuli consisting of oriented gratings, obtained by averaging 165 image frames. Panel (B) shows a single frame obtained during a spontaneous recording session (no visual stimulus was presented). Panel (C) shows a single frame recorded during the presentation of a grating with vertical orientation. Note the similarity between all three panels, particularly the spontaneous and evoked response patterns in (B) and (C). Reproduced from Kenet et al. (2003) with permission.

While the experiments of Kenet et al. were carried out in anesthetized animals, observations in the visual cortex of the alert ferret provide additional support for the idea that spontaneous cortical activity exhibits patterns that resemble those seen during visual stimulation (Fiser et al., 2004). In fact, Fiser et al. (2004) noted that the correlation structure of spontaneous neural firing was only weakly modified by visual stimulation. Ongoing fluctuations in neural activity in the absence of visual input also occur in the primate visual cortex (Leopold et al., 2003). Coherent slow fluctuations in local field power were found to occur independently of behavioral context, including during task states and rest. Consistent with these experiments, functional neuroimaging studies of human visual cortex showed spontaneous slow fluctuations of the BOLD signal in the absence of visual stimuli (Nir et al., 2006) that were spatially correlated and exhibited characteristic neuroanatomical distributions. Once visual input was provided, these fluctuations were replaced by spatially less coherent and input- or task-specific patterns of functional connectivity. Thus, transitions between rest and task state were associated with changes in the spatial pattern of functional connectivity rather than with the presence or absence of neural activity (see chapter 9).

What all these observations have in common is that they reveal cortex as spontaneously active, with ongoing fluctuations that exhibit characteristic spatiotemporal patterns shaped by recurrent structural connectivity.[7] The complex dynamics and rich patterning of spontaneous network activity at the cellular scale is a remarkable example of how anatomy and cellular physiology can combine to generate a set of dynamic network states in the absence of external input or stimulus-evoked cognitive processing. Sensory inputs "awaken" or modulate intrinsic cortical dynamics rather than instruct central brain activity or transfer specific information that is then processed in a feedforward manner. Many open questions remain. The effect of extrinsic inputs on intrinsic network states is still incompletely understood, and several current studies suggest a nonlinear interaction, in particular in relation to UP or DOWN states, rather than linear superposition. So far, most of the dynamic structure of ongoing neural activity has been demonstrated within local patches of cortex—how much additional structure exists between cells separated by greater distances or located in different cortical regions is still unknown. The anatomical and physiological factors that govern the slow temporal dynamics of coordinated transitions between UP and DOWN states in cortical neurons require further study. The topology of cellular cortical networks remains largely uncharted as network analysis techniques have yet to be widely applied in this experimental domain. How UP/DOWN states relate to fluctuations of neural activity measures in EEG/MEG or fMRI is yet to be determined. Finally, the possible relationship of spontaneous cortical activity with sequences of cognitive or mental states of the organism urgently awaits further empirical investigation.

Most of these studies on spontaneous activity in cellular networks have been obtained from neurons in visual cortex, a part of the brain that would be expected to be largely inactive at rest under a feedforward, reflexive model of neural processing. Recent work in cognitive neuroscience has provided evidence that spontaneous, ongoing cortical activity is not restricted to sensory areas—instead, observations of large-scale patterns of functional connectivity suggest that such patterns are widespread, involve the whole brain, and are shaped by structural brain networks.

Large-Scale Functional Networks in the Resting State

Functional connectivity can be observed with a large number of neural recording techniques, noninvasively and over several time scales (see chapter 3). Spontaneous activity during quiet waking can be noninvasively recorded from the human brain with functional neuroimaging (fMRI) and electrophysiological and magnetoencephalographic techniques (EEG, MEG). While these techniques differ in their spatial and temporal resolution, sensitivity, and signal origin, they reveal functional networks that show a number of consistent topological features. We will first turn to the topology of functional networks of spontaneous brain activity obtained with fMRI.

Most classical neuroimaging studies employ a subtractive methodology to identify brain regions that are differentially activated in the context of specific cognitive tasks. The subtractive paradigm has delivered many important insights into localized neural substrates of cognition. It is based on the assumption that task-specific neural activity can be identified by comparing the task state to a suitable control state, an approach that traces its origins to Donders's mental chronometry. Cognitive subtraction presupposes that the neural correlates of different components of a cognitive task do not show significant interactions (the hypothesis of "pure insertion"), thus rendering them amenable to subtractive analysis. This view has been challenged, and alternative approaches to the mapping of cognitive anatomy have been suggested (Friston et al., 1996), for example, the use of experimental designs that probe for significant interactions among cortical regions. Further important developments include the application of modeling tools to go beyond descriptive approaches to brain mapping and answer mechanistic questions about how observed patterns of regional activation and coactivation are generated (see chapters 3 and 9).

However, neural correlates of cognition are not limited to the appearance of task-related activations. Particularly puzzling from the perspective of classical subtractive studies was the observation that, compared with a passive control condition such as visual fixation, activity in a particular set of brain regions showed task-induced decreases (Shulman et al., 1997). It appeared that cognitive tasks not only were associated with specific activations of circumscribed brain regions but also modified the activity pattern present in the control condition, when the brain was cognitively "at rest." Closer analysis of the pattern of activity decreases revealed that they comprised a specific set of brain regions, including the precuneus/posterior cingulate cortex, medial frontal cortex, and lateral parietal cortex. This raised the possibility that these regions formed a previously unknown coherent system that operated during the resting state. PET studies of brain metabolism carried out by Marc Raichle and colleagues established a "default mode" of brain function, an organized state corresponding to a physiological baseline that is suspended during attention-demanding goal-directed cognitive tasks (Raichle et al., 2001; Gusnard and Raichle, 2001). Notably, within this default mode, the precuneus/posterior cingulate cortex exhibits extremely high rates of tonic metabolic activity (see figure 6.11). Interestingly, recent studies of structural brain networks have shown this region to be highly connected and central, forming one of the main structural hubs of the cortex (see chapter 6; Parvizi et al., 2006; Hagmann et al., 2008).

In 1995, Bharat Biswal and colleagues demonstrated that slow fluctuations in fMRI signal recorded from regions of motor cortex showed robust patterns of correlations, which were observed between contralateral patches of motor cortex and other functionally linked regions (Biswal et al., 1995). The amplitude of these signal fluctuations was found to be within the same dynamic range as typical task-specific "cognitive" activations. Numerous subsequent studies have recorded significant low-frequency correlations in fMRI time series at rest between functionally related areas of cortex (see figure 8.3). Greicius et al. (2003) examined the hypothesis that brain regions that participated in the brain's default mode and were commonly deactivated during goal-directed cognitive tasks formed an interconnected network. Analysis of fMRI time series data showed that nearly all areas previously identified as commonly deactivated during goal-directed processing were also dynamically correlated (functionally connected). This functionally linked "default mode network" persisted during a sensory task with low cognitive demand but was attenuated during a working memory task. The network exhibited anticorrelations with brain regions such as the prefrontal cortex that were activated during more demanding cognitive operations. The precuneus/posterior cingulate cortex was identified as playing a central role within the default mode network, as its functional connectivity robustly spanned the entire default pattern and displayed strong inverse correlations with task-related brain regions.

More recent studies have confirmed and greatly extended these initial observations. A central role for the precuneus/posterior cingulate cortex within the default mode network was recently confirmed by Fransson and Marrelec (2008; see figure 8.4, plate 9). Further studies have shown

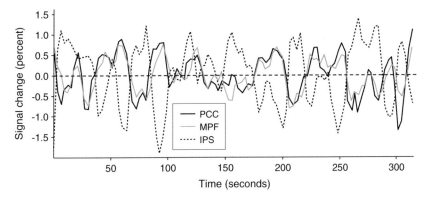

Figure 8.3
Correlated functional magnetic resonance imaging (fMRI) signal fluctuations in the resting state. Traces show time series of fMRI signals recorded from the posterior cingulate cortex/precuneus (PCC), the medial prefrontal cortex (MPF), and the intraparietal sulcus (IPS) of a participant who is quietly awake and cognitively at rest. There is a strong temporal correlation between two of the traces (PCC and MPF, both core regions of the default mode network) and an anticorrelation of these two traces with the IPS. Note the slow time course of the fluctuations and the magnitude of the signal change (about one percent to two percent of baseline). This figure is adapted and redrawn from data shown in Fox et al. (2005).

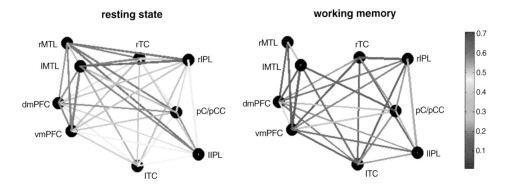

Figure 8.4 (plate 9)
Central role of precuneus/posterior cingulate cortex in the default mode network. Plots show the strengths of the pairwise or marginal correlations between nine distinct brain regions, all part of the default mode network. The data were recorded during the resting state (left panel) and during the performance of a working memory task (right panel). Note that the strongest and most consistent pattern of correlations is found for node pC/pCC (precuneus/posterior cingulate cortex). Note also that many of the correlations persist in the transition from rest to task, albeit at reduced levels. rMTL, right medial temporal lobe; lMTL, left medial temporal lobe; dmPFC, dorsomedial prefrontal cortex; vmPFC, ventromedial prefrontal cortex; rTC, right temporal cortex; lTC, left temporal cortex; rIPL, right inferior parietal lobe; lIPL, left inferior parietal lobe. Reproduced from Fransson and Marrelec (2008) with permission.

that task-related (task-positive) and default mode (task-negative) regions form internally coherent but mutually anticorrelated large-scale networks (Fox et al., 2005; see figure 8.5, plate 10). Functional connectivity within the default mode network was shown to be highly reliable and reproducible (Shehzad et al., 2009), and, as I will discuss shortly, the topology of the pattern has been linked to underlying long-range structural connections between brain regions. The neural mechanisms underpinning the slow rhythmicity of the BOLD signal are not yet clearly understood (Fox and Raichle, 2007). Some physiological observations suggest that BOLD signal fluctuations are driven by fluctuations in neural activity (Shmuel and Leopold, 2008), particularly in neural firing rate and high frequency (40–100 Hz) power modulations of local field potentials (Nir et al., 2008). The identification of a neuronal origin for slow spontaneous fluctuations in BOLD signals is important because such signal fluctuations could in principle arise from filtering of neural noise or from nonneuronal vascular dynamics. Recent electrocorticographic recordings of fast electrical activity provide strong and direct evidence for a neuronal basis of default mode brain activity (He et al., 2008; Miller et al., 2009).

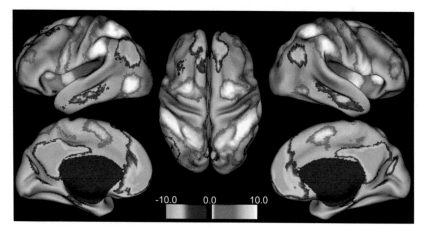

Figure 8.5 (plate 10)
Anticorrelated task-positive and task-negative networks in the human brain. Networks are defined on the basis of resting-state functional magnetic resonance imaging recordings. Positively correlated nodes (red/yellow) correspond to a set of brain regions that are jointly activated during tasks demanding focused attention and working memory. Anticorrelated nodes (blue/green) largely correspond to task-negative regions, including the default mode network, that are deactivated during goal-directed processing. Reproduced from Fox et al. (2005) with permission.

The default mode network is not the only set of functionally linked brain regions that is present in resting-state fMRI data. While the default network is often extracted by placing seed ROIs in some of its known key components, other methods such as independent component analysis (ICA) allow the objective identification of resting-state networks from spontaneous brain activity. ICA has revealed at least half a dozen resting-state networks that are superimposed and partly overlapping (Beckmann et al., 2005; De Luca et al., 2006; Mantini et al., 2007). Several of these resting-state networks correspond to sets of interconnected brain regions that cooperate in specific cognitive domains such as vision, motor planning, or episodic memory. The remarkable consistency with which these patterns of spontaneous brain activity appear across individuals (Biswal et al., 2010) raises this question: What shapes the correlation structure of the default mode network in resting-state fMRI?

A main candidate is large-scale white matter pathways or, more generally, structural brain connectivity. A growing number of empirical and modeling studies support the idea that patterns of endogenous neural activity are sculpted by cortical anatomy. Vincent et al. (2007) found that cortical patterns of coherent spontaneous BOLD fluctuations in macaque monkey were similar to those of anatomical connectivity. Zhang et al. (2008) mapped resting-state BOLD signal correlations between human thalamus and cortex and noted significant agreement between BOLD correlations and connectional anatomy within the same cortical hemisphere. Johnston et al. (2008) performed a resting-state fMRI study on a young patient before and directly after a complete section of the corpus callosum. Postsurgery, interhemispheric functional connectivity was dramatically reduced, suggesting an important role for the callosum in generating functional connectivity across the two cerebral hemispheres. In addition to these studies of specific pathways and fiber bundles, direct comparisons of whole-brain structural and functional connectivity provide additional support for the idea that functional connections are shaped by anatomy.

Comparing Structural and Functional Connectivity

The persistence and reproducibility of functional networks measured during the brain's resting state provide a unique opportunity for comparing functional connectivity to structural connectivity. Specifically, we can ask how much of the pattern of functional connections is accounted for or predicted by the pattern of structural connections. Such a comparison can also offer insight into the possibility of inferring structural connections from functional connections—an attractive possibility since functional connections are currently much more easily obtained from empirical data. The studies reviewed in this section have been carried out using cross-correlation of BOLD time series as the measure of functional connectivity and a variant of diffusion MRI for deriving fiber anatomy.

A first study was undertaken by Koch et al. (2002), who collected both DTI and fMRI data from a single brain slice. Functional connectivity was obtained from cross-correlation of BOLD-signal fluctuations between pairs of voxels, and structural connectivity was estimated from DTI data using a probabilistic "particle jump" algorithm. The study reported a positive correlation between structural and functional connections. Low functional connectivity was rarely found between voxels that were structurally linked. However, high functional connectivity was found to occur between voxels that were not linked by direct structural connections, presumably a result of indirect or unobserved anatomical links.

Two central regions within the default mode network, the precuneus/posterior cingulate cortex and the medial frontal cortex, are known to be connected via the cingulum bundle, a dense white matter tract running along the cortical midline. Van den Heuvel et al. (2008a) extracted these two cortical areas and the connecting cingulum bundle from fMRI and DTI scans of 45 participants obtained during the resting state. The magnitude of the functional connection between the two regions and the average value of the fractional anisotropy of the cingulum bundle, a measure reflecting the microstructural organization of the fiber tract, were found to be significantly and positively correlated. Greicius et al. (2009) performed structural imaging to search for and map anatomical pathways linking known components of the default mode network, specifically the posterior cingulate cortex, the medial prefrontal cortex, and the bilateral medial temporal lobe. DTI tractography revealed the presence of anatomical connections linking the posterior cingulate cortex and medial prefrontal cortex, as well as posterior cingulate cortex and medial temporal lobe. Despite the absence of direct structural links between medial temporal lobe and medial prefrontal cortex, these areas were found to be functionally connected as part of the default mode network. These data suggest that medial temporal lobe and medial prefrontal cortex become functionally connected via the posterior cingulate cortex or another unobserved intermediate brain region. In a similar study, van den Heuvel et al. (2009a) extracted a total of nine resting-state networks, including the default mode network, in a cohort of 26 healthy participants and then examined structural connections between those regions found to be functionally linked. Cortical regions participating in eight out of nine resting-state networks were found to be structurally interconnected by anatomical fiber tracts, thus providing a structural basis for their dynamic coupling.

More recently, several studies have appeared that performed direct comparisons of structural and functional connectivity across the whole brain in the same cohort of participants (Skudlarski et al., 2008; Hagmann et al., 2008; Honey et al., 2009). Skudlarski et al. performed a voxel-wise comparison of structural and functional connectivity using global connection matrices for 5,000 brain voxels. There was significant overall agreement between fiber counts and BOLD-signal cross-correlations, with highly connected voxels showing the strongest relationship between structural and functional measures. Hagmann et al. (2008) reported significant positive correlations between DSI-derived structural connectivity and resting-state fMRI cross-correlations of pairs of brain regions across the entire cortex (see figure 8.6, plate 11). The presence of a

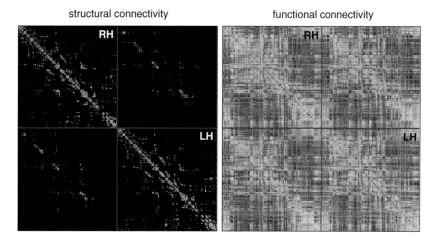

Figure 8.6 (plate 11)
Comparison of structural connectivity derived from diffusion imaging (Hagmann et al., 2008) and resting-state functional connectivity derived from fMRI (Honey et al., 2009) from the same set of five participants. Maps show connectivity among 998 ROIs shown here in an anterior–posterior–temporal arrangement (the same ordering as in figure 5.8) to emphasize spatial organization. The structural connectivity matrix is sparse and has only positive entries (fiber densities). The functional connectivity matrix has both positive (hot colors) and negative entries (cool colors). See figure 8.7 for a matching statistical comparison and figure 8.8 for a computational model. RH, right hemisphere; LH, left hemisphere. Data replotted from Honey et al. (2009).

structural connection between two regions quantitatively predicted the presence of a functional connection. A high-resolution analysis of pairwise structural and functional connectivity between 998 ROIs, uniformly covering the two cerebral hemispheres (Honey et al., 2009) confirmed this statistical relationship (see figure 8.7). Additional strong functional connections often exist between ROIs with no direct structural connections, making it impractical to infer structural connections from functional connections by simple means such as thresholding. Further analysis revealed that many functional connections between unconnected region pairs can be explained by the existence of indirect structural connections.

While each study used somewhat different imaging protocols and tractography algorithms, the convergent message is that structural connections, when present, are indeed highly predictive of the presence and strength of functional connections. However, structural connections cannot reliably be inferred on the basis of observed functional coupling since strong functional connections may also exist between regions that are not directly anatomically linked. An intuitive argument suggests that the correspondence between structural and functional connectivity should become less direct as brain networks are acquired from finer and finer anatomical partitions. As structural nodes approach the level of single neurons, structural connectivity becomes increasingly sparse, and indirect couplings are likely to dominate the topology of functional networks. Thus, recent successes in relating empirical structural to functional connectivity should not lead to the mistaken conclusion that their relationship is simple or even trivial (Damoiseaux and Greicius, 2009). A more refined understanding of this structure–function relationship may come from computational models of endogenous neural activity.

Computational Models of the Brain's Resting State

The relationship between structural and functional connectivity in large-scale brain systems can be investigated with the help of computational modeling. Such models are useful because they allow the precise specification of structural coupling and the recording of complete neural time series data that can then be processed similarly to empirical data sets.[8] Structural and functional connectivity can then be compared, and their relationship can be interpreted without the need to account for many of the potential confounds present in experimental data such as physiological noise, imaging artifacts, or problems with coregistration. Recent

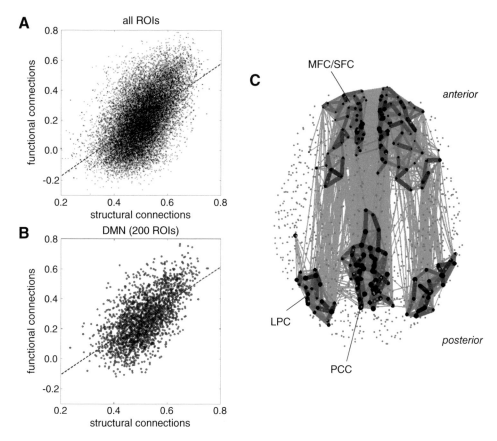

Figure 8.7
Structural and functional connectivity in whole brain and default mode network (DMN).
(A) Scatterplot of structural connections and corresponding functional connections (r =
0.54, p < 10⁻⁶). (B) Scatterplot of structural connections and corresponding functional connections (r = 0.61, p < 10⁻⁶) for 200 regions of interest (ROIs) that form the DMN. These
200 ROIs were derived by placing seeds in the posterior cingulate/precuneus (PCC), medial
frontal cortex (MFC), and lateral parietal cortex (LPC) and then selecting the 200 ROIs
that were most strongly functionally correlated. (C) Anatomical location of the 200 DMN
ROIs and their structural interconnections. While there are dense structural pathways
between the MFC and superior frontal cortex (SFC) and both the PCC and LPC, few
connections are seen between the LPC and PCC (see also van den Heuvel, 2009a). All data
shown here represent averages over five participants originally reported in Honey et al.
(2009).

models of endogenous neural activity in primate cerebral cortex informed by neuroanatomical data sets have made significant progress toward clarifying the complex relationship between structural connectivity and dynamics.

Honey et al. (2007) investigated the relationship between structural and functional connectivity in a large-scale model of the macaque monkey cortex. The model was based on a structural network of segregated regions and interregional pathways collated using the CoCoMac database (see chapter 2, figure 2.6) and on a nonlinear dynamic model of spontaneous neuronal activity. The dynamic model, based on the observed physiological characteristics of cortical neuronal populations (Breakspear et al., 2003), was capable of chaotic behavior and transient synchronization. Modeled millisecond resolution voltage time series were used to estimate synthetic BOLD signals from a nonlinear model of the brain's hemodynamic response (Friston et al., 2003). Cross-correlations between these BOLD signals then yielded functional connectivity patterns. Over longer time periods (several minutes), BOLD-derived functional connectivity showed significant agreement with the underlying structural connectivity. This relationship was also seen for other measures of functional connectivity that were applied directly to the modeled voltage time series, for example, the information-theoretic measures of mutual information and transfer entropy (see chapter 3). Consistent with experimental findings, modeled BOLD responses showed slow spontaneous fluctuations. Importantly, these fluctuations were not due to the convolution of noisy time series with a (low-pass) hemodynamic response function but reflected transient synchronization between varying sets of brain regions. Fluctuations in synchrony reliably preceded fluctuations in the BOLD response. Thus, the model predicted that BOLD fluctuations in the real brain originate from transients of neuronal population dynamics.[9] Some recent results regarding the origin of fluctuating fMRI signals are consistent with this prediction (Shmuel and Leopold, 2008; Nir et al., 2008; Schölvinck et al., 2010).

The availability of human structural brain connectivity from diffusion MRI (Hagmann et al., 2008) allowed an extension of the model to the scale of the entire human cerebral cortex. Honey et al. (2009) implemented the dynamic model just described on a human structural connection matrix linking 998 nodes. Functional connectivity patterns were again derived from cross-correlations of synthetic BOLD time series data. Comparison of these modeled patterns to the empirically obtained functional connectivity revealed significant similarity (see figure 8.8,

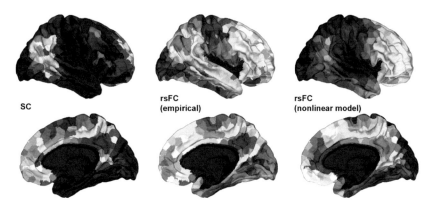

Figure 8.8 (plate 12)
Modeling and prediction of functional connectivity. The plots show cortical surface maps
for structural connectivity (SC), empirical resting-state functional connectivity (rsFC), and
modeled functional connectivity. The maps were created by placing seeds in the posterior
cingulate/precuneus (PCC), medial frontal cortex, and lateral parietal cortex (LPC; see
figure 8.7). High connection/correlation is indicated by hot colors, low connection/correla-
tion by cool colors. Note substantial agreement between modeled and empirical FC along
the cortical midline but lack of functional connectivity to LPC in the model, most likely
due to weak structural connections detected between PCC and LPC. Data were replotted
from Honey et al. (2009).

plate 12). The model could account for much of the empirically observed
functional coupling strengths present between structurally linked node
pairs. The model also was able to partially predict the strength of empirical functional connections on the basis of indirect structural coupling.
Prediction accuracy was especially high for many components of the
default mode network, particularly structures along the cortical midline.
The model strongly suggests that much of the patterning of the brain's
functional connectivity in the resting state can be explained by the
pattern of structural connections linking regions of the cerebral cortex.

Ghosh et al. (2008a; 2008b) constructed a model of spontaneous neural
activity by combining a large-scale structural connectivity matrix of
macaque cortex and a neural mass model based on the dynamic equations of FitzHugh–Nagumo. Importantly, the model equations included
estimates for neural conduction delays that varied with the spatial distances between connected region pairs, as well as a noise term modeling
Gaussian fluctuations of each node's membrane potential. Ghosh et al.
varied conduction velocity and coupling strengths to map regions of the
model's parameter space where the model displayed dynamically stable
or unstable behavior. A spatiotemporal analysis of the model dynamics
was performed to identify dominant subnetworks that underlie the

ongoing oscillatory dynamics observed during spontaneous activity. Simulated BOLD signals were computed from neural activity time series, and modeled functional connectivity patterns were derived. The correlation structure of these patterns was found to be largely consistent with those in empirically observed resting-state fMRI. In the model of Ghosh et al., conduction delays within a physiologically realistic range as well as physiological noise are found to be two important ingredients for generating rich spatiotemporal patterns in spontaneous dynamics that resemble those seen in the brain at rest.

Another model of spontaneous neural activity also incorporated conduction delays and noise within a structural connection matrix of the macaque cortex (Deco et al., 2009). The model focused on the sensitivity of interregional synchronization to variations in conduction velocity, coupling strength, and noise level. Deco et al. reported anticorrelated clusters of regions that corresponded closely to the anatomical and functional clustering previously reported by Honey et al. (2007). Additionally, the model demonstrated "stochastic resonance," with anticorrelations between clusters that depended on the presence of a low level of noise. The level of synchronization between different brain regions was found to be associated with the amplitude of the BOLD response.

Taken together, these modeling studies reinforce the idea that within large-scale cortical networks structural and functional connectivity are related.[10] However, they also suggest that the degree to which this correspondence manifests itself depends on spatial resolution and time scales. The relationship is particularly robust for functional networks obtained at low frequencies (as in resting-state fMRI) and over long sampling periods (on the order of minutes). Despite constant coupling between network nodes, the models of Honey et al. (2007; 2009), Ghosh et al. (2008a; 2008b), and Deco et al. (2009) demonstrate that the collective spontaneous dynamics of a large-scale neural system can give rise to a rich and diverse set of spatiotemporal patterns. Thus, we should not think of the brain's endogenous neural activity as a static time-invariant pattern of interneuronal or interregional coupling. Instead, spontaneous dynamics exhibits significant shifts, transitions, and nonstationarity, allowing for rapid reconfigurations of functional interactions at fast time scales of hundreds of milliseconds, even in the absence of exogenous perturbations. The resulting dynamic diversity requires us to revisit the temporal aspect of functional networks later in the book (see chapter 12). However, first I will turn to a simpler question. In chapter 6 I discussed the specific topological features of structural brain networks—

do functional networks exhibit similar topologies, characterized by a modular architecture interlinked by highly central hub regions?

Topology of Resting-State Functional Connectivity

If structural and functional connectivity are indeed related, we might expect to see correspondences between their network topology and architecture. Modularity and hubs are consistently found within the large-scale organization of mammalian cortical anatomy (see chapter 6). Does the topology of functional networks derived from observed brain dynamics mirror the topology of the underlying anatomy? Over the past decade, numerous studies of functional brain connectivity have indeed demonstrated that functional interactions within large-scale structural networks exhibit characteristic patterns that resemble those seen in the anatomy.

One of the earliest studies to report on modular functional connectivity was based on empirical data collected decades ago using strychnine neuronography in the macaque cortex (Stephan et al., 2000). As discussed in chapter 3, the localized application of strychnine to the cortical surface results in disinhibition and spread of epileptiform neural activity which is propagated along corticocortical pathways (see figure 3.3). Collation of published data on activity propagation from a number of experiments resulted in a matrix of functional connectivity between 39 cortical regions within a single hemisphere.[11] Stephan and colleagues found that this matrix exhibited robust small-world attributes, including high levels of clustering and short path lengths, and thus their study is one of the first reports of small-world organization in a dynamic brain network. Using hierarchical clustering algorithms, they also demonstrated that this functional connectivity matrix contained a number of distinct modules. Three main modules contained primarily visual, somatomotor, and orbito–temporo–insular regions, respectively. The composition of each module revealed regions that were generally considered to be functionally related, for example, areas in the occipital and parietal cortex involved in different aspects of vision. Stephan et al. (2000) noted the potential relationship of their functional connectivity patterns with similar small-world features of structural connectivity in the macaque cortex (Hilgetag et al., 2000; Sporns et al., 2000a). A companion paper presented a computational model of activity propagation in the cat cortex based on known anatomical projections and compared the performance of the model to empirical data from strychnine neuronography

(Kötter and Sommer, 2000). The model incorporating empirical connection data clearly outperformed random or nearest-neighbor architectures and thus provided early support for the notion that the topology of corticocortical pathways shaped the flow of neural activations.

Salvador et al. (2005) applied hierarchical cluster analysis to human resting-state neural activity acquired with fMRI and demonstrated its modular and small-world organization. Within a parcellation of 90 cortical and subcortical regions, resting-state functional connectivity exhibited small-world attributes and formed 6 major clusters, each containing regions that had previously been described as anatomically and functionally related. Other resting-state fMRI studies have lent additional support to the idea that the basic architecture of large-scale dynamic brain networks is both small-world and modular (Achard et al., 2006; Meunier et al., 2009a; Valencia et al., 2009). Consistently, functional modules contain regions that are known to be more strongly connected via white matter pathways, as well as related in terms of their known functionality. A small set of brain regions maintains functional connections that extend across multiple modules, thus enabling system-wide dynamic interactions and ensuring short path length. These highly connected and highly central hub nodes were found primarily within multimodal association cortex, including the inferior parietal lobule, the precuneus, the angular gyrus, and portions of the superior frontal gyrus (Achard et al., 2006). Clustering and physical connection distance were negatively correlated for hub regions, indicating that hubs were connecting physically remote regions that did not directly connect to each other. Other studies of resting-state fMRI functional connectivity have confirmed the modular organization of the human cerebral cortex. He et al. (2009) performed a modularity analysis on functional connectivity derived from resting-state fMRI signals. Modules in spontaneous brain activity again reflected known functional subsystems, such as visual, auditory, attention, and default networks.[12]

To what extent does the network structure depend on the spatial resolution of the individual network nodes?[13] Most fMRI-based analyses of resting-state functional connectivity employ various cortical parcellation schemes that result in networks comprising between 50 and 90 nodes. Very few studies have attempted to perform network analyses on the basis of time series data from single voxels. Eguíluz et al. (2005) provided the first example of such a study and not only reported the coexistence of high clustering and short path length, that is, a small-world architecture, but also presented evidence for a scale-free distribution of functional connections when nodes were defined at the scale of single voxels. A scale-free degree distribution in voxel-based human functional networks was also described in a more recent study by Van den Heuvel et al. (2008b). In contrast, degree distributions of regional functional networks typically show an exponentially truncated power law (e.g., Achard et al., 2006), that is, they contain highly connected nodes in proportions above those of equivalent random networks but below those of scale-free networks. This discrepancy may be due to differences in data averaging, preprocessing, or the correlation pattern of the hemodynamic signal for voxel-based as compared to region-based functional networks. Further work is needed to determine if indeed the increased spatial resolution provided by voxel-level networks reveals additional features of network organization that are not detected in networks based on coarser cortical parcellations.

Networks of functional connections obtained from electrophysiological recordings also display characteristic patterns providing further support for the highly ordered nature of spontaneous brain activity. One of the very first demonstrations of small-world topology in a human brain functional network came from MEG recordings obtained from a group of five healthy participants (Stam, 2004). Across several frequency bands, patterns of synchronous coupling displayed small-world attributes, including high clustering and short path lengths. Other studies confirmed these findings in healthy subjects and compared small-world measures in healthy controls with those of subjects with various forms of brain disease (e.g., Stam et al., 2007; Micheloyannis et al., 2006; Rubinov et al., 2009a). We will return to these comparisons and their implications for our understanding of the network aspects of brain disease in more detail in chapter 10.

In one of the most comprehensive studies to date using wavelet correlations to estimate frequency-dependent functional connectivity between MEG sensors, Bassett et al. (2006) showed that functional networks across different frequencies exhibit self-similarity, scale-invariance, and fractal patterning (see chapter 12). Small-world attributes were identified at all frequency scales, and global topological parameters were conserved across scales. Highest clustering and shortest path lengths were found at higher frequencies, which have been associated with integrative processes supporting perception and cognition (see chapter 9). Importantly, the topology of these functional networks remained largely unchanged during transitions from a state of cognitive rest to the performance of a motor task, despite significant spatial reconfiguration.

Hubs in Functional Connectivity

A comprehensive network analysis of resting-state functional connectivity identified locations of cortical hubs in several heteromodal association areas, including posterior cingulate, lateral temporal, lateral parietal, and medial/lateral prefrontal cortex (Buckner et al., 2009). The locations of these hubs were largely consistent across different task states, such as a passive fixation task (similar to an "eyes open" resting state) as well as an active word-classification task, suggesting that hubs are stable features of functional networks. Hubs were identified on the basis of their high degree of connectivity, and the data were processed at single-voxel resolution. Buckner and colleagues compared the locations of cortical hubs with distributions, obtained through PET imaging, of the amyloid-β protein, a key marker of cellular pathology in Alzheimer's disease (AD). A striking degree of overlap between hubs in functional connectivity and amyloid-β accumulation suggests a possible link between network topology and pathology (see chapter 10).

While several studies have identified highly connected and highly central hubs in the human brain, it is at present unclear what features of neural dynamics discriminate between hub and nonhub regions. By definition, hubs are well connected, and within the modular architecture of the brain they link communities that otherwise do not directly interact. Thus, hubs are in a privileged position of influence and control. They enable functional interactions between distinct communities and help to integrate specialized information. In information and social networks, hubs often promote navigability and searchability. What is it like, in neural terms, to be a hub? In most other types of networks (social, transportation, economic), hubs tend to be nodes that are exceptionally "busy" at all times, that is, nodes that participate in unusual levels of traffic, information flow, or signal fluctuations. In the brain, hub regions may be expected to share in the variance of multiple segregated modules and thus engage in more variable dynamics. Increased dynamic variability may cause an elevated baseline metabolism. Consistent with this hypothesis, high metabolism was found to be associated with high centrality in the large-scale structural network of the cortex (Hagmann et al., 2008; see figure 6.11).

Are hubs in functional networks also structural hubs in the underlying anatomy? Empirical data, although not yet obtained from the same individual participants, suggests this is indeed the case. Structural network analyses have consistently found a highly central role of the posterior cingulate/precuneus as well as various parietal and frontal regions.

Buckner et al. (2009) identified hubs in functional networks whose positions largely coincided with those of structural hubs identified in diffusion imaging data (see chapter 6; figure 6.11). The modeling study of Honey et al. (2007) reported a similar correspondence when comparing structural connectivity to functional connectivity averaged over a long time interval (see figure 8.9). Interestingly, significantly less agreement was seen on short time scales. For example, while the centrality of nonhub regions remains consistently low across time, the centrality of regions that were identified as network hubs on the basis of long-time averages displayed significant variations. Under spontaneous dynamics, hubs can engage and disengage across time, as they link different sets of brain regions at different times. These fluctuations in network parameters result from fluctuations in the strengths of functional connections and

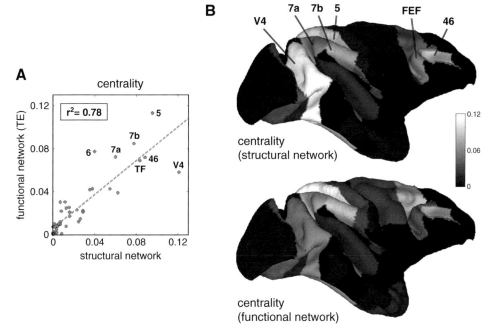

Figure 8.9
Comparison of structural and functional hubs in macaque cortex. These data are derived from a simulation study of the macaque visual and somatomotor cortex. Structural connections were obtained from a neuroanatomical database (connection matrix shown in figure 2.6), and functional connections were derived from long-time samples of simulated endogenous neural activity. The centrality of nodes in the structural and functional network is highly correlated. Panel (A) shows a scatterplot of the betweenness centrality for structural and functional connectivity, and panel (B) shows a distribution of centrality on the macaque cortical surface. Data were replotted from Honey et al. (2007). For abbreviations of anatomical areas see figure 2.6. TE, transfer entropy.

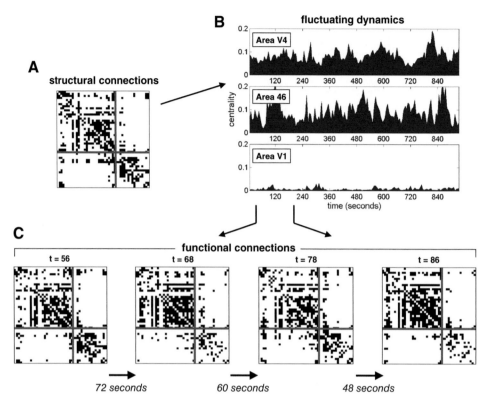

Figure 8.10
A repertoire of functional networks in spontaneous neural activity. Fixed structural connectivity (A; cf. figure 2.6) gives rise to fluctuating neural dynamics that results in time-dependent patterns of functional connectivity. Panel (B) shows the time evolution of betweenness centrality computed from samples of functional dynamics obtained from overlapping 30-second windows of neural activity. Nodes that have high centrality in long-time average functional networks (e.g., area V4 and area 46; see figure 8.9) exhibit significant fluctuations in centrality over shorter time periods. Panel (C) shows that the pattern of functional connectivity exhibits time-dependent changes on a time scale of seconds to minutes (t = time in seconds). Data replotted from Honey et al. (2007).

lead to changes in the topology of functional networks over time (see figure 8.10). These fluctuations support the creation of diverse dynamic states in the brain (see chapter 12) and constitute a functional repertoire of varying network topologies.

Spontaneous Brain Activity, Behavior, and Cognition

Does endogenous network activity have a functional role in the brain? Do these dynamic patterns contribute to cognitive and behavioral responses, or are they nothing but "physiological noise" without function? Despite the long history of spontaneous neural activity in electrophysiology, tracing back to the 1920s, the cognitive role of such activity remains very much a matter of debate and controversy. The functional meaning of the brain's default mode has been questioned (Morcom and Fletcher, 2007; see responses by Raichle and Snyder, 2007; Buckner and Vincent, 2007).[14] Some authors have pointed to nonneuronal components in resting brain fluctuations. Others have criticized the significance of endogenous brain activity, a point that stems from the idea still prevalent within cognitive science that most of human cognition is about computing purposeful responses to specific processing demands posed by the environment. At the time of writing, the neuronal origin of default mode or resting brain activity appears firmly established (e.g., Miller et al., 2009), and the reappraisal of the role of intrinsic brain activity in perception and cognition has ushered in a paradigm shift in brain imaging (Raichle, 2009, 2010).

Endogenous activity has key functional roles to play, not only in the adult organism but also in the neural development of sensory and motor systems (see chapter 11). In the mammalian nervous system, spontaneous neural activity is essential for the early patterning and refinement of synaptic connectivity of the visual system (Feller, 1999; Torborg and Feller, 2005), long before sensory and motor structures have fully matured and are capable of receiving or generating specific sensory inputs. Spontaneous activity of networks of spinal neurons generates embryonic limb movements in the developing chicken embryo (O'Donovan et al., 1998; Bekoff, 2001). Embryonic motility driven by spontaneous neural activity has multiple roles, from calibrating developing sensorimotor circuits to generating correlated sensory inputs. Just as processes of neuroplasticity extend from development into adulthood, the developmental roles of spontaneous neural activity may hint at their functional contributions in the adult organism,[15] possibly related to the need for maintaining functional homeostasis (see chapter 4).

The metabolic cost of endogenous default mode neural activity far exceeds that of evoked activity (Raichle and Mintun, 2006), with perhaps as little as a few percent of the brain's total energy budget associated with momentary processing demands. The large cost of endogenous activity does not by itself reveal its functional role, but it presents a compelling argument for its physiological importance. Equally significant are observations that highlight fundamental relationships between endogenous and evoked brain activity, many of which have been reviewed in this chapter. Endogenous activity is functionally organized and shaped by the same set of anatomical connections that are engaged in the context of cognitive tasks. As is borne out by empirical study of both cellular and large-scale systems, patterns of endogenous activity resemble evoked responses, revealing functional brain architecture at rest that reflects sets of dynamic relationships that are expressed in different configurations during cognitive processing.

The relationship of patterns of task-evoked brain activations with resting-state networks has been documented in several meta-analyses of large numbers of brain activation experiments (Toro et al., 2008; Smith et al., 2009). For example, a meta-analysis of a number of fMRI studies of social cognition revealed a significant overlap between brain regions identified as centrally involved in social cognitive processes and the brain's default network (Schilbach et al., 2008). This suggests the idea that the physiological baseline of the brain is related to a "psychological baseline," a mode of cognition that is directed internally rather than being externally driven and that is concerned with self and social context. Along the same lines, Malach and colleagues have suggested that the cortex can be partitioned into two coherently active systems, an "extrinsic system" associated with the processing of external inputs and an "intrinsic system" (overlapping with the default mode network) dealing with self-related signals and processes (Golland et al., 2007; 2008).

Synchronized patterns of resting-state functional connectivity persist during the execution of cognitive tasks and may affect behavioral outcomes. A significant fraction of the observed trial-to-trial variability of the BOLD response can be accounted for by these persistent ongoing fluctuations (Fox et al., 2006). Spontaneous fluctuations in the BOLD response are also highly correlated with behavioral variables (Fox et al., 2007) as shown in experiments where task-related and spontaneous activity were separated by comparing left and right motor cortex, which are known to be highly correlated at rest. Neural fluctuations may thus account for at least some of the variability of human behavior. The dependence of neural responses to sensory stimuli on an internal "network state" (Fontanini and Katz, 2008), modulated by spontaneous dynamics, attention, or experience, represents a fundamental aspect of sensory processing. Variable sensory responses are more fully accounted for by the interaction of an input and an intrinsic context generated from the dynamic repertoire of network states (see figure 8.11).

Correlated activity within the brain's default mode network has been described by some authors as the physiological basis of conscious spon-

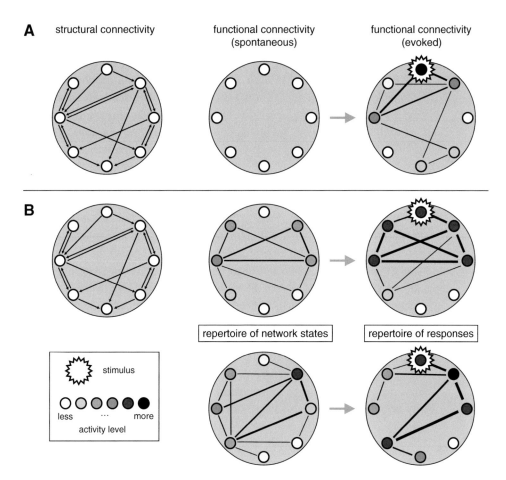

Figure 8.11
Functional repertoire of network states and variability in evoked responses. The schematic
diagram shows structural connectivity on the left, patterns of spontaneous activity (network
states) in the middle, and neural response patterns to sensory stimulation on the right.
Panel (A) depicts the "traditional" or reflexive model of sensory processing. Sensory
responses act on a quiescent brain, and thus a given sensory stimulus should evoke stereotypical responses. Panel (B) shows a repertoire of intrinsic functional connectivity due to
dynamic diversity (see figure 8.10; see also chapter 12) as well as dependence on the internal state of the organism. An identical sensory stimulus results in variable neural responses.
Modified and redrawn after a diagram in Fontanini and Katz (2008).

taneous cognition as manifested in "daydreaming" or "mind wandering" (Mason et al., 2007). However, studies of humans transitioning from waking to sleep (Larson-Prior et al., 2009) and under light sedation (Greicius et al., 2008), as well as anaesthetized nonhuman primates (Vincent et al., 2007), have shown that correlated default mode activity persists even in the absence of consciousness. Thus, it does not appear that all correlated spontaneous activity reflects conscious mental states. Instead, the continued presence of correlated fluctuations outside of consciousness suggests a more basic, but no less fundamental, role and does not exclude its participation in unconscious mental processes.

Computational modeling studies reviewed in this chapter suggest that endogenous fluctuations give rise to temporal sequences of network states that collectively form a diverse functional repertoire (see chapter 12). The idea has gained considerable empirical support from comparisons of thousands of brain activation maps acquired during cognitive studies and resting-state networks extracted by objective pattern discovery methods (Smith et al., 2009). Such comparisons indicate that functional networks deployed during task-related processing are continually active even when the brain is cognitively at rest. This ongoing rehearsal of functional couplings may be a requirement for the continued maintenance of the cognitive architecture, or it may serve to prepare the brain for adaptive responses to intermittent environmental stimuli by continually replaying the past or imagining the future (Schacter et al., 2007).

9 Networks for Cognition

If we make a symbolic diagram on a blackboard, of the laws of association between ideas, we are inevitably led to draw circles, or closed figures of some kind, and to connect them by lines. When we hear that the nerve-centres contain cells which send off fibres, we say that Nature has realized our diagram for us, and that the mechanical substratum of thought is plain. In *some* way, it is true, our diagram must be realized in the brain; but surely in no such visible and palpable way as we at first suppose. [...] Too much anatomy has been found to order for theoretic purposes, even by the anatomists; and the popular-science notions of cells and fibres are almost wholly wide of the truth. Let us therefore relegate the subject of the *intimate* workings of the brain to the physiology of the future.[1]
—William James, 1890

William James' skepticism regarding the relation of cognition to the anatomy of the human brain may strike many of us as old-fashioned. After all, modern neuroscience continues to yield a plethora of empirical data that reveal the neural basis of cognition in ever greater detail, and the "physiology of the future" must surely have arrived by now. And yet, the relationship between brain and cognition is still only poorly understood. Great progress notwithstanding, neuroscience still cannot answer the "big questions" about mind and intelligence. Consequently, most cognitive scientists continue to hold the position that intelligence is fundamentally the work of symbolic processing, carried out in rule-based computational architectures whose function can be formally described in ways that are entirely independent of their physical realization. If cognition is largely symbolic in nature, then its neural substrate is little more than an inconsequential detail, revealing nothing that is of essence about the mind.[2] Naturally, there is much controversy on the subject.

The idea that mental life can be explained as a set of computational processes has undeniable power and appeal. Yet, the nature of these processes must in some way depend on the biological substrate of brain and body and on their development and natural history. There have been many false starts in the attempt to link brain and cognition. One such failure is neuroreductionism, a view that fully substitutes all mental phenomena by neural mechanisms, summarized in the catchphrase "You are nothing but a pack of neurons," or, put more eloquently, "'You', your joys and your sorrows, your memories and your ambitions, your sense of personal identity and free will, are in fact no more than the behavior of a vast assembly of nerve cells and their associated molecules" (Crick, 1994). The problematic nature of this statement lies not in the materialist stance that rightfully puts mental states on a physical basis but rather in the phrase "no more than," which implies that the elementary properties of cells and molecules can explain all there is to know about mind and cognition. Reductionism can be spectacularly successful when it traces complex phenomena to their root cause, and yet it consistently falls short as a theoretical framework for the operation of complex systems because it cannot explain their emergent and collective properties (see chapter 13).

In this chapter, I will attempt to move beyond reductionist models of cognition and view the subject from the more integrative perspective of complex networks. I will focus on some of the main architectural principles that underlie various forms of cognitive processing in the mammalian brain—in particular, the dichotomy between functional segregation and integration, and the hierarchical organization of brain networks. These principles emerge naturally from a close consideration of anatomical connections and neural dynamics. First, I will briefly lay out a few current theories of how cognition may result from the action of neurocognitive networks that span large portions of the mammalian thalamocortical system. The problem of functional integration is central to all neural accounts of how coherent cognitive and behavioral states are generated in the brain, and I will consider two ways in which integration is achieved in the brain, convergence and synchrony. Next, the central role of hierarchical processing demands an analysis of its structural and physiological basis and of its relationship to the modularity of brain networks. Finally, I will turn to the rapid reconfiguration of functional and effective brain networks in response to varying demands of the environment, which provides a dynamic basis for the flexible and adaptive nature of cognition.

Cognition as a Network Phenomenon

Cognition is a network phenomenon. It does not exist in synapses or single neurons. Instead, it is a collective property of very large numbers of neural elements that are interconnected in complex patterns.[3] The search for elementary principles of how cognition emerges from network interactions has led to several proposals that approach network function from different angles and perspectives. One of the most influential movements in modern cognitive science built on a set of models collectively named "parallel distributed processing" (PDP; Rumelhart et al., 1986). What many of these models had in common was that they viewed cognition as a process of cooperative computation, carried out in parallel across distributed networks. The activity of nodes in these networks formed representations about perceptual or conceptual entities such as letters, words, visual shapes, and motor commands. The weights of connections between nodes encoded knowledge about how these perceptual or conceptual entities related to one another. The network as a whole transformed a set of inputs into outputs, with outputs often consisting of stable configurations of activated nodes that represented the network's response to the input and expressed its encoded knowledge. PDP models provided many powerful examples of how cooperative processes could yield "good" computational results within specific problem domains— for example, in visual recognition. Yet, their utility as models of actual neural processes was limited since their computational paradigms often imposed narrow constraints on the types of network structures and dynamics that could be implemented.

In parallel to PDP studies of neural computation, the interconnected and dynamic nature of large-scale brain networks became of central concern in cognitive neuroscience, fueled by increasingly detailed data on the anatomical connectivity and functional activation of the cerebral cortex. The tension between models that relied on hierarchical versus distributed processing soon became apparent in anatomical and functional accounts of the visual cortex (Zeki and Shipp, 1988) and the prefrontal cortex (Fuster, 1980; Goldman-Rakic, 1988), as well as a variety of other systems of the brain. Functional integration was soon recognized as a central problem for neural accounts of cognition, and the problem was approached from fundamentally different perspectives. Many cognitive studies suggested the operation of a "central executive," a process exerting supervisory control over mental resources and decision making, often thought to be affiliated with the prefrontal cortex

(Goldman-Rakic, 1995). Instead, decentralized accounts of neural and cognitive function emphasized the recurrent, recursive, and reentrant nature of neural interactions and the complexity of their dynamics (Edelman, 1978; 1987).

Marcel Mesulam proposed that the physical substrate of cognition is a set of distinct large-scale neurocognitive networks that support different domains of cognitive and behavioral function (Mesulam, 1990). He conceptualized brain–behavior relationships as both localized and distributed, mapping complex cognition and behavior to a "multifocal neural system" rather than a circumscribed set of specialized anatomical regions. He noted the absence of simple one-to-one correspondences between anatomical regions and cognitive functions and instead argued that specific domains of cognition or behavior are associated with *networks* of regions, each of which individually may support a broad range of functions. Mesulam (1998) envisioned sensory processing to unfold along a "core synaptic hierarchy" consisting of primary sensory, upstream unimodal, downstream unimodal, heteromodal, paralimbic, and limbic zones of the cerebral cortex (see figure 9.1). The last three subdivisions together constitute transmodal areas that bind signals across all levels and form integrated and distributed representations. Crosscutting this hierarchical scheme, Mesulam distinguished five large-scale neurocognitive networks, each concerned with functions in a specific cognitive domain: spatial awareness, language, explicit memory/emotion, face/object recognition, and working memory/executive function. These networks do not operate in isolation, instead they engage in complex interactions partly coordinated by transmodal areas.

Steven Bressler put the notion of distinct neurocognitive networks in a more dynamic context when he defined a complex function of the brain as "a system of interrelated processes directed toward the performance of a particular task, that is implemented neurally by a complementary system, or network, of functionally related cortical areas" (Bressler, 1995, p. 289). According to this view, the structural networks of the cerebral cortex, or the entire brain, serve as a substrate for the system-wide dynamic coordination of distributed neural resources (Bressler and Tognoli, 2006). An implication of this definition is that different complex functions are accomplished by transient assemblies of network elements in varying conditions of input or task set. In other words, different processing demands and task domains are associated with the dynamic reconfiguration of functional or effective brain networks. The same set of network elements can participate in multiple

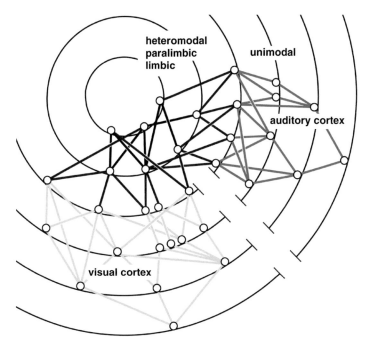

Figure 9.1
A schematic diagram for representing different levels of cortical processing, after Mesulam (1998). Each concentric circle represents a synaptic level, and cortical regions (represented as nodes) are arranged on these circles depending on their interconnections and response characteristics. The continuous arcs represent connections between nodes at the same level. Additional connections are indicated as lines between different levels. Unimodal sensory cortices are integrated by heteromodal and limbic regions in temporal, parietal, and frontal cortex, arranged on the innermost circles of the diagram. Modified and redrawn after Mesulam (1998).

cognitive functions by rapid reconfigurations of network links or functional connections.

The multifunctional nature of the brain's network nodes leads to the idea that functions do not reside in individual brain regions but are accomplished by network interactions that rapidly reconfigure, resulting in dynamic changes of neural context (McIntosh, 1999; 2000; 2008). Regional activation is an insufficient indicator of the involvement of a given brain area in a task, since the same pattern of regional activations can be brought about by multiple distinct patterns of dynamic relationships. Randy McIntosh suggested that the functional contribution of a brain region is more clearly defined by the neural context within which it is embedded. This neural context is reconfigured as stimulus and task conditions vary, and it is ultimately constrained by the underlying structural network. Comparison of regional activation patterns in a variety of cognitive paradigms strongly suggests that a given brain region can take on more than one functional role depending on the pattern of interactions with other regions in the brain (McIntosh et al., 1997; McIntosh et al., 2003; Lenartowicz and McIntosh, 2005; Bressler and McIntosh, 2007). McIntosh hypothesized that a special class of network nodes is instrumental in fast and dynamic reconfigurations of large-scale networks—for example, during task switching. These so-called "catalysts" facilitate the transition between large-scale functional patterns associated with cognitive processing (McIntosh, 2004; 2008). Catalysts may be identifiable on the basis of their embedding in structural or functional networks.

Network theories of cognition place an emphasis on cooperative processes that are shaped by anatomical connectivity. The mapping between neurons and cognition relies less on what individual nodes can do and more on the topology of their connectivity. Rather than explain cognition through intrinsic computational capacities of localized regions or serial processing within precisely specified or learned connections, network approaches to cognition aim for defining relationships between mental states and dynamic neural patterns of spontaneous activity or evoked responses. One of the most important features of these large-scale system dynamics is the coexistence of opposing tendencies toward functional segregation and integration.

Functional Segregation and Integration

Segregation and integration are two major organizational principles of the cerebral cortex (Zeki, 1978; Zeki and Shipp, 1988; Tononi et al., 1994; 1998; Friston, 2002; 2005a; 2009b) and are invoked in almost all cognitive domains. This dichotomy results from the need to reconcile the existence of discrete anatomical units and regional specialization with the phenomenological unity of mental states and behavior.[4] For example, the construction of a perceptually coherent visual image requires both segregation and integration. It requires the activation of cells with specialized receptive field properties, as well as the "unification" of multiple such signals distributed around the brain (Zeki, 1993).[5] This unification or "binding together" of object attributes has to be carried out quickly and reliably and on a virtually infinite set of objects that form part of a cluttered and dynamic visual scene. This so-called "binding problem" (see below) represents just one example of the general need to rapidly and efficiently integrate specialized and distributed information.

Evidence for anatomical and functional segregation comes from multiple levels in the brain, ranging from specialized neurons to neuronal populations and cortical areas. For example, maps of cortical regions, such as those assembled by Ungerleider and Mishkin (1982), Van Essen and Maunsell (1983), Zeki and Shipp (1988), and Felleman and Van Essen (1991), have provided increasingly refined network diagrams of multiple anatomically and functionally distinct areas of the primate visual cortex. These specialized and segregated brain regions contain neurons that selectively respond to specific input features (such as orientation, spatial frequency, or color) or conjunctions of features (such as objects or faces). Segregation can be defined in a purely statistical context as the tendency of different neurons to capture different regularities present in their inputs. The concepts of functional localization (see chapter 4) and segregation are therefore somewhat distinct from one another. Segregation implies that neural responses are statistically distinct from one another and thus represent specialized information, but it does not imply that segregated neural populations or brain regions become functionally encapsulated or autonomously carry out distinct mental faculties. Furthermore, segregation is a multiscale phenomenon, found not only among cortical areas but also among local populations of neurons or single cells. Structural connectivity supports functional segregation. For example, some intraregional (Gilbert and Wiesel, 1989; Tanigawa et al., 2005) and interregional (Angelucci et al., 2002) anatomical connections are arranged in patches or clusters that link populations with similar responses, thus preserving segregation.

Most complex cognitive processes require the functional integration of widely distributed resources for coherent behavioral responses and mental states. There are at least two ways by which neuronal architectures can achieve functional integration in the brain, convergence and phase synchrony.[6] Integration by convergence creates more specialized neurons or brain regions by conjunction of inputs from other less specialized neurons. Convergence can thus generate neurons whose activity encodes high-level attributes of their respective input space, increasing the functional segregation and specialization of the architecture.[7] There is abundant evidence that the convergence of neural connectivity within hierarchically arranged regions can yield increasingly specialized neural responses, including neurons that show selective modulations of firing rate to highly complex sensory stimuli (e.g., Quiroga et al., 2005). It should be noted that these localized responses depend on widely distributed network processes, including feedforward and feedback influences.

Network interactions endow even simple "feature detectors," for example, cells in primary visual cortex, with extremely rich response properties that are particularly evident when these responses are recorded during natural vision (Gallant et al., 1998; Vinje and Gallant, 2000). These complex response properties reflect contextual influences from outside of the cell's classical receptive field that subtly modulate its neural activity. Thus, network interactions contribute to complex and localized neuronal response properties encountered throughout the brain.

Integration by convergence is also found within large-scale neurocognitive networks. Mesulam suggested that a special set of "transmodal nodes" plays a crucial role in functional integration (Mesulam, 1998). These regions bind together multiple signals from unimodal areas and create multimodal representations. Graphically, they serve as articulation points between networks supporting different cognitive domains. A somewhat different idea was proposed by Antonio Damasio, starting from the premise that the integration of multiple aspects of external and internal reality depends on the phase-locked coactivation of neural patterns in distinct and spatially remote areas of cortex (Damasio, 1989). This integration is supported by "convergence zones" (see figure 9.2) that can trigger and synchronize distributed neural patterns through feedback projections but are not themselves the locus of integration or encoders of integrated mental content. Convergence zones are thought to occur throughout the forebrain, and their distinguishing feature is their mode of connectivity that supports binding and integration. In this sense, convergence zones are reminiscent of hubs placed throughout the neurocognitive skeleton, whose coordinating activity ensures distributed functional integration but that do not represent the endpoint of integration in a serial processing architecture. Damasio's model effectively combines aspects of convergence and distributed interactions, and it is supported by a broad range of physiological studies (Meyer and Damasio, 2009).

A rich set of models suggests that functional integration can be achieved even without convergence, through dynamic interactions, for example, resulting in phase locking or synchronization between distant cell populations. This mechanism depends on reciprocal structural connections linking neurons across segregated brain regions. This alternative model has been most fully explored in the context of the binding problem in vision (Treisman, 1996). The visual binding problem arises because the different attributes of visual objects are analyzed in a large number of segregated brain regions and yet must be perceptually integrated. Exper-

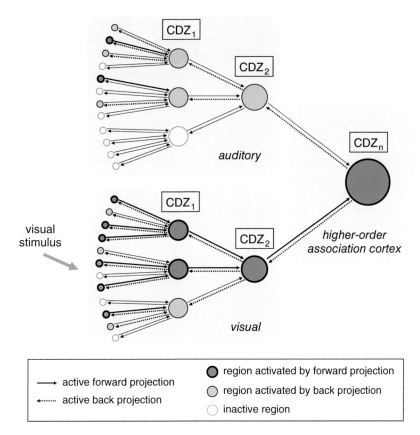

Figure 9.2
Convergence zones. Schematic diagram of a response pattern unfolding within a hierarchical neural architecture containing multiple levels of convergence/divergence zones (CDZs). The presentation of a visual stimulus results in activation of specialized visual regions and visual CDZs, as well as a CDZ in higher order association cortex, because of convergent forward projections. Divergent projections lead to retroactivation of additional regions in visual cortex as well as auditory cortex, which reconstruct activation patterns that were previously experienced together with the visual stimulus, for example, the sound of a voice accompanying the visual image of a lip movement. Modified after Meyer and Damasio (2009).

iments by Wolf Singer and colleagues have provided evidence for stimulus-dependent neural synchrony within and between cortical regions (Gray and Singer, 1989; Gray et al., 1989; Engel et al., 1991) and for its potential role in perceptual processes such as grouping and figure–ground segregation (Singer and Gray, 1995; Phillips and Singer, 1997; Singer, 1999). Intra- and interregional synchronization, particularly of neuronal activity in the gamma frequency band (~20–80 Hz), is encountered in a great number of vertebrate species, including primates, and in the context of a broad range of behavioral and cognitive tasks (Ward, 2003; Fries, 2009).[8] Synchronization has distinct effects on neural processing by enabling the detection of coincident spikes in areas that receive convergent synchronized signals, as well as rhythmic modulations of local inhibition and sensitivity to input. Coherent phase-synchronized activity between neurons facilitates their mutual communication and modulates their interaction strength (Fries, 2005; Womelsdorf et al., 2007). Spontaneous or evoked changes in phase coherence and synchronization can therefore rapidly reconfigure networks of functional and effective connectivity, while the underlying structural connectivity remains relatively constant.

Task-dependent modulation of synchrony has been demonstrated in a wide spectrum of human and animal experiments. One of the most compelling and thoroughly studied examples comes from local field potential recordings of macaque cortex during the execution of a visual discrimination task (Bressler et al., 1993). Monkeys were trained to respond to brief visual presentations of one type of pattern and to withhold responding to another type of pattern. Broadband coherence of cortical potentials was observed during specific stages of the task, reflecting time-dependent cooperative interactions of cortical regions. Patterns of dynamic coupling were created and dissolved within hundreds of milliseconds, in accordance with momentary demands on sensory and motor processing. Time series analysis tools capable of detecting directed influences revealed a task-dependent network of causal relationships between recording sites (Brovelli et al., 2004; see figure 9.3). The role of phase synchronization in perception and cognition was further explored by Francisco Varela and colleagues, who stressed the transient nature of coherence and functional integration (Rodriguez et al., 1999; Varela et al., 2001). Perception of faces, but not of meaningless shapes, was associated with intermittent periods of long-distance synchronization. These transient episodes of coherence are a reflection of the brain's metastable dynamics (see chapter 12) and of an ongoing process of coordination among widely distributed populations of neurons. The work of Bressler and Varela, among others, strongly suggests that large-scale integration is a dynamic process that is essential for perceptual and cognitive performance and that time-dependent networks of phase synchronization unfolding within the anatomical substrate of the cerebral cortex are one of its key mechanistic ingredients. We note that the repertoire of functional interactions between brain regions is significantly expanded

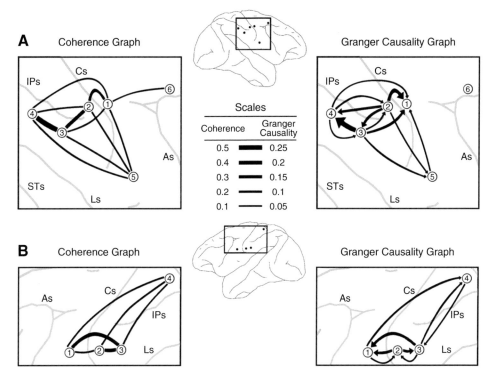

Figure 9.3
Sensorimotor networks in macaque cortex. Graphs show coherence (left) and Granger causality (right) between recording sites on the cerebral cortex. Recordings were obtained with implanted surface microelectrodes during the monkey's execution of a task requiring sensorimotor integration. Panels (A) and (B) show significant pairwise coherences and directed interactions between sites in frontal and parietal cortex. Cs, central sulcus; IPs, intraparietal sulcus; STs, superior temporal sulcus; Ls, lateral sulcus; As, arcuate sulcus. Reproduced from Brovelli et al. (2004) with permission.

by a variety of asynchronous (nonlinear) interactions that are not captured by linear measures of functional connectivity.

The integrative role of phase synchrony in perception and cognition has been explored in a large number of computational models. Temporal correlations between distributed neural signals (functional or effective connectivity) can express relations that are essential for neural encoding of objects, figure–ground segregation, and perceptual grouping (von der Malsburg, 1981; von der Malsburg and Schneider, 1986; Sporns et al., 1989; 1991). Anatomically based computational models demonstrated that fast synchronization and cooperative interactions within and among segregated areas of the visual cortex can effectively solve the binding problem and enable coherent behavioral responses (Tononi et al., 1992). While the role of phase synchrony in visual perception continues to be a subject of much debate, network oscillations are now considered to be a common and prominent feature of neuronal activity with putative functional roles that range from representing relational information to regulating patterns of information flow and supporting information retrieval (Sejnowski and Paulsen, 2006).

In summary, the coexistence of segregation and integration is indispensible for the proper functioning of large-scale neurocognitive networks. All coherent perceptual and cognitive states require the functional integration of very large numbers of neurons within the distributed system of the cerebral cortex. It is likely that both mechanisms for integration covered in this section, convergence and synchrony, make important contributions. The capacity of the network to sustain high levels of both segregation and integration is crucial for its efficiency in cognition and behavior, and in an information-theoretic context it forms the origin of brain complexity (see chapter 13).

Hierarchy and Recurrent Processing in Cognition

An important concept in the architecture of neurocognitive networks is that of a processing hierarchy, an arrangement of neural units and brain regions where information flows from lower (sensory) to higher (multimodal and associative) levels and is gradually elaborated from simple to more complex responses. Many cognitive accounts of brain function are built on the notion that sensory information is sequentially processed on several different levels, mostly in a feedforward manner. According to these accounts, sensory inputs trigger sequences of discrete representations, constructed from neurons with increasingly complex response properties. Physiological recordings of individual neurons in the central visual system initially supported the idea that vision was carried out in a mostly serial hierarchy (Hubel and Wiesel, 1962). However, the prevalence of reciprocal anatomical connections throughout the cerebral cortex soon cast doubt on the strictly serial nature of hierarchical processing and triggered efforts to extract stages of the cortical hierarchy from data on interregional anatomical connectivity (Van Essen and Maunsell, 1983; van Essen et al., 1990; Felleman and van Essen, 1991). Based mostly on laminar termination patterns of axonal pathways, Felleman and Van Essen proposed a hierarchical scheme for the macaque visual cortex consisting of around ten separate levels linked by feedforward, lateral, and feedback connections. The scheme reconciled information on hundreds of interregional pathways and included connections that spanned single or multiple levels in either direction. Similar hierarchical schemes could be constructed for other sensory systems in the macaque monkey and the cat. Complementing the hierarchical arrangement of areas, Van Essen and colleagues described segregated streams that were arranged in parallel and relayed different types of visual information, most notably the dorsal and ventral visual cortex (Van Essen et al., 1992).

Building on the data set assembled by Felleman and Van Essen, Hilgetag et al. (1996) searched for an optimal hierarchical arrangement that contained minimal violations of the set of anatomical constraints imposed by laminar termination patterns. A large number of hierarchical orderings were found that contained an equally minimal number of constraint violations, suggesting that a unique optimal solution for the visual hierarchy did not exist. Consistent hierarchical ordering emerged mostly at lower levels of the architecture, with primary and secondary visual cortex always placed at the very bottom, while arrangements of higher visual areas exhibited much greater ambiguity. Recently, a more refined automated optimization approach which used a continuous metric for the assignment of hierarchical levels resolved some of the remaining inconsistencies and confirmed many of the features of the visual hierarchy as originally proposed (Reid et al., 2009). Thus, anatomical data support the idea of a hierarchical ordering of visual regions, not in the form of a strict serial sequence but with some overlap in the definition of hierarchical levels.

These anatomical studies do not take into account physiological effects or functional interactions. In fact, the relation of the anatomical hierarchy to visual function is far from simple (Hegdé and Felleman, 2007). Some physiological properties of visual areas accurately reflect their position in the anatomical hierarchy, such as receptive field sizes, complexity of response tuning, or onset latency of response. However, when one is probing visual responses in different areas with a uniform set of tests—for example, for shape selectivity—areas placed at distinct levels display overlapping tuning characteristics that violate the serial nature of the hierarchy. The notion of serial hierarchies and fully segregated functional streams is further undermined by mounting empirical evidence for cross- and multisensory processing even in "lower" and thus presumably unisensory cortical regions (Ghazanfar and Schroeder, 2006). For example, neurons in what is generally considered unimodal visual cortex often have both visual and auditory receptive fields. Standard models of the cortical hierarchy predict that such multisensory response properties appear only at later stages of processing, as a result of multimodal convergence. However, multisensory influences are pervasive at all levels and form an integral part of both simple and complex sensory processing. Recurrent feedback from "higher" to "lower" visual areas, thalamocortical interactions, and multisensory integration during natural vision all contribute to a loosening of the strictly serial hierarchical order.[9]

Feedforward and feedback connections have different physiological and computational roles. Forward connections drive neural activity at short latencies, while feedback connections mediate a broad range of modulatory synaptic effects (Salin and Bullier, 1995; Büchel and Friston, 2000). The distinct dynamic effects of feedback can be quantified with modeling and time series analysis tools applied to electrophysiological or neuroimaging data. Dynamic causal modeling shows that long latency stimulus-evoked potentials are due to recurrent dynamics meditated by feedback connections (Garrido et al., 2007). Granger causality analysis of fMRI data sets reveals top-down control signals sent from frontal and parietal cortex to visual cortex during an attention-demanding spatial task (Bressler et al., 2008). The specific contributions of feedforward and feedback connections in stimulus- and task-evoked neural dynamics can be further assessed with models that extract effective connectivity (see chapter 3 and below).

In the visual system, several authors have suggested that top-down (feedback) connections may provide predictions about bottom-up sensory inputs (Rao and Ballard, 1999) and thus support visual recognition and categorization. The role of expectation in the visual process has also been explored by Young (2000) and Bressler (2004). Hierarchical models are central to a theoretical framework proposed by Karl Friston (Friston, 2005b; 2010). A major tenet of the theory is that the main computational problem for the sensory brain is the inference of the causes that underlie its inputs. A central role for inference in cortical processing makes predictions about the arrangement of cortical connectivity. An architecture supporting the generation of dynamic predictions and causal inference should consist of hierarchical levels that are reciprocally interconnected, with both driving and modulatory connections. Prediction and inference must occur on multiple time scales since most natural environments exhibit rich temporal structure. Kiebel et al. (2008) have proposed that the brain represents causal changes unfolding at different time scales within different levels of the cortical hierarchy, with fast environmental processes primarily involving lower levels. Empirical studies by Hasson et al. (2008) have indeed provided evidence for a cortical hierarchy of temporal receptive windows in the human brain.

These models and observations all suggest that recurrent processing plays an important role in hierarchical accounts of the brain and that it is compatible with hierarchical ordering of the anatomical organization. The prominence of recurrent connectivity also implies that each hierarchical level may have only limited functional autonomy and that feedforward and feedback projections are always concurrently engaged. Gerald Edelman proposed that the actions of feedforward and feedback connections should be considered as part of a unified dynamic process, called reentry, that recursively links neural populations within the thalamocortical system (Edelman, 1978; 1987). Models have demonstrated that reentry can support a broad range of functions from conflict resolution and the construction of new response properties (Finkel and Edelman, 1989) to intra- and interregional synchronization, feature binding, and perceptual grouping (Sporns et al., 1989; 1991). Reentrant dynamics select and unify distributed resources while at the same time relaying contextual influences that modulate local responses as appropriate under a given set of environmental conditions. A reentrant system operates less as a hierarchy and more as a heterarchy, where super- and subordinate levels are indistinct, most interactions are circular, and control is decentralized.[10]

Hierarchical Modularity

There is a subtle link between hierarchical accounts of neural processing and the existence of modules and hubs previously identified as key ingredients of the brain's small world (see chapters 6 and 8). The hierarchical arrangements of cortical connectivity described so far are not easily revealed with standard graph-theoretical algorithms since the specification of the hierarchical order generally requires taking into account details of laminar termination patterns, topographic mappings, receptive field properties, or other physiological properties. Nevertheless, the term "hierarchy" is also used in graph theory and network analysis, albeit in a somewhat different sense from that discussed so far. Network hierarchy is often invoked in the context of modularity. Here, instead of a processing hierarchy, hierarchical levels are defined as levels of modularity, or nested arrangements of modules within modules. Systems with hierarchical modularity can be recursively subdivided into ever smaller and denser modules. The brain's anatomic organization, with individual neurons that are grouped into local populations, which are in turn grouped into brain regions and large-scale systems, resembles a network with hierarchical modularity. Hierarchical modularity has important implications for the temporal structure of brain dynamics (see chapter 12).

Hierarchical modularity can be measured with network analysis tools, defined on the basis of structural or functional connectivity. In some cases, modules detected by these methods correspond to "functional streams," for example, the dorsal and ventral streams of the visual system (Sporns et al., 2007; Hagmann et al., 2008). Hub regions that interconnect these network modules are often identified as multimodal or transmodal regions previously thought to be located at the highest levels of a serial hierarchy. Thus, modularity and hub analysis can identify regions of high intermodal convergence (functional integration) and distinct processing streams (functional segregation). Evidence for the existence of hierarchical modularity in the functional networks of the human brain comes from two recent studies by Ferrarini et al. (2009) and Meunier et al. (2009b). Using a decomposition algorithm capable of revealing hierarchically arranged modules (Blondel et al., 2008) and resting-state fMRI data from 18 participants, Meunier et al. detected five major functional modules (see figure 9.4, plate 13). These modules were fairly consistent

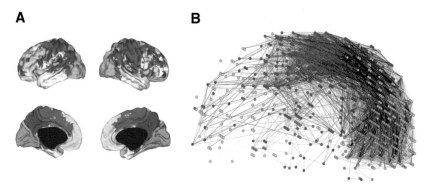

Figure 9.4 (plate 13)
Modules in functional connectivity. Modularity is derived from resting-state fMRI recordings of 18 participants. Both plots show five major modules (blue, lateral occipital module; red, central module; dark blue, parietofrontal module; green, medial occipital module; and yellow, frontotemporal module). (A) Cortical surface map. (B) Plot of all nodes in anatomical space (lateral view, anterior to the left). Reproduced from Meunier et al. (2009b).

across individual participants, suggesting that they have a basis in underlying patterns of structural connectivity. Several of these modules could be further decomposed into submodules, thus indicating the presence of a hierarchical modular organization in functional connectivity.

The application of pattern extraction techniques to functional imaging data sets has revealed a number of coherently active networks, many of which resemble known neurocognitive networks involved in sensory or motor function, memory, executive control, or attention (Calhoun et al., 2001; van de Ven et al., 2004; Beckmann et al., 2005; Perlbarg and Marrelec, 2008). Since these networks can be extracted from endogenous resting-state neural activity, they are likely shaped by structural connectivity. Some of these networks can be further decomposed, as is the case for the dorsal and ventral stream within the visual resting-state network, consistent with the concept of hierarchical modularity. Acute task or stimulus effects can modify the composition or configuration of neurocognitive networks, and at least some of the connections within and between these networks are altered in neuropathology (Buckner et al., 2008; see chapter 10).

How does the modularity of structural brain connectivity (or its functional counterparts) relate to the concept of "modularity of mind" in cognitive science (Fodor, 1983)? Structural and functional modules identified by network analysis have little in common with the putative cognitive modules proposed by Fodor and others. Fodor's mental modules are defined as "informationally encapsulated," that is, they are dissociable and can carry out their distinct functional roles without making reference to other modules. Such modules are computational systems whose informational resources are restricted to what is available to its (innate) database, and that are cognitively impenetrable by other extramodular processes. Fodor acknowledges that while computational theories of cognition apply well to such modules, the more "holistic" or "inferential" capacities of the mind defy such computational accounts and are not well captured with mental models based on modules. In fact, functional integration in the brain must be able to cut across cognitive domains and is thus essentially intermodular in character. Brain modules must therefore be able to influence each other, through "weak ties" (in Granovetter's terminology) that enable globally efficient information flow. Modules of brain networks define communities of structurally and functionally related areas, but they do not represent or support discrete mental faculties.

Task Dependence and Dynamic Reconfiguration

Structural, functional, and effective brain networks change on different
time scales. Structural networks remain relatively stable over shorter
time periods, while functional and effective networks undergo rapid
dynamic changes in the course of spontaneous activity or in response
to varying demands imposed by input or task. Temporal modulation
of functional connectivity patterns has been documented across a wide
range of conditions and in many systems of the brain. Electrophysiological studies in animals have shown that specific and highly dynamic
(short-lasting) patterns of temporal correlations (functional connectivity) between different regions of the thalamocortical system are engaged
during different behavioral tasks. Patterns of interregional cross-
correlations have been found to accompany the performance of specific
behavioral tasks in monkey (Bressler et al., 1993; Liang et al., 2002;
Brovelli et al., 2004) and cat cortex (e.g., Roelfsema et al., 1997; von Stein
et al., 2000).

In the human brain, early reports on changes in functional connectivity related to task performance came from experiments using PET data.
Analysis of correlations in regional cerebral blood flow in visual cortex
during a face-matching and a dot-location task revealed different patterns of associations between segregated components of the visual
system (Horwitz et al., 1992). Task-related changes in interregional interactions have also been recorded with covariance structural equation
modeling (see chapter 3), a method that attempts to explain the observed
covariance of a set of functional data on the basis of a structural model
that incorporates features of the anatomy (see chapter 3). Different task
demands in vision (McIntosh et al., 1994; see figure 9.5), working memory
(McIntosh et al., 1996), and sensory learning in aware and unaware
subjects (McIntosh et al., 1999) recruit different functional networks
within the same cortical architecture. Effective coupling between visual
regions can be modulated by attention in a task-dependent manner
(Büchel and Friston, 1997; 2000). Changes in functional connectivity
measured from fMRI time series data have been observed in virtually
all cognitive domains, including sensory, motor, memory, planning, and
executive control paradigms. For example, functional connectivity
between Broca's and Wernicke's areas is increased relative to cognitive
rest when subjects are engaged in a listening task (Hampson et al., 2002),
while viewing motion stimuli modulated the functional connectivity of
visual area MT/V5 (Hampson et al., 2004), and cognitive interference

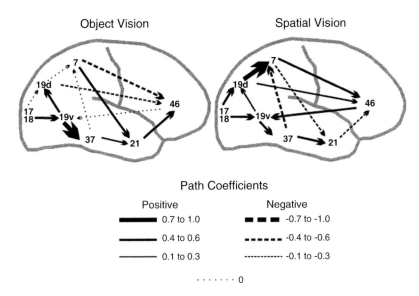

Figure 9.5
Networks of brain regions supporting different visual tasks. PET imaging data of subjects engaged in object and spatial vision tasks were processed with covariance structural equation modeling to obtain estimates of path coefficients for directed interactions between a set of mostly visual brain regions. Note that the two tasks engage different networks. Reproduced from McIntosh et al. (1994) with permission.

generated during a Stroop task induced changes in the functional connectivity of the inferior frontal cortex (Kemmotsu et al., 2005). These observations of task-dependent large-scale patterns of functional connectivity in fMRI are consistent with results from EEG/MEG and electrophysiological studies indicating that changes in cognitive or behavioral state are associated with changes in distributed coherent patterns of neural activity (e.g., Srinivasan et al., 1999; von Stein et al., 1999; Schnitzler and Gross, 2005).

In chapter 8, I reviewed the evidence for consistent patterns of functional connectivity during the resting state, recorded in the absence of stimulus input or task demands. How similar or how different are these resting-state patterns from those generated by networks that are engaged during specific cognitive tasks? Hampson et al. (2004) measured functional connectivity in fMRI data obtained while subjects were at rest and during presentation of visual motion stimuli. Such stimuli are known to activate an area in extrastriate cortex homologous to macaque monkey MT/V5. During rest, area MT/V5 was found to display a wide range of correlations within the visual cortex. The range of correlations was reduced during visual motion input as a more specific and task-related network became activated.

An analysis of MEG data by Bassett et al. (2006) examined the topology of functional brain networks sampled at rest and during the performance of a motor task. Resting-state functional networks exhibited robust small-world attributes across multiple frequency ranges (see chapter 8). This topology did not change significantly with the imposition of a specific behavioral task. Bassett et al. observed that functional networks were spatially reconfigured in the transition from rest to task, particularly with the appearance of new long-range functional connections in higher frequency bands. Changes in behavioral state were also associated with the appearance of new highly connected and highly central nodes. These results suggest that varying task demands can rapidly and transiently reconfigure functional networks while maintaining some of their topological characteristics.

How does external task demand modulate the functional interactions among regions within the default mode network? Cognitive load results in deactivation of most default mode network components and attenuates, but does not completely abolish, their functional coupling (Fransson, 2006; Fransson and Marrelec, 2008; see figure 8.4). These results suggest that cognitive load modulates and reorganizes intrinsic network activity without completely suspending neural processes that are predominantly expressed during rest. The relationship between spontaneous and task-evoked functional connectivity is also documented by the consistency of major hub regions and functional modules (Buckner et al., 2009). The consistency of these patterns suggests the hypothesis that resting-state activity is composed of a succession of patterns drawn from an intrinsic functional repertoire and that these individual patterns resemble those seen under cognitive load.

Steve Petersen and colleagues have demonstrated that the reconfiguration of functional brain networks based on the momentary demands of the environment is an active process involving regions that are specialized for task control (Dosenbach et al., 2006). These regions deliver signals for initiating and maintaining functional networks that are appropriate in the context of current environmental stimuli and instructions. Control signals can be time locked to task onset or offset or to signal performance or error feedback. Core regions that become engaged across many different types of cognitive tasks are the dorsal anterior cingulate cortex/medial superior frontal cortex as well as the left and right anterior insula/frontal operculum. Network analysis revealed that these regions form two distinct networks, comprising frontoparietal and cinguloopercular regions, each supporting different aspects of task control (Dosenbach et al., 2007; 2008; see figure 9.6). These task-control networks have little overlap with the default mode network, which is prominently engaged during the resting state, in the absence of external task set.

Individual Differences

Brain anatomy and connectivity show significant individual variability (see chapter 4). If patterns of brain connectivity are associated with cognition, then individual variations in brain networks should also be associated with variable cognitive performance. This should be the case for disturbances of cognition observed in clinical pathology (see chapter 10), and it should also explain individual differences among healthy human subjects.

Hampson et al. (2006a) found that the strength of functional connectivity between two core regions of the default mode network, the posterior cingulate cortex and the medial prefrontal cortex, was correlated with the performance level of individual subjects in a working memory task. In a separate study, Hampson et al. (2006b) found that the strength of the functional connection between the left angular gyrus and Broca's area, both regions known to be involved in lexical processing, was correlated with reading skill in individual healthy subjects. These findings are consistent with earlier reports of disrupted functional connectivity of the angular gyrus in people with dyslexia (Horwitz et al., 1998). Seeley et al. (2007) reported that the strength of functional connectivity in specific networks extracted from resting-state fMRI time series was correlated with several independently measured behavioral and cognitive characteristics. For example, anxiety ratings provided by individual subjects before the MRI scan were found to be tightly correlated with the functional connectivity between voxels in the dorsal anterior cingulate gyrus and other brain regions. In a study that combined structural and functional imaging as well as behavioral testing, Boorman et al. (2007) demonstrated correlated individual variations in measures of structural connectivity, functional connectivity, and behavior in a task requiring subjects to select motor actions on the basis of visuomotor associations. These examples support the idea that individual variations in specific structural or functional connections are expressed in variable behavior. These structure–function relations become even more significant in light

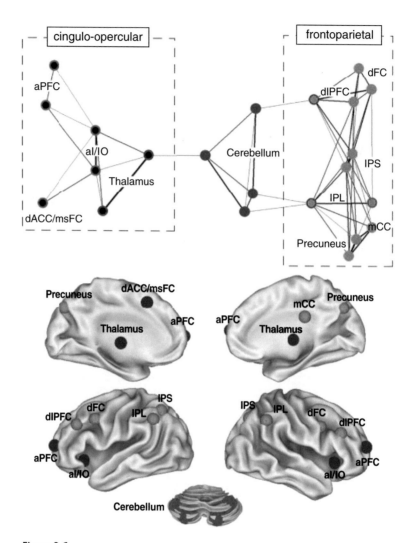

Figure 9.6
Distinct task-control networks, identified as modules in functional connectivity. The graph at the top shows resting-state functional connections between a total of 22 brain regions. Line thickness indicates the strength of each functional connection, and the graph layout was derived from a spring embedding algorithm. Two distinct and largely segregated networks are shown, the cingulo-opercular and the frontoparietal network, each engaged in different aspects of task performance. aPFC, anterior prefrontal cortex; aI/fO, anterior insula/frontal operculum; dACC/msFC, dorsal anterior cingulate cortex/medial superior frontal cortex; dFC, dorsal frontal cortex; dlPFC, dorsolateral prefrontal cortex; IPL, inferior parietal lobule; IPS, intraparietal sulcus; mCC, middle cingulate cortex. Modified and reproduced from Dosenbach et al. (2008), with permission.

of emerging evidence that many facets of brain connectivity are under tight genetic control (Glahn et al., 2010).

Methods for measuring "general intelligence" have had a long and controversial history in the behavioral sciences. Attempts to link simple indices such as the intelligence quotient (IQ) to human genetic or social factors have led to prolonged and often contentious debate. In parallel to the ongoing controversy about the value and interpretation of measures of general intelligence, cognitive neuroscience has recently begun to draw relationships between structural and functional brain measures and individual differences in the level of cognitive performance. Functional neuroimaging studies have suggested a link between intelligence and the way specific "higher" brain regions become functionally engaged (Duncan et al., 2000), brain volume and regional gray matter/white matter distribution (Haier et al., 2004), and the strength of resting-state functional connectivity of a subset of frontal and parietal regions (Song et al., 2008).

The global organization of structural and functional brain networks has also been linked to individual differences in cognitive performance (Bassett et al., 2009) and intelligence. Li et al. (2009) extracted whole-brain structural networks from 79 individual subjects using DTI and computational tractography. These subjects also received scores on a Chinese version of the Wechsler Adult Intelligence Scale, a standard and widely used test for general intelligence. Their intelligence scores were compared against several network measures, for example, the network's path length and global efficiency. Li et al. (2009) reported significant negative correlations between path length and IQ and positive correlations between IQ and global efficiency. These results suggest that more efficient parallel information flow is associated with higher levels of general intelligence.

Support for this idea also comes from analyses of functional brain networks derived from single voxel resting-state fMRI time series (van den Heuvel, 2009b; see figure 9.7). IQ scores showed no significant correlation with either the total number of functional connections or the functional network's clustering coefficient. Significant negative correlations were found for the network's path length, indicating that an increased capacity of the network to efficiently integrate information may promote higher levels of cognitive performance. A regional analysis identified several cortical regions that showed particularly strong negative correlations between IQ and regional path length. These regions included the precuneus/posterior cingulate cortex, the medial prefrontal

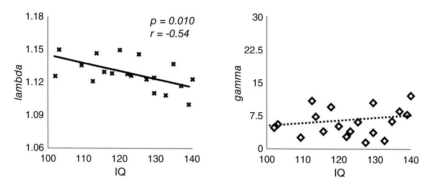

Figure 9.7
Individual variations in small-world properties and general intelligence. Across 18 subjects, the normalized characteristic path length ("lambda") was found to be negatively correlated with the intelligence quotient ("IQ") while the normalized clustering coefficient ("gamma") showed no significant correlation. Reproduced from van den Heuvel et al. (2009b) with permission.

gyrus, and the lateral inferior parietal cortex, all core regions of the default mode network and hub regions in human functional brain networks (see chapter 8). This regional specificity suggests that hub regions are particularly important in promoting efficient information flow and enabling high intellectual performance.

Brain structure is partly determined by genetic influences, and some structural characteristics of cortical gray matter are known to be correlated with general intelligence (Thompson et al., 2001). Connectional anatomy appears to be under strong genetic control, and common genetic factors may affect intelligence as well as white matter integrity in specific central pathways (Chiang et al., 2009). Consistent with genetic influences on structural connectivity, Smit et al. (2008) reported that the small-world organization of functional brain networks is more highly correlated for monozygotic twins than for dizygotic twins. Genetic factors shaping brain connectivity are important not only for uncovering structural bases of normal individual variability in cognitive performance but also as markers for clinical conditions such as schizophrenia or autism (see chapter 10).

In addition to genetic factors, differences in developmental and experiential histories contribute to intersubject variability in neural responses and behavioral performance. Most neuroimaging studies focus on task-evoked effects that are common to all (or most) individuals within a cohort of subjects, and "idiosyncratic activations" are generally treated as random errors, or as inconsistent and therefore nonessential manifestations of the neural response. However, individual differences in cognitive activations or covariance patterns may also reflect real differences in neurocognitive substrates—the same mental process may be carried out with different combinations of structural elements, an example of degeneracy (Tononi et al., 1999; Price and Friston, 2002). Individual differences in brain function will likely receive increased attention as more structural and functional brain mapping, genetic, and behavioral data from single subjects are collected.

Modeling Neurocognitive Networks

The sheer volume and complexity of brain imaging data demand the use of computational and modeling approaches to test hypotheses about the nature and neural origin of observed patterns of brain dynamics (Horwitz and Sporns, 1994; Horwitz et al., 1999; Horwitz et al., 2000; Friston, 2004). At least two different types of approaches to modeling large-scale human brain data sets can be distinguished. One approach attempts to create large computational models that allow the user to explain and predict empirical neural response patterns. Another approach is to use modeling techniques to infer causes of observed neural responses and thus test specific hypotheses about their neural origin. Both approaches have made significant contributions to our understanding of neurocognitive networks.

The construction of large-scale models constrained by anatomy and physiology mainly aims at capturing empirically observed neural activations and time series. This "large-scale neural modeling" allows the simulation of neural responses at multiple time scales and across multiple levels of spatial resolution. These types of models typically involve the simulation of several interconnected brain regions, and their elementary neural units may be spiking neurons or larger neural populations (neural fields or masses). Models can be stimulated in ways that replicate experimental conditions or tasks, or their spontaneous activity can be sampled and analyzed (see chapter 8). Their neural time series can be fully recorded and analyzed, and the modeling environment allows for manipulations such as lesions, anatomical rewiring, or changes to local biophysical properties of neurons and connections that would be difficult if not impossible to carry out empirically. Large-scale neural models can even be interfaced with robotic hardware to simulate the interactions between neural states, environment, and behavior (see chapter 14).

Among the earliest examples of large-scale neural modeling were simulations of rhythmic activity in hippocampal networks (Traub et al., 1989) and of visual circuits involved in binding and figure–ground segregation (Sporns et al., 1989; 1991; Tononi et al., 1992). As discussed earlier in this chapter, these models incorporated some key patterns of connectivity within and between visual cortical regions and investigated the role of these anatomical connections in creating patterns of temporal correlations seen in empirical recordings. These models demonstrated the important role of structural connectivity between cell populations for shaping stimulus-dependent synchrony.[11] Barry Horwitz and colleagues designed a large-scale model of multiple segregated regions of the visual and prefrontal cortex to simulate neural interactions that underlie working memory in a delayed match-to-sample task (Tagamets and Horwitz, 1998). The connectivity of the model was based on anatomical and physiological data and showed neural responses that were similar to those found in neurophysiological recordings. Furthermore, simulated PET signals computed from the model's neural time series showed regional and temporal patterns that were consistent with those obtained in human neuroimaging experiments. One of the challenges for large-scale modeling is the design of models that show realistic behavior across several tasks and task domains. Addressing this challenge, Horwitz and colleagues extended their previous model to the domains of recognition and working memory in the auditory modality (Husain et al., 2004) and to investigation of the role of anatomical connectivity in functional connectivity as measured by fMRI (Horwitz et al., 2005). Numerous other examples of large-scale neural modeling have been proposed, several of which have studied the role of structural brain networks in shaping endogenous modes of functional connectivity (see chapter 8).[12]

A different approach to neural modeling aims at inferring neural causes for observed regularities in physiological responses. The goal is to use objective quantitative tools to select neural models that best explain observed neural patterns as measured in neuroimaging or electrophysiological recordings. The result is a model of effective connectivity that describes a causal (or directed) network of interactions between neural regions or populations. Models of effective connectivity are often preferable to functional connectivity. Functional connectivity, while usually quite straightforward to record, only captures deviations from statistical independence among neural nodes; it cannot reveal causal influences of one region over another (see chapter 3). DCM uses an explicit model of regional neural dynamics as well as a model for transforming neural responses to BOLD signals to capture changes in regional activation and interregional coupling in response to stimulus or task demand (Friston et al., 2003; Penny et al., 2004). Parameters of the model are estimated from empirically obtained BOLD data, and multiple structural models can be compared using an objective model selection procedure that balances model fit and model complexity. Since its original formulation, DCM has been applied in a great variety of experimental contexts, and the modeling framework has been extended to deal with nonlinear interactions that might result, for example, from modulatory influences (Stephan et al., 2008).

As this extremely brief overview shows, computational models of neurocognitive networks differ in their implementation and design, but they have a common goal of revealing neural processes in complex brain networks responding to changing environmental and task demands. Each modeling approach faces significant challenges. For example, even the most comprehensive "synthetic" large-scale neural models inevitably contain only a fraction of the details present in a complete nervous system or organism. Their design thus requires careful selection of relevant anatomical and physiological parameters. In fact, models that replicate the structure and dynamics of every neuron and synapse in a complex nervous system, if feasible at all, may well turn out to be as incomprehensible and unmanageable as the real brain. Modeling necessarily involves a reduction of the complexity of the real system to reveal principles of organization.[13] Important constraints for such reduced models will likely be provided by data-driven models of causal neural dynamics.

Cognition: Pattern Formation in Networks

Several themes have emerged in this brief discussion of the network basis of cognition. First, cognition has an anatomical substrate. All cognitive processes occur within anatomical networks, and the topology of these networks imposes powerful constraints on cognitive architectures. The small-world attributes of large-scale structural and functional networks, as well as their hierarchical and modular arrangement, naturally promote functional segregation and integration across the brain. Much of cognitive processing can be characterized in terms of dynamic integration of distributed (segregated) resources. Second, integration involves dynamic coordination (synchrony, coherence, linear and nonlinear coupling) as well as convergence. Recurrent connectivity enables system-wide patterns of functional connectivity, while highly central network nodes play specialized roles in coordinating information flow. These hub nodes are invoked in the context of association, transmodal processing, or dynamic convergence. Third, stimuli and cognitive tasks act as perturbations of existing network dynamics. Patterns of functional connectivity due to spontaneous neural activity are reconfigured in response to changes in sensory input or environmental demands.

Viewed from a network perspective, cognition is nothing more (and nothing less) than a special kind of pattern formation, the interplay of functional segregation and integration and the continual emergence of dynamic structures that are molded by connectivity and subtly modified by external input and internal state. The shape of cognition, the nature of the information that can be brought together and transformed, is determined by the architecture of brain networks. The flow of cognition is a result of transient and multiscale neural dynamics, of sequences of dynamic events that unfold across time. The variety of cognition, the seemingly endless diversity of mental states and subjective experiences, reflects the diversity and differentiation made possible by the complexity of the brain.

The network perspective differs radically from serial, representational, and symbolic accounts of cognition. Perhaps network thinking will eventually allow us to move beyond neural reductionism and cognitive functionalism and formulate a theoretical framework for cognition that is firmly grounded in the biology of the brain.

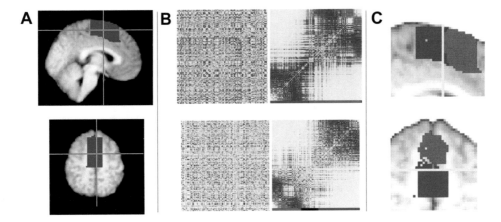

Plate 1 (figure 4.3)

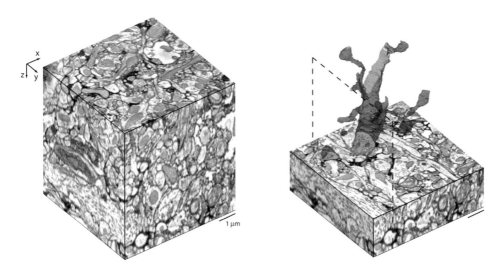

Plate 2 (figure 5.2)

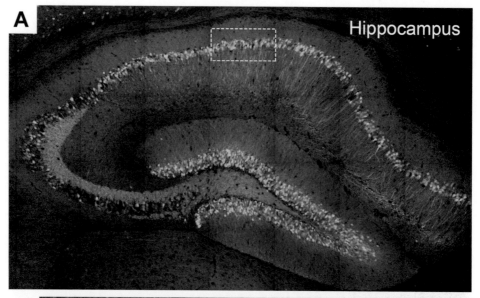

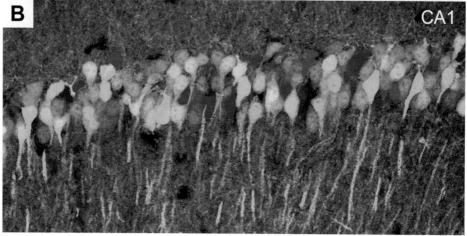

Plate 3 (figure 5.4)

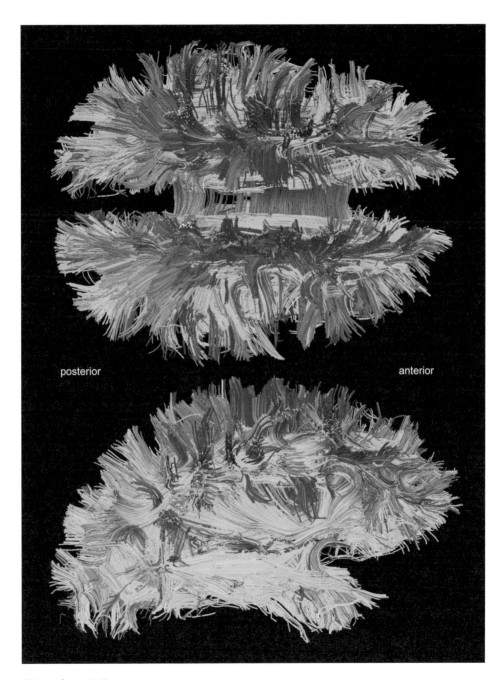

posterior

anterior

Plate 4 (figure 5.7)

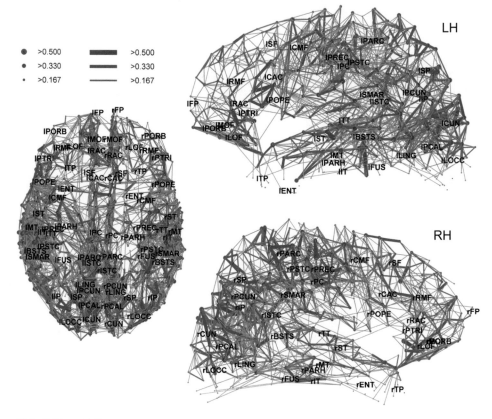

Plate 5 (figure 5.9)

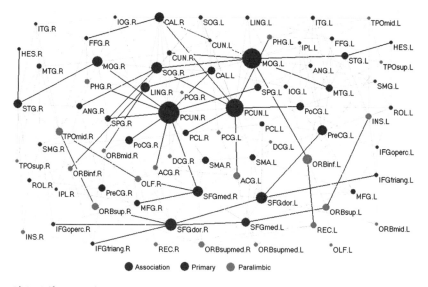

Plate 6 (figure 6.9)

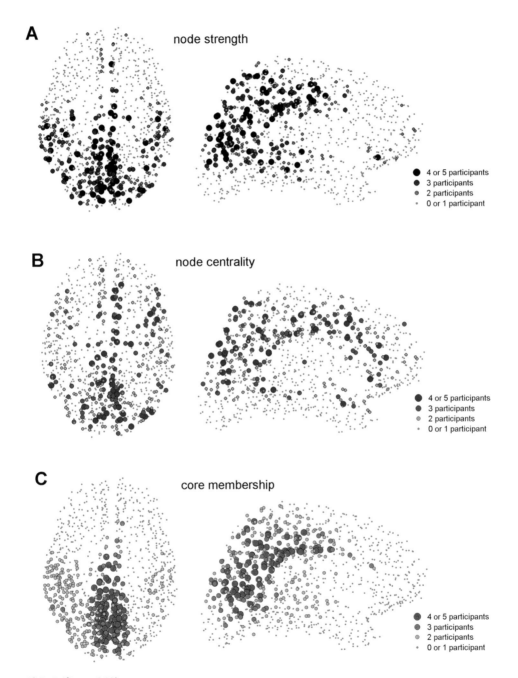

A   node strength

● 4 or 5 participants
● 3 participants
● 2 participants
· 0 or 1 participant

B   node centrality

● 4 or 5 participants
● 3 participants
● 2 participants
· 0 or 1 participant

C   core membership

● 4 or 5 participants
● 3 participants
● 2 participants
· 0 or 1 participant

Plate 7 (figure 6.10)

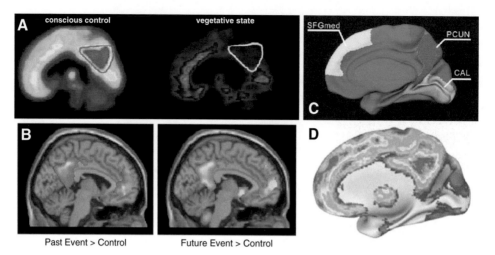

Plate 8 (figure 6.11)

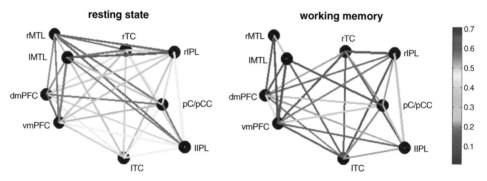

Plate 9 (figure 8.4)

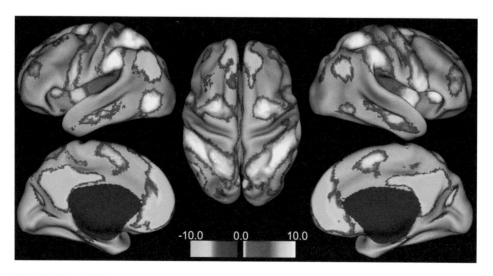

Plate 10 (figure 8.5)

structural connectivity

functional connectivity

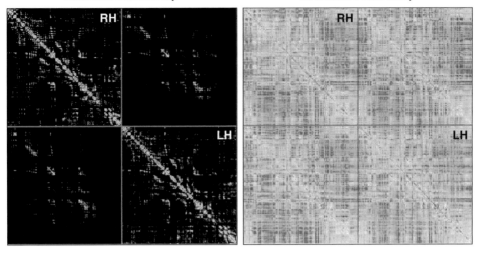

Plate 11 (figure 8.6)

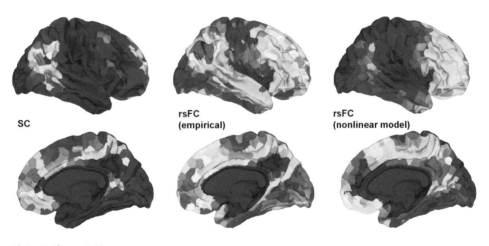

SC

rsFC
(empirical)

rsFC
(nonlinear model)

Plate 12 (figure 8.8)

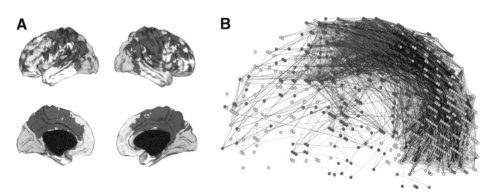

Plate 13 (figure 9.4)

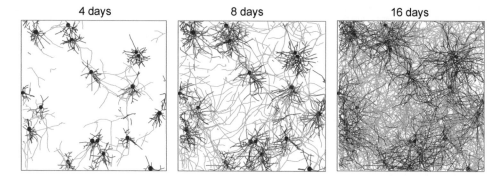

4 days   8 days   16 days

Plate 14 (figure 11.3)

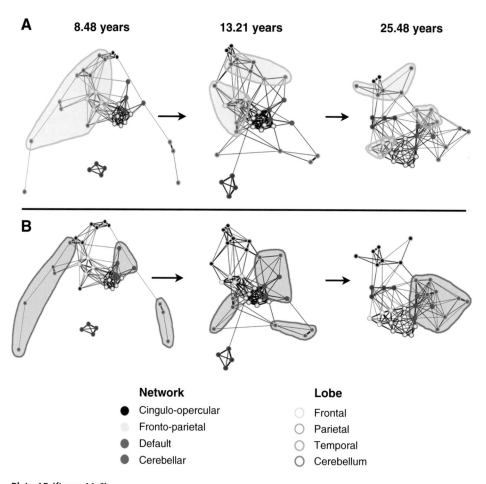

A   8.48 years   13.21 years   25.48 years

B

Network
- Cingulo-opercular
- Fronto-parietal
- Default
- Cerebellar

Lobe
- Frontal
- Parietal
- Temporal
- Cerebellum

Plate 15 (figure 11.6)

There is [...] nothing surprising in considering the functional mental disorders as fundamentally diseases of memory, of the circulating information kept by the brain in the active state, and of the long-time permeability of synapses. Even the grosser disorders such as paresis may produce a large part of their effects not so much by the destruction of tissue which they involve and the alteration of synaptic thresholds as by the secondary disturbances of traffic—the overload of what remains of the nervous system and the re-routing of messages—which must follow such primary injuries.[1]
—Norbert Wiener, 1948

Norbert Wiener's 1948 volume *Cybernetics* laid the foundation for a new scientific discipline, "the entire field of control and communication theory, whether in the machine or in the animal" (Wiener, 1948, p. 11). Among the far-ranging subjects touched upon in this slim volume, Wiener discusses the causes of mental illnesses such as schizophrenia, depression, and paranoia (which he terms "functional mental disorders") in a chapter entitled "Cybernetics and Psychopathology."[2] Rather than attributing mental illnesses to the loss of specific anatomical substrates, Wiener saw these illnesses as disorders of "circulating information," a notion that is consonant with more recent ideas of recurrent dynamics and functional integration in the brain. In Wiener's terminology, circulating information is a form of online memory, contained in impulses that travel along circular paths within the nervous system and maintain a record of past events. In the human brain, these circular paths are traced by long "neuronic chains" that can become overloaded, to the point of mental breakdown, "either by an excess in the amount of traffic to be carried, by the physical removal of channels for the carrying of traffic, or by the excessive occupation of such channels by undesirable systems of traffic" (Wiener, 1948, p. 151). This cybernetic view of mental disorders traces the causes of mental disturbances to disruptions of information flow and system dynamics. In this chapter I will advance the view that network disturbances and the disruptions in the dynamics of "circulating information" they entail may indeed underlie the deficits of cognition and behavior in neurological and psychiatric disorders.

When networks fail, bad things happen. We directly experience the negative outcomes of an overstressed or malfunctioning network when we navigate through clogged hubs of the air transportation system during peak travel times, lose electricity in a cascading failure of the power grid, or witness the destruction of great wealth in a near-collapse of the world's financial system.[3] Network failures like these are common occurrences in complex interconnected systems. By quantitatively characterizing complex networks, we aim to gain insights into the robustness or vulnerability of the corresponding complex systems. The hope is that these insights will allow us to avoid, or at least anticipate, catastrophic failure.[4] Graph theory predicts that different network architectures present different patterns of vulnerability. For example, network studies on the topology of the Internet revealed a scale-free organization that is highly resilient against the removal of randomly selected nodes but vulnerable to attacks that target a few, highly connected network hubs (Barabási and Albert, 1999; Albert et al., 2000). Deletion of hub nodes can result in the disintegration of the network by seriously disrupting the flow of information.

In molecular systems biology, researchers are beginning to establish links between patterns of failure in biological networks (e.g., protein–protein interaction networks or genetic regulatory networks), on the one hand, and neurodegenerative disorders (Goehler et al., 2004; see figure 10.1) and various forms of cancer (Ergün et al., 2007; Altieri, 2008) on the other hand. For example, the widely expressed cellular protein p53 acts as a tumor suppressor by shutting down the replication of stressed or damaged cells. The inactivation or mutation of p53 is known to increase the risk of cell malignancy. Remarkably, the p53 protein is also one of the most highly connected proteins in the cell, with a very large number of known activating signals, binding partners, and downstream regulators (Vogelstein et al., 2000). In other words, p53 may be thought of as a highly central hub in a molecular interaction network. The deletion of hub proteins is more disruptive than the deletion of peripheral proteins (Jeong et al., 2001). The topological embedding of proteins may thus be at least partly predictive of the functional impact of their inactivation, deletion, or mutation.[5] These considerations have, in some cases, led to clinical applications: for example, protein subnetworks extracted from

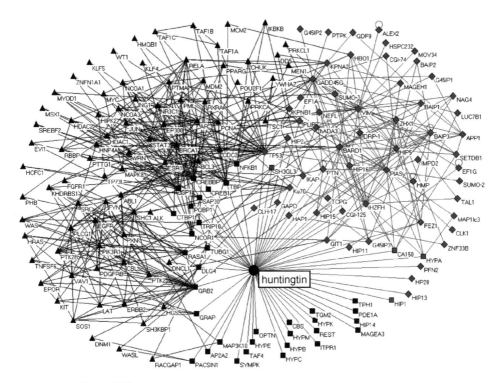

Figure 10.1
A protein network involved in a brain disease. The diagram shows the protein interaction network of huntingtin, a major molecular component involved in the neurodegenerative disorder Huntington's disease. Symbols (triangles, squares, diamonds) refer to interactions compiled from different studies and databases. Modified and reproduced from Goehler et al. (2004) with permission.

proteomics databases are more reliable and more accurate markers of metastatic tumors, compared to individual proteins (Chuang et al., 2007). The quantitative analysis of failure modes in biological networks may thus become an important ingredient in the molecular characterization, diagnosis, and treatment of a broad range of human diseases (Ideker and Sharan, 2008; Auffray et al., 2009), including numerous forms of cancer.[6]

Compared to the explosive growth of network analysis methods in systems biomedicine, the application of network approaches to brain disease or brain injury is still in its infancy. In this chapter, I will argue that complex network approaches can contribute to a deeper understanding and more effective treatment of acute brain injury and degenerative disease. Many forms of brain dysfunction can be conceptualized as a network disease, an impairment of the normal functionality of brain networks. In many cases, brain injury or disease involves the irreversible loss of neuronal elements (cells and their axonal connections, nodes and edges)—for example, through acute events such as traumatic brain injury and stroke or through gradual processes such as neurodegeneration or abnormal neurodevelopment. Disturbances of connectivity are not limited to the loss of specific nodes and edges but also involve significant "nonlocal effects" as expressed, for instance, in changes of global network parameters. As is the case in other complex systems, networks of the brain display characteristic patterns of robustness and vulnerability. These patterns will be discussed in the context of focal brain lesions, neurodegenerative diseases such as AD, mental disorders such as schizophrenia, and some neurodevelopmental disorders, including autism. Each of these conditions involves specific patterns of network failure that can be quantitatively characterized with the tools of network science.

Origins of Biological Robustness

Most engineered technological systems currently in existence do not rely on network mechanisms to ensure their functional robustness or protect them against failure. Instead, they rely on redundancy, the duplication and segregation of critical components. For example, the electrical flight control ("fly-by-wire") systems of a modern passenger jet are essential for the positioning of its flight control surfaces and thus for flight path stability and modification. Computers, actuators, and hydraulic controls in these systems are redundant to ensure system survivability.

In contrast to engineered systems, biological systems rely on network mechanisms for robustness to extrinsic and intrinsic perturbations (Kitano, 2004). One way to visualize robustness is to imagine a system in a stable state (an attractor) perturbed by a stochastic input or an internal fluctuation (see figure 10.2). A robust system will return to its original attractor or, if the perturbation is sufficiently large, transition to a new attractor. Network mechanisms may make the system more robust by limiting the effects of potentially disruptive perturbations and by preserving the attractor in the face of structural damage. Of the many mechanisms that support robustness in biological systems, the mechanisms of modularity and degeneracy are particularly relevant in a neural context.

Modularity limits the spread of, and helps to contain, the potentially disruptive effects of noisy perturbations. Structural and functional modules are key architectural ingredients in networks of highly evolved

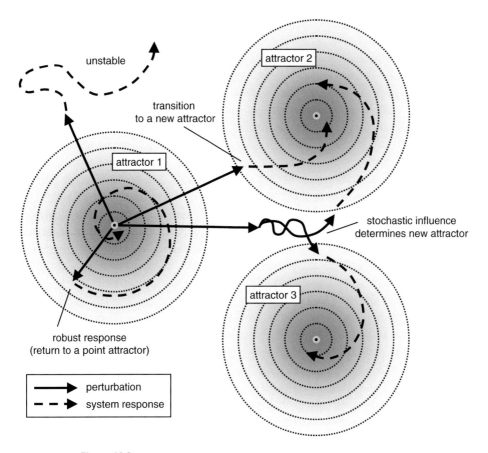

Figure 10.2
Dynamic effects of perturbations and robustness. This schematic diagram represents the state of a system as a point in (two-dimensional) state space. Three different point attractors (see chapter 2) are shown, and their basins of attraction are indicated by concentric circles. Initially, the system is at rest in the center of attractor 1. A small perturbation leaves the system within the original attractor, and it robustly returns to its previous state. Larger perturbations that place the system outside of its original basin of attraction can result in a transition to a new attractor or in an unstable response pattern. Transitions between attractors can be subject to stochastic influences. Modified and redrawn after Kitano (2004).

nervous systems (see chapter 6). Modules are also ubiquitous in many other biological networks, such as networks of cellular regulatory elements or metabolic pathways. The importance of modularity in robustness extends to evolutionary and developmental processes (see chapter 7).

Degeneracy is the capacity of a system to perform an identical function with structurally different sets of elements (Tononi et al., 1999; Edelman and Gally, 2001). Thus, a degenerate system can deliver constant performance or output even when some of its structural elements are altered, compromised, or disconnected. Unlike redundancy, degeneracy does not require duplication of system components. Degeneracy is ubiquitous in complex networks with sparse and recurrent structural connectivity. For example, communication patterns in such networks can occur along many alternative paths of equivalent length, a property that protects the network from becoming disconnected if nodes or edges are disrupted.

Jointly, modularity and degeneracy make brain networks functionally robust, by ensuring that the networks are stable to small structural perturbations. In addition, these concepts may underlie the remarkable capacity of the brain to withstand larger perturbations in the course of injury or disease. Clinical observations of patients suggest that individual brains have different degrees of "reserve" to counter degradations in their structural and functional networks. One theory of the concept of reserve suggests that passive reserve should be distinguished from active compensation (Stern, 2002). Passive reserve invokes an intrinsic capacity of the brain to withstand, up to an extent, the effects of structural damage. Individual brains may differ in their reserve capacity, due to differences in size or wiring pattern, with "high-reserve individuals" displaying more resilience against damage. In contrast to passive reserve, active compensation involves the capacity to engage in many different processing modes and to distribute functional networks to new locations in the brain if their structural substrates are compromised. Active compensation is closely related to the earlier discussed notion of degeneracy. Both passive reserve and active compensation are likely associated with efficient small-world network topologies and high dynamic diversity (see chapter 12). It is an intriguing hypothesis that higher variability and degeneracy may predict greater robustness to injury or disease.

Brain Injury and Brain Lesions

Lesions have been used to infer localized substrates of brain function for a long time. The descriptions of two cases of profound loss of speech production by Paul Broca in 1861 provided one of the earliest and most suggestive examples of the link between a localized region of cerebral cortex and a specific cognitive function (Broca, 1861a; 1861b; see chapter 4). Both of Broca's patients had lesions in approximately the same region of the left inferior frontal lobe, a finding that established an association between a circumscribed brain region and speech as a segregated mental faculty. The nature of brain damage in these patients was originally described as a relatively small and circumscribed surface lesion of cortex. However, a recent reexamination of the preserved brains with high-resolution MRI revealed much more widespread damage to cortical gray and white matter, including damage to more medial frontal areas and disruption of major corticocortical fiber pathways (Dronkers et al., 2007). Had the true extent of these lesions been known at the time, the interpretation of Broca's findings in terms of cortical localization might have been less compelling.[7]

Other studies of anatomical lesions and their impact on cognitive and behavioral capacities cast doubt on the idea that the functional impact of cortical lesions could solely be attributed to the lost tissue. The British neurologist Hughlings Jackson advocated a careful consideration of nonlocal effects of lesions giving rise to aphasia, writing that "destructive lesions cause loss of function of some nervous arrangements, and thereby over-function of others is permitted" (Hughlings Jackson, 1879, p. 337). Constantin von Monakow developed the concept of diaschisis to explain nonlocal effects of brain lesions. In 1914, he wrote the following:

The generally accepted theory according to which aphasia, agnosia, apraxia, etc. are due to destruction of narrowly circumscribed appropriate "praxia, gnosia, and phasia centres" must be finally discarded on the basis of more recent clinical and anatomical studies. It is just in the case of these focal symptoms that the concept of complicated dynamic disorders in the whole cortex becomes indispensable. (von Monakow, 1969, p. 35)

The precise definition of this concept turned out to be a great challenge that was not easily met given the anatomical and physiological knowledge of the time. Consequently, nonlocal concepts for "action at a distance" like diaschisis lacked a solid mechanistic foundation and could never quite dispel the uncertainty surrounding the variable and unpredictable effects of brain lesions on behavior.

The study of the anatomical substrates of aphasia, almost from its very beginnings, revealed that speech results from associative linkages between several cortical centers. Carl Wernicke and Ludwig Lichtheim developed some of the first "network models" of a higher cognitive function (see figure 10.3). Their work revealed that speech depends on the integrity of corticocortical pathways as well as on the cortical gray matter (Catani and Mesulam, 2008). Building in part on these early models of "conduction aphasia," Norman Geschwind formulated a theory of "disconnection syndromes" that attributed numerous cognitive deficits to

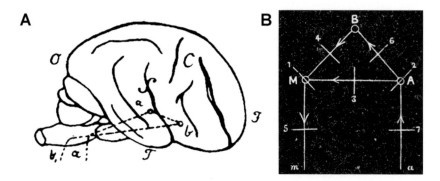

Figure 10.3
Early "network models" of speech. (A) Carl Wernicke's diagram of cortical centers involved in speech. The letter "a" designates the termination point of the acoustic nerve, "b" corresponds to the cortical region necessary for the production of sound (shown here on the right hemisphere), and association fibers link the two centers. From Wernicke (1874). (B) In Ludwig Lichtheim's diagram, areas "A," "M," and "B" corresponded to a "center for auditory images" (today called Wernicke's area), a "center for motor images" (Broca's area), and a "concept center" (*Begriffszentrum*), respectively, and lines between them are connection pathways. Lichtheim hypothesized that each lesion of an area or disconnection of a pathway was associated with a specific disruption of language or speech processing. As he pointed out, the concept center, "B," was indicated as a single spot "for simplicity's sake" and was thought in reality to involve "the combined action of the whole sensorial sphere" (Lichtheim, 1885, p. 477).

damage of association pathways, either within or between the cerebral hemispheres (Geschwind, 1965).[8] Today, the development and refinement of diffusion MRI enables the detection and mapping of such disturbances with unprecedented resolution (Catani, 2006). Modern methodologies strongly support the idea that the significance of a lesion is increasingly determined not only by the local function but also by the connectivity pattern of the lesioned brain area (Catani and Mesulam, 2008; see figure 10.4).

Cognitive and behavioral effects of brain lesions are highly variable, and their mechanistic origins, despite the efforts of von Monakow, Geschwind, and others, remain difficult to discern. Effects of lesions include damage to structural brain networks, as well as a subsequent impact on functional brain networks that extends across time. In patients, the immediate impact of the lesion is often followed by a complex time course of brain reorganization and functional recovery (Geschwind, 1985). In many cases, the remarkable plasticity of the nervous system allows for substantial long-term improvement and sometimes complete restoration of functional deficits. These recovery processes represent a major challenge to network theories of the brain as they are the result

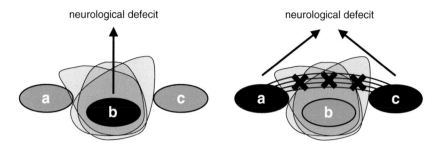

Figure 10.4
Anatomical interpretations of neurological deficits. The schematic diagram shows three brain regions (a, b, c) and three overlapping lesions (irregular shaded areas). On the left, the resulting neurological deficit is attributed to the loss of region b, which is removed by all three lesions. On the right, the disconnection of an anatomical pathway between regions a and c results in a different interpretation of the anatomical basis of the observed neurological deficit. Even more complex interpretations are possible if nonlocal dynamic consequences of lesions—for example, the disturbance of interactions of remote brain areas (not shown here)—are considered. Modified and redrawn after Catani and Mesulam (2008).

of a complex interplay of physiological and behavioral processes and possibly deploy "brain reserve" to increase network resilience. Despite these complex structural and functional substrates, lesions of specific brain regions are often associated with specific cognitive and behavioral disturbances, and lesions of some areas tend to have more widespread effects than others (Damasio and Damasio, 1989; Mesulam, 2000).

Brain lesions are perturbations of structural brain networks that have physiological effects. Some of these effects are the direct consequence of the loss of nodes and edges while other effects involve the disruption of functional interactions between nonlesioned structures. Studies of functional brain networks in patients with specific cognitive deficits support this model. For example, He et al. (2007a) examined BOLD functional connectivity in patients with spatial neglect following a stroke in the right cerebral hemisphere (see figure 10.5). Acute disruptions of functional connections within a network of brain regions involved in spatial attention outside of the primary lesion location are strongly correlated with an impairment of attentional processing. These results support a network approach to understanding complex neurological disorders such as spatial neglect and document the contributions of nonlocal lesion effects to disruptions of behavior and cognition (He et al., 2007b). Hence, explanations of lesion effects cast exclusively in terms of local information processing in the lesioned area are at best incomplete.[9]

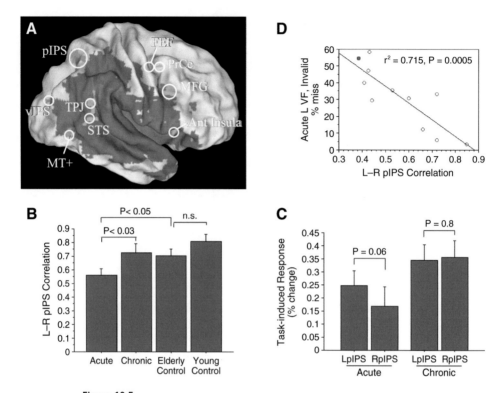

Figure 10.5
Breakdown and recovery of functional connectivity following brain lesions. All data are
from He et al. (2007a). (A) Overlay of lesion extent for a cohort of 11 patients who had
sustained damage to the cerebral cortex in the right hemisphere, including portions of the
right parietal and temporal lobe, following a stroke. All patients exhibited significant cognitive deficits including spatial neglect. (B) Functional connectivity between the left and right
intraparietal sulcus (IPS) is significantly decreased in the acute (approximately 30 days)
and chronic (approximately 40 weeks) stages of recovery. (C) Task-evoked responses of
both left and right IPS are diminished in the acute stage, and they recover as well as rebal-
ance in the chronic stage. (D) Across all 11 acute patients, the magnitude of the left–right
IPS functional connectivity is significantly correlated with task performance (the detection
of visual targets in the left visual field, which is typically impaired in spatial neglect). The
patient with the largest lesion (filled dot) has the weakest left–right IPS functional connection and is among the most strongly impaired. FEF, frontal eye field; pIPS, posterior intraparietal sulcus; vIPS, ventral intraparietal sulcus; MT+, middle temporal area; TPJ,
temporoparietal junction; STS, superior temporal sulcus; PrCe, precentral sulcus; MFG,
middle frontal gyrus. Panel (A) modified, all panels from He et al. (2007a), reproduced
with permission.

One way to gauge the possible consequences of localized brain lesions is to model the effects of deleting subsets of nodes and edges on the structure and function of the remaining brain. Several such studies have been carried out on structural networks of the mammalian cerebral cortex. The link between patterns of connections in the thalamocortical system and the behavioral effects of localized brain lesions was first explored by Young et al. (2000) with the aid of a simple computational model to illustrate nonlocal network-mediated lesion effects. The model consisted of an anatomically based coupling matrix derived from the cat thalamocortical system and neural units that represented the mean activity levels of entire brain regions. The pattern of decreased activity seen across the remaining brain after lesion of a single brain region served as an indicator of lesion impact. The model clearly demonstrated that the effects of lesions could propagate to structures that were not directly connected with the lesion itself. Furthermore, lesioning of highly connected regions resulted in larger effects on the remaining brain than lesioning of less highly connected regions. Finally, highly connected regions were affected by lesions in a more diverse set of locations. Young and colleagues argued that conventional means by which functions of brain regions are inferred from structural lesions have to be revised in light of more precise formulations of the meaning of function within the cortical network. A more formal framework, "functional contribution analysis," was suggested by Aharonov et al. (2003) for assessing functional contributions of brain areas or, indeed, any node in a biological network. Functional contribution analysis attempts to attribute function from observed effects of multiple lesions, thus circumventing the limitations of the single lesion paradigm.

Kaiser and Hilgetag (2004c) investigated the vulnerability of cortical networks of cat and macaque monkey, as well as a number of other biological and technological networks, by performing single edge deletions on the structural connectivity and calculating the resulting network-wide effects on the remaining graph. For example, the deletion of an edge lengthens communication paths and may even disconnect the network entirely. The lengthening of communication paths can be summarized by comparing the network's path length before and after the lesion. Kaiser and Hilgetag found that given the clustered, modular architecture of the mammalian cortex, loss of intercluster edges caused more severe disruptions while loss of intracluster edges had much less of an effect. Thus, the modular small-world architecture of the mammalian cortex showed a vulnerability pattern similar to that of a scale-free network such as the World Wide Web, with relative resilience to lesions of intracluster edges and relative vulnerability to lesions of intercluster edges, which are comparatively few in number. A subsequent study (Kaiser et al., 2007b) of node lesions in cat and macaque cortex confirmed that the pattern of structural damage of brain networks resembles that of scale-free networks, likely as a result of their modular architecture. A vulnerability analysis carried out by Achard et al. (2006) also indicated significant resilience or resistance to damaging network-wide effects in a large-scale human functional brain network. Sequential deletion of randomly selected nodes had little effect on network integrity, while targeted deletion of high-degree nodes had greater impact, though not as great as that seen in comparable scale-free networks.

A model of lesion effects on the macaque cortex attempted to establish relationships between structural centrality and functional impact, through simulated neural activity (Honey and Sporns, 2008). Neural dynamics were simulated using a neural mass model which engages in transient and metastable patterns of interregional phase locking and information flow (Breakspear et al., 2003; see chapter 8). The model demonstrated that lesions of highly connected and highly central hub nodes produced the largest nonlocal lesion effects and that the extent of these lesion effects was largely determined by the modularity or community structure of the network. Lesions of connector hubs (see chapter 2) had the largest effects on functional connectivity and information flow as measured by patterns of interregional transfer entropy. Connector hubs had effects that extended beyond their immediate neighborhood and affected regions to which they were not directly connected. In contrast, lesions of provincial hubs (hubs whose central role was limited to a single module) had effects on other regions within the module, but not beyond. Lesions of peripheral nodes had little effect on information flow elsewhere in the network.

The neural mass model in the above study was extended to the human cortex, first in an analysis of spontaneous ("resting-state") functional connectivity (Honey et al., 2009) and then to a model that probed for the functional impact of structural lesions (Alstott et al., 2009). The structural connectivity matrix was derived from diffusion MRI data sets discussed previously (see chapters 5, 6, and 8; Hagmann et al., 2008) and comprised 998 ROIs covering the entire cortical surface on both hemispheres. This structural connection matrix was lesioned in two ways. The first method involved sequential deletion of single nodes, which were selected randomly or on the basis of high degree or centrality. The structural effect of the lesion on the remaining network was assessed using procedures analogous to those of other network vulnerability studies (e.g., Barabási and Albert, 1999; Achard et al., 2006). The second method involved the placement of localized lesions around selected central locations defined by a standard brain coordinate. Around this central point, a fixed number of nodes (ROIs) and their attached edges were removed from the structural matrix, and the spontaneous dynamics of the remaining brain were recorded and compared to the dynamic pattern of the intact brain (see figure 10.6). The functional impact of localized lesions

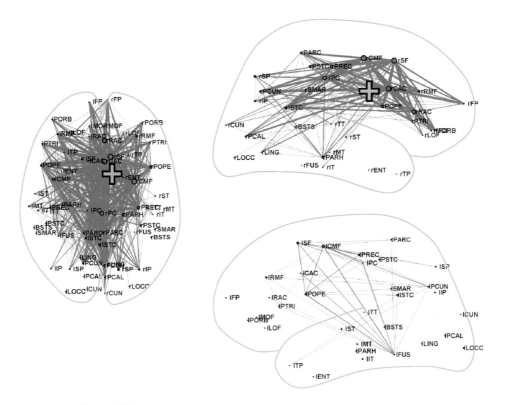

Figure 10.6
Dynamic consequences of lesions in a model of the human brain. Lesions were centered approximately at the location of the cross, comprising about five percent of the cortical surface around the right hemisphere anterior cingulate cortex. Functional connections across the brain that were significantly changed (increased or decreased) are shown in a dorsal view of the brain (plot on the left) as well as within the left and right hemispheres. Note that the lesion, while limited to only one hemisphere, results in disruptions of functional connectivity in both ipsilateral and contralateral hemispheres, including disruptions of functional connectivity between remote region pairs. For abbreviations, see figure 5.8. Modified from Alstott et al. (2009).

was then quantified by determining the difference between the spontaneous functional connectivity of the intact and lesioned brain. Sequential node deletion revealed that the human brain structural network was resilient to random node deletions and deletion of high-degree nodes, but much less resilient to deletion of high-centrality nodes. Localized lesion analysis showed that the centrality of the removed nodes was highly predictive of the functional impact of the lesion. Among the most disruptive were lesions of structures along the cortical midline, including the anterior and posterior cingulate cortex, as well as those in the vicinity of the temporoparietal junction. Lesions of areas in primary sensory and motor cortex had relatively little impact on patterns of functional connectivity.

The general picture that emerges from these computational models is that the functional impact of lesions can be partially predicted from their structural embedding in the intact brain. Lesion of highly central parts of the network (network hubs) produces larger and more widely distributed dynamic effects. Furthermore, lesions of some particularly disruptive areas in our model are known to produce profound disturbances of behavior, cognition, and consciousness in vivo. Models such as these must be further refined to include lesions of white matter pathways and neuroplasticity-mediated recovery. Since these models cannot currently be tested for specific behavioral or cognitive deficits, the assessment of lesion impact is based on the assumption that spontaneous network activity is a diagnostic marker of global dynamic differences. This idea has to be further explored and validated in empirical studies of brain injury and damage. Nonetheless, all these models reveal distributed structural and dynamical effects of localized structural lesions.

Network Damage in Alzheimer's Disease

Alzheimer's disease (AD) is the most common neurodegenerative disorder, affecting millions of people worldwide. Clinical symptoms include progressive dementia, confusion, irritability, and memory loss. The characteristic neuropathology of AD, first described by Alois Alzheimer (1906), entails progressive neuronal degeneration and neuronal death due to aggregations of intra- and extracellular protein and deposits of neuritic plaques and neurofibrillary tangles. Despite the fact that plaques and tangles are formed by distinct and well-characterized proteins (amyloid and tau, respectively), the molecular mechanisms causing AD are still only incompletely understood. The time course and spatial distribution of amyloid and tau deposition suggest that the progression of AD shows some regional specificity. In early stages of AD, atrophy of neuronal structures is first seen in the medial temporal lobe, a region of the brain known to be important for memory formation.

AD results in disruptions of structural and functional connectivity and has thus been described as an example of a cortical disconnection syndrome (Delbeuck et al., 2003). Reduced activity and hypometabolism in the posterior cingulate cortex are among the most consistently observed findings in brains of patients at early stages of AD (Minoshima et al., 1997). More recent studies of functional connectivity have shown that AD not only compromises the metabolic activity of specific brain structures but also disrupts the global pattern of cortical functional interactions. PET imaging in patients with AD suggests that AD involves a functional disconnection between the prefrontal cortex and the hippocampus (Grady et al., 2001). A resting-state fMRI study confirmed that patients with AD show decreased activity in the posterior cingulate and the hippocampus compared to healthy controls (Greicius et al., 2004). These results also suggest that AD compromises the connectivity between these regions and that the integrity of the default mode network may provide a biomarker for the onset of the disease. Sorg et al. (2007) confirmed the loss of functional connectivity between components of the default mode network and the hippocampus in patients with mild cognitive impairment that were at high risk for developing AD. Wang et al. (2007) found significantly reduced functional connectivity in resting-state fMRI between frontal and parietal regions, as well as a disorganization of functional relationships of individual areas such as the posterior cingulate cortex, in AD patients.

The first characterization of functional brain networks in a clinical population demonstrated disease-related differences in EEG data recorded in the beta frequency band (15–35 Hz) from a set of 15 patients with AD and from 13 control subjects (Stam et al., 2007). Functional networks were computed using synchronization likelihood, a measure of statistical dependence that is sensitive to linear and nonlinear coupling. Significant differences between subject groups were seen in the characteristic path length, but not in the clustering coefficient. Functional networks of AD patients had longer path lengths, indicating a less efficient organization of the connectivity. Test scores from the Mini Mental State Examination, a standard test for assessing a person's level of cognitive function, were negatively correlated with path length, thus demonstrating a link between a graph measure obtained from a whole-brain functional network and a clinical measure of cognitive performance.

More recently, a resting-state fMRI study examined the large-scale organization of functional brain connectivity in a cohort of 21 patients with AD and a group of 18 age-matched control subjects (Supekar et al., 2008). Wavelet analysis of fMRI time series allowed the estimation of frequency-dependent functional connectivity across 90 nodes covering cortical and subcortical regions. Functional networks in patients with AD showed significantly reduced global clustering as well as regional differences in clustering—for example, in the case of the hippocampus. There was no difference in global efficiency between the two groups. The global clustering measure was able to discriminate patients with AD from age-matched healthy control subjects with high specificity and sensitivity, which potentially makes it a useful diagnostic marker. Both studies of functional networks in AD (Stam et al., 2007; Supekar et al., 2008) demonstrated a disruption of small-world measures in AD, although one study found significant differences in path length, while the other reported differences in clustering. These discrepancies may be due to methodological differences (EEG vs. fMRI), differences in spatial resolution, or different sensitivities in the measure of functional connectivity (Supekar et al., 2008).

MEG recordings from groups of AD patients and control subjects confirmed the disruption of small-world attributes in functional networks computed from the phase lag index, a measure of synchrony which is relatively insensitive to volume-conduction effects (Stam et al., 2009). The mean value of synchrony was found to be significantly decreased in patients with AD. In the lower alpha frequency band (8–10 Hz), AD functional networks exhibited a combination of lower clustering and shorter path length, interpreted as increased randomization of the diseased network. Modeling of disease effects suggested that this change was largely due to loss of connectivity at high-degree network hubs rather than being due to more diffuse loss of connectivity throughout the brain.

Buckner et al. (2005) noted that neuropathology, atrophy, and metabolism all display similar profiles on the cortical surface in patients with AD. Key regions of the default mode network showed high levels of amyloid deposition in these patients, and, more recently, high levels of amyloid were also found to be associated with reduced functional connectivity among default mode regions in clinically normal older adults

(Hedden et al., 2009; see figure 10.7). This suggests the idea that neural activity within the default mode network may provide regional conditions conducive to amyloid deposition. Particularly vulnerable to atrophy and amyloid deposition are regions of the brain that were identified as highly central in structural network studies (e.g., Hagmann et al., 2008), for example, the precuneus, posterior cingulate, and retrosplenial cortex. Buckner et al. (2009) have extended their studies to examine functional networks obtained during resting-state fMRI for highly connected and highly central hubs and explore the relationship of these hubs to locations of high amyloid deposition in AD. Cortical hubs and amyloid deposition were found to be highly correlated, suggesting that hub regions are particularly vulnerable to AD, possibly because of their high rates of baseline metabolic activity (see chapter 8; see also figure 6.11). Buckner et al. (2009) emphasized that cortical hubs in functional networks appear to be stable features of functional anatomy as they are found to be present during the brain's resting state as well as during goal-oriented

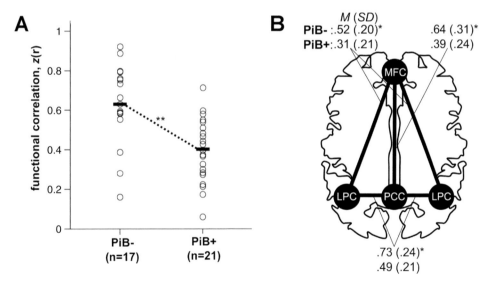

Figure 10.7
Altered functional connectivity and amyloid deposition. Amyloid protein deposits can be quantified with positron emission tomography imaging of a labeled compound (PiB) that binds to fibrillar amyloid. (A) Brains of clinically normal older adults are divided into two classes, those with (PiB+) and without (PiB–) substantial amyloid burden. There is a significant group difference in functional connectivity within the default mode network. (B) Significantly reduced functional correlations among default regions (MFC, medial frontal cortex; LPC, lateral parietal cortex; PCC, posterior cingulate cortex) in PiB+ brains. Reproduced from Hedden et al. (2009) with permission.

activity. Thus, their disruption would have effects on both resting and task-evoked neural processing.

Seeley et al. (2009) presented evidence suggesting that several neurodegenerative diseases, including AD, target different large-scale brain networks. Thus, the hypothesis that degenerative brain disease involves the disruption of structural and functional connectivity may not be limited to AD but may include a number of dementia syndromes distinguished by specific clinical profiles. Causes for the selective vulnerability of different large-scale brain networks remain to be determined (Mesulam, 2009).

In summary, there is convergent evidence that neurodegenerative diseases such as AD manifest as a disturbance of functional, and thus presumably structural, cortical networks. This disturbance may potentially be assessed by estimating small-world attributes—such attributes have the potential to become a sensitive diagnostic tool. There is an intriguing correlation between the location of network hubs and the progression of at least one neuropathological component of the disease, the deposition of amyloid protein. The devastating consequences of AD may thus result from a "targeted attack" on cortical hubs by a disease process unfolding at the cellular and molecular level.[10]

Schizophrenia—A Disconnection Syndrome?

The term "schizophrenia," or "split mind," was coined in 1908 by the Swiss psychiatrist Eugen Bleuler (Bleuler, 1908) to name a psychiatric disorder whose most characteristic sign is the disintegration of psychological functions resulting in the loss of unity of mind and consciousness. "Of the thousands of associative threads which guide our thinking, this disease seems to interrupt, quite haphazardly, sometimes such single threads, sometimes a whole group, and sometimes even large segments of them. In this way, thinking becomes illogical and often bizarre" (Bleuler, 1950, p. 13). Despite a century of research, the biological cause or causes of schizophrenia have remained obscure. Genetic and environmental factors contribute to the disease, and its many behavioral and cognitive symptoms are associated with numerous pathological changes in the structure and function of the nervous system. Even a cursory review of the causes of schizophrenia is beyond the scope of this chapter, given the complexity of the disease and its variable manifestations.

Disrupted patterns of large-scale structural and functional connectivity of the brain may illuminate the origin of the various cognitive and behavioral symptoms of schizophrenia. PET studies of interactions between cortical and subcortical regions of the brain revealed abnormalities in the degree and pattern of functional coupling in patients with schizophrenia compared to healthy controls (Volkow et al., 1988). A number of more recent studies using EEG, PET, or fMRI (Calhoun et al., 2009) data sets have provided additional evidence of disruptions in functional and effective connectivity, involving both increased and decreased coupling and likely reflecting a mixture of directly disease-related and compensatory effects. Abnormal functional connectivity between regions of the frontal and temporal lobes has been documented with PET and fMRI, while EEG and MEG studies have shown abnormal patterns of cortical synchronization within and across cortical areas during rest, sensory processing, and cognitive tasks.

Recent research in diffusion imaging, as well as histological and genetic studies, has shown that schizophrenia is also associated with structural disturbances of the subcortical white matter (Kubicki et al., 2005a; 2005b). Cerebral white matter of people with schizophrenia exhibits differences in volume, structural integrity, myelination, and density and coherence of axonal cortical fibers. While it is an open question whether these structural disturbances are directly linked to primary risk factors for schizophrenia or constitute secondary manifestations of the disease (Konrad and Winterer, 2008), they are a likely substrate for at least some of the disconnection and disintegration of mental processes.

Several authors have suggested that the many symptoms of psychic disintegration that accompany schizophrenia are the result of the disconnection of cognitive networks in the brain (Friston and Frith, 1995; Friston, 1998b; Tononi and Edelman, 2000).[11] Friston and Frith (1995) argued that a distinction should be made between regionally specific neuropathology and pathological disruptions of regional interactions and that complex symptoms of schizophrenia such as hallucinations and delusions are better understood in terms of disruptions of interactions and of large-scale integrative processes. Their "disconnection hypothesis" of schizophrenia suggests that abnormal functional integration of distributed neural systems is caused by aberrant regulation of synaptic plasticity by ascending modulatory neurotransmitter systems (Friston, 1998b; Stephan et al., 2006).[12] Such dysregulation may occur in the absence of any overt anatomical differences in white matter pathways by affecting the physiological efficacy of corticocortical connections, which, in turn, would alter patterns of (resting and task-evoked) functional and effective connectivity. Tononi and Edelman (2000) advanced the idea that schizophrenia results from a disruption of reentrant interactions responsible for the functional integration of the activities of distributed brain areas that give rise to conscious experience. This proposal framed schizophrenia as a "disease of reentry" (Edelman, 1989), the result of a disturbance of cortical mechanisms of integration that underlie conscious mental processes. Tononi and Edelman used computer simulations of cortical integration to identify numerous physiological factors, including altered patterns of synaptic plasticity, that may lead to functional disconnection.

If schizophrenia is associated with profound disruptions of large-scale functional interactions within the thalamocortical system, then patients with the disease should exhibit altered brain network topologies. The application of network measures is beginning to reveal the effects of schizophrenia on the topology of structural and functional brain networks. The first examination of brain-wide functional connectivity obtained from resting-state fMRI indicated that functional connectivity was diminished among many pairs of regions throughout the brain (Liang et al., 2006). Similar studies of larger cohorts of patients with schizophrenia have investigated the regional distribution of differences in functional connectivity in greater detail (Zhou et al., 2007b; Liu et al., 2008). Several topological attributes of large-scale brain networks in patients with schizophrenia were disturbed relative to those of healthy controls, including a diminished level of connectivity, as well as lower clustering and longer path length, indicative of a disruption of the brain's small-world architecture. The degree to which the topology was disrupted was found to be correlated with the duration of the disorder, suggesting a progressive time course for these network changes. Small-world attributes of brain nodes in sections of the frontal, parietal, and temporal lobes exhibited significant differences, indicating that the disruption of large-scale networks in schizophrenia shows a regionally specific pattern.

Two studies of resting-state fMRI activity in patients with schizophrenia have noted that the deactivation of default mode network activity during task-related neural processing was impaired (Pomarol-Clotet et al., 2008; Whitfield-Gabrieli et al., 2009). This "failure to deactivate" was accompanied by increased resting-state functional connectivity of major components of the medial portion of the default mode network, including the medial prefrontal cortex and the posterior cingulate cortex. The degree to which the default network was hyperconnected correlated with the severity of the psychopathology of the patients as measured by a quantitative assessment of behavioral symptoms (Whitfield-Gabrieli et al., 2009; see figure 10.8). Disturbances of the default network were also seen in relatives of persons with schizophrenia, suggesting that these abnormal functional patterns may have a genetic basis. Further evidence supports the dysregulation of default network activity in schizophrenia and suggests additional disruption of functional coupling in other resting-state networks (Kim et al., 2009).

Consistent with resting-state fMRI studies, functional connectivity derived from EEG data also exhibits disturbed small-world attributes (Micheloyannis et al., 2006; Rubinov et al., 2009a). Micheloyannis et al. reported a reduction in small-world attributes of functional brain networks in the course of a working memory task. Rubinov et al. extended this analysis to resting-state brain activity and confirmed that clustering, path length, and the centrality of hub regions differed between patient and control groups. Rubinov and colleagues interpreted their finding as a "subtle randomization" of connectivity resulting in altered cluster boundaries and between-clusters communication and resulting in a disturbance of the balance of segregation and integration at the scale of the whole brain. Both of these EEG studies used a nonlinear measure of synchronization and thus accounted for changes in both linear and nonlinear interactions.

Schizophrenia has also been shown to disrupt the topology of large-scale structural networks of the brain. Bassett et al. (2008) derived structural networks linking 104 gray matter regions of the brain, including 48 cortical regions in both cortical hemispheres, from correlations in cortical

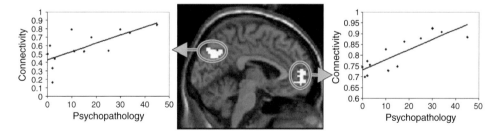

Figure 10.8
Resting-state functional connectivity and correlation with psychopathology in schizophrenia. Functional connectivity of two regions within the default mode network (located in the precuneus/posterior cingulate cortex and medial prefrontal cortex, middle plot) with a seed region in medial prefrontal cortex is shown in relation to a composite score of positive symptomology in schizophrenia. Reproduced from Whitfield-Gabrieli et al. (2009) with permission.

thickness measurements across large cohorts of healthy control subjects and people with schizophrenia. Comparison of the inferred structural connectivity patterns revealed a significant degradation of the hierarchical arrangement of multimodal cortical nodes, as well as longer connection distances between regions indicative of a loss of efficiency in axonal wiring. In people with schizophrenia, frontal hubs were diminished while other, nonfrontal hub regions emerged. In contrast to findings in EEG and fMRI functional networks, global small-world attributes were found to be largely unchanged between control and clinical subject groups.

In summary, network approaches are beginning to be applied to the study of schizophrenia. However, the prolonged time course of the disorder, the heterogeneity of symptoms, the lack of simple diagnostics, and the variable medication use render any systematic and well-controlled study of its neural substrates particularly challenging. Nevertheless, empirical evidence from a number of independent studies using different methodologies indicates that schizophrenia is associated with disturbances of large-scale structural and functional brain connectivity. Future work needs to identify specific patterns of disturbance, particularly for structural networks where current data are still very incomplete. Whatever the actual causes of the disease, knowledge of underlying disconnectivity will help to achieve a better understanding of the neurological origin of its characteristic symptoms and potentially lead to much-needed objective diagnostic tests.

Neurodevelopmental Disorders

Autism (or, more broadly, autism spectrum disorders) is a relatively common neurodevelopmental disorder with almost entirely unknown causes. People with autism typically show abnormal social interactions, deficits in verbal and nonverbal communication, lack of empathy, and a behavioral pattern of stereotypy and preoccupation. Some accounts have characterized the cognitive symptoms of autism as due to "weak central coherence," reflecting a dominance of cognitive strategies that emphasize detail-focused processing and a parallel loss of integrative power. The relationship between local and global coherence likely has complex origins and manifestations and can be explained on the basis of different computational and neural models (Happé and Frith, 2006). Children with autism exhibit various abnormal features of brain structure, most notably an increase in cerebral volume in both gray and white matter, possibly due to accelerated growth in early childhood. In addition, postmortem neuropathology has revealed abnormalities in cortical cytoarchitecture, and diffusion MRI results point to disorganization of white matter pathways (Keller et al., 2007), although comprehensive whole brain tractography has not yet been carried out.

Belmonte et al. (2004) advanced a hypothesis about the origins of autism based on the abnormal development of brain connectivity. Summarizing a large number of empirical findings on changes in cortical activations, synchrony, and anatomical connectivity, Belmonte and colleagues suggested that autism may result from an overabundance of short-range or local cortical pathways that interfere with the functional differentiation of brain regions, as well as a selective loss of specific long-range pathways that support global integrative processes. Loss of functional connectivity during task and rest conditions has been reported (Cherkassky et al., 2006; Just et al., 2007)—for example, between regions of frontal and parietal cortex.

Functional MRI studies have revealed that people with autism fail to show the characteristic deactivation of midline default network areas such as the medial prefrontal cortex and posterior cingulate cortex when transitioning from a state of cognitive rest to an attention-demanding cognitive task (Kennedy et al., 2006). The amount of deactivation in the medial prefrontal cortex was inversely correlated with a clinical measure of social impairment. This lack of deactivation may be explained by the low level of default activity during rest in autism. Thus, abnormal self-referential thought processes that occur during rest in people with autism may be due to a functional impairment of endogenous neural activity within the default network, particularly along the cortical midline (Lombardo et al., 2007).

Other neurodevelopmental disorders are also associated with disruptions of functional connectivity. People with attention-deficit/hyperactivity disorder (ADHD) exhibit abnormally low functional coupling between midline structures of the default mode network, specifically between anterior and posterior cingulate cortex (Castellanos et al., 2008). Functional brain networks in ADHD showed altered patterns in local efficiency, with some nodes exhibiting increased and others decreased efficiency (Wang et al., 2009b).

Networks in Clinical and Translational Neuroscience

As this brief survey has shown, network approaches and measures may offer new insights into disruptions of structural and functional brain networks in the damaged or diseased brain (see also Bassett and Bullmore, 2009; Zhang and Raichle, 2010). Convergent evidence from studies that employ different methodologies for the recording and analysis of brain data indicates that AD and schizophrenia, as well as a range of neurodevelopmental disorders including autism, are associated with abnormal topological organization of structural and functional brain networks.[13] These abnormalities are revealed in analyses of specific fiber pathways or in functional connectivity studies undertaken in the course of task-evoked neural processing. In addition, an increasing number of studies utilize spontaneous brain dynamics, in particular resting-state functional connectivity, to gauge the effects of brain damage and disease on functional couplings within the cerebral cortex (Greicius, 2008). In a clinical context, resting-state fMRI studies offer a number of advantages. Since they do not require the performance of a specific task, they can be carried out in patients and control subjects alike without the need to communicate task instructions. Several large-scale cortical networks activated during rest can be identified and, in many cases, mapped onto known cognitive functions and domains. To the extent that task- or stimulus-evoked activation can be monitored, the use of methods that extract effective brain networks, such as DCM, offers important additional information about which brain networks are compromised and how the remaining brain compensates.

Network measures have the potential to become sensitive and objective diagnostic and monitoring markers, as well as markers of the effectiveness of pharmacological or psychological therapies, thus expanding on the study of pharmacologically induced modulation of cognitive activations (Honey and Bullmore, 2004). Clinical applications of network approaches are still in their infancy, but initial results are encouraging. For example, drugs acting on the dopaminergic system can modulate functional brain network measures in animal (Schwarz et al., 2007) as well as human fMRI (Honey et al., 2003). Application of a dopamine D2 receptor antagonist has been shown to decrease the efficiency of human resting-state fMRI functional networks (Achard and Bullmore, 2007). Network measures might also help to understand brain recovery. Monitoring the recovery of damaged brain networks by measuring the time evolution of specific network attributes may reveal commonalities between individual recovery profiles. If functional recovery is shown to be related to specific network measures, novel therapeutic agents and strategies could be devised that promote the restoration of these measures. Future investigation of brain disorders may utilize multimodal imaging approaches that seek to combine information about structural differences as well as alterations in brain dynamics (Jiang et al., 2008). The additional combination of multimodal imaging and genetic information may allow the identification of new biomarkers for specific brain diseases that will facilitate early detection and treatment (Schmitt et al., 2008).

These are just a few of the many avenues for clinical applications of network analysis in the brain. In health and in disease, human cognition rests on the structural arrangement of brain connectivity and its expression in rich patterns of neural dynamics. Hence, it is not surprising that so many cognitive disorders are associated with the localized or global failure of brain networks. Whatever biological factors contribute to a given cognitive disorder, from genetic mutations to alterations in gene expression to disrupted developmental processes, ultimately result in abnormal brain connectivity.[14] Conversely, variations in molecular, cellular, or developmental processes that leave brain connectivity undisturbed are unlikely to result in any major disruption of cognitive function. Patterns of network failure in the brain will become of increasing importance as network analysis gains ground in clinical and translational medicine.

11 Network Growth and Development

The brain structure has to be one which can be achieved by the genetical embryological mechanism, and I hope that this theory that I am now working on may make clearer what restrictions this really implies. What you tell me about growth of neurons under stimulation is very interesting in this connection. It suggests means by which the neurons might be made to grow so as to form a particular circuit, rather than to reach a particular place.[1]
—Alan Turing, 1951

Throughout his life, Alan Turing was fascinated by two major problems: the problem of mechanical computation leading to the construction of intelligent machines and the problem of biological growth, the "taking shape" or morphogenesis of biological matter (Hodges, 1983). The theory referred to in this letter to the neurobiologist J. Z. Young[2] was later published under the title "The Chemical Basis of Morphogenesis" and laid the foundation for mathematical models of biological pattern formation (Turing, 1952). Turing's theory of morphogenesis demonstrated how an initially homogeneous substrate of chemicals, consisting in the simplest case of just two compounds, an activator and an inhibitor, could "self-organize" into complex spatial patterns. Pattern formation was driven by two processes (Gierer and Meinhardt, 1972), the autocatalytic production of the activator and the differential diffusion of activator and inhibitor, resulting in the emergence of distinct spatial regions where one or the other compound prevailed. Turing developed his theory without ever having performed a single biological experiment. Given Turing's lifelong interest in the logical operations of the brain and in biological growth, it may have been only a matter of time for him to turn to a neural theory of circuit formation or network growth. Alas, a victim of prejudice and persecution that led to his premature death in 1954, Turing was not to see the coming revolution in modern biology with its stunning advances in the embryology and development of body and brain.

Turing's work on morphogenesis demonstrated the power of self-organizing developmental processes in shaping biological organisms. Self-organization is found throughout the natural world, including in such diverse phenomena as the pigmentation patterns of seashells (see figure 11.1), cloud formation, sand ripples on a shallow sea floor, the symmetry of snowflakes, the branching patterns of rivers, or Jupiter's great red spot (Ball, 1999). Self-organization, the formation of patterns without any overt prespecification, also plays an important role in neural development. Morphogenetic mechanisms combine features of Turing's original proposal of reaction–diffusion systems with more recently discovered principles of gene regulation and transcriptional control. Gradients of morphogens can exert concentration-dependent effects that determine expression levels of proteins at the cellular level and thus influence elementary developmental processes such as cell migration, differentiation, and adhesion. Computational models of neural development have addressed processes operating at different stages, from the formation of the neural tube to neurite outgrowth, the formation of topographic maps, and the refinement and remodeling of synaptic connections (van Ooyen, 2003). The combination of growth processes operating during embryonic development and a multitude of mechanisms of

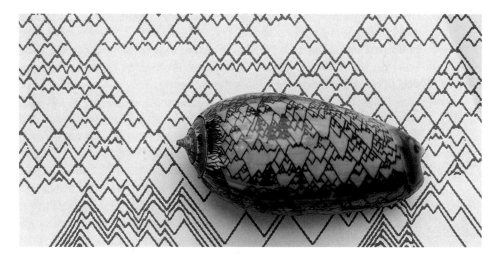

Figure 11.1
Pattern formation in seashells. The image shows an example of the seashell *Oliva porphyria* and its characteristic pigmentation pattern. Chemical reaction–diffusion models, descendants of Turing's original proposal for the chemical basis of morphogenesis, are capable of producing similar patterns, plotted here in the background. Reproduced from Meinhardt (2009) with permission.

neuronal plasticity that continue throughout the lifetime of the organism shapes the topology of brain networks. It is impossible to fully understand or interpret the structure of brain networks without considering their growth and development (see chapter 7).

Any attempt to summarize the vast literature on neuronal development is much beyond the scope of this book. Rather, we will focus on growth processes that are relevant to the topology and spatial patterning of brain networks. Network growth focuses on how networks come to be, how nodes and edges are added, deleted, or rewired. Neural models of network growth address how developmental changes in structural connections give rise to changes in dynamic patterns of neural activity. A number of models have been proposed for the growth of the Internet or certain social networks. These more abstract models of network evolution can explain some of the statistical properties of real-world networks. Yet, their straightforward application to the brain is problematic because in most of these models growth processes do not explicitly depend on network dynamics or on the network's spatial embedding. In brain networks, however, structural and functional connectivity are highly interrelated. Not only does the topology of structural connections shape neuronal activity but structural networks are also subject to change as a result of dynamic patterns of functional connectivity. These ongoing changes in the strength or persistence of structural links underlie developmental patterns of functional connectivity observed in the human brain from childhood to senescence.

Abstract Models of Network Growth

All networks, whether they are social, technological, or biological, are the result of a growth process. Many of these networks continue to grow for prolonged periods of time, continually modifying their connectivity structure throughout their entire existence. For example, the World Wide Web has grown from a small number of cross-linked documents in the early 1990s to an estimated 30 billion indexed web pages in 2009.[3] The extraordinary growth of the Web continues unabated and has occurred without any top-down design, yet the topology of its hyperlink structure exhibits characteristic statistical patterns (Pastor-Satorras and Vespignani, 2004). Other technological networks such as the power grid, global transportation networks, or mobile communication networks continue to grow and evolve, each displaying characteristic patterns of expansion and elaboration. Growth and change in social and organizational networks likely involve complex processes of social cognition, individual learning, decision making, or sociodemographic factors, to name but a few.

Network growth can be modeled in several different ways, either by starting with a fixed number of nodes and then gradually adding edges or by adding both nodes and edges simultaneously. Models of network growth have been formulated within graph theory (where network growth is often referred to as "graph evolution," even for nonbiological graphs) as well as within specific application domains. One of the simplest abstract models of network growth was described and analyzed by Paul Erdös and Alfred Rényi in their seminal paper entitled "On the Evolution of Random Graphs" (Erdös and Rényi 1960; see chapter 2). In this model, the growth process starts with a fixed (and very large) number of n nodes. Edges are added by sequentially selecting at random pairs of nodes. Erdös and Rényi's analysis revealed sudden changes in network properties as the number of edges grew beyond certain thresholds. One such network property is the size of the largest component, defined as the largest set of nodes in which every pair of nodes is connected by at least one path. Initially all nodes are unconnected. As edges are added to the graph, several small components will begin to form. When the number of edges exceeds n/2, a single large component emerges, which quickly encompasses the entire network (see figure 11.2). This emergence of a single giant component is an example of a phase transition involving the sudden appearance of a new network property in the course of graph evolution. Importantly, this phase transition occurs in the course of a continuous process of network growth where edges are added one by one.[4] The occurrence of phase transitions in network growth is significant because the sudden appearance of new structural network properties may have consequences for the network's dynamic behavior. Phase transitions have been suggested as important steps in the spontaneous emergence of collectively autocatalytic sets of molecules in the origin of life (Kauffman, 2000). Their potential role in neural development is still entirely unexplored.

Adding connections between node pairs with fixed probability represents one of the simplest possible growth rules, one that is unlikely to be a realistic approximation for most real-world growth processes. Erdös and Rényi were aware of this fact, and at the beginning of their paper on random graph evolution they remarked that "the evolution of graphs may be considered as a rather simplified model of the evolution of certain communication nets [...]. (Of course, if one aims at describing

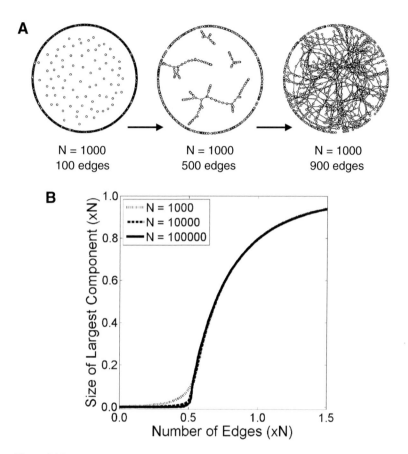

Figure 11.2
Random growth model and phase transition. (A) Growth of an Erdös–Rényi random graph consisting of 1,000 nodes, displayed using a force-spring layout algorithm. This algorithm places disconnected nodes equidistant from the center of the plot and connected components closer to the center. When 100 edges have been added, there are a few small components, mostly consisting of 2–4 nodes, and they remain disconnected from one another. When 500 edges have been added, a few larger components have appeared. After 900 edges have been added, there is a single large component consisting of approximately 750 nodes. (B) The size of the largest connected component as a function of the number of edges added during random growth. A single large component appears suddenly, in a phase transition, when N/2 edges have been added.

such a real situation, one should replace the hypothesis of equiprobability of all connections by some more realistic hypothesis.)" (Erdös and Rényi, 1960, p. 19). Cohen (1988), in his discussion of random graph models, speculated that the consideration of new growth rules for the addition of nodes and edges might allow the Erdös–Rényi growth model to be extended to the evolution of biochemical or neuronal networks. I will discuss several such models later in this chapter.

One of the most widely studied network growth models generates networks with power-law degree distributions—so-called scale-free networks (Barabási and Albert, 1999; Barabási et al., 2000; see chapter 2). The model requires only two basic mechanisms, the continual addition of new nodes ("growth") and the creation of new edges between the new node and the existing nodes with probabilities proportional to the node degree ("preferential attachment").[5] Analytic treatment of the model reveals that the network's degree distribution will converge to a power law if both growth and preferential attachment mechanisms are implemented. In contrast, growth without preferential attachment yields an exponential degree distribution. The preferential attachment model displays interesting patterns of error and attack tolerance, with resilience against random node deletions and vulnerability to loss of hub nodes.[6] More recently, other network growth models have been proposed that also produce scale-free organization but employ a different set of growth rules, for example, rules that involve merging or aggregating nodes (Alava and Dorogovtsev, 2005) or duplicating nodes, edges, or entire subgraphs.

While the universality of the preferential attachment model is appealing, the growth of networks in different domains of nature and technology likely involves more specific sets of rules for the addition of nodes and edges and usually depends on patterns of network dynamics and signal traffic. The random growth and preferential attachment models do not offer a plausible mechanism for the growth of brain networks, largely because they fail to take into account neural activity and the spatial embedding of the brain. Spatial embedding of networks has important implications for their topology and growth because the addition of new nodes or new connections consumes limited resources such as space and metabolic energy (see chapter 7).

Growth of Spatially Embedded Networks

Many complex networks are spatially embedded, a fact that has significant and still largely unexplored implications for their topology and function. Examples include all transportation networks (air travel, rail, urban commuting), power distribution grids, the (physical) Internet, and many social and ecological networks, as well as cellular or metabolic networks once the association of molecules with cellular compartments is taken into account. Clearly, the spatial arrangement of nodes in the brain and their connection distances are of great importance for understanding brain network structure and dynamics (see chapters 6 and 7). Realistic models of network growth in the brain must incorporate these factors.

Kaiser and Hilgetag proposed a spatial growth model to account for the observed small-world architecture of cortical networks (Kaiser and Hilgetag, 2004a,b; 2007). The model started with a single node and no connections. Nodes were added over time, and connections between newly added nodes and existing nodes were established with a probability that decreased exponentially with the Euclidean internode distance. Two parameters of this exponential governed the overall density and the spatial range of the connectivity. Some settings of these parameters yielded networks that resembled cortical small-world networks, while others resulted in networks that are also spatially embedded but follow growth rules different from those in cortex or in nonspatially embedded networks such as those of cellular metabolism. Interestingly, this spatial growth model could generate wiring length distributions similar to those found in cortical networks without the need to impose an explicit wiring minimization rule.

More recently, Kaiser et al. (2009) created a model that did not use an exponential law for distance-dependent connection probability but instead generated realistic connection length distributions by modeling axonal outgrowth. The model postulated that axons would grow in random directions until potential neuronal targets are encountered. They would continue their linear growth trajectory if the target was already occupied by another competing connection. This simple model was able to generate distributions for connection lengths that showed an exponential decay of connection length with distance. Competition for axonal space on dendritic trees was found to generate realistic values for the proportion of established synapses relative to all possible synapses, the so-called filling fraction.

The modular small-world architecture of the brain is not readily obtained with growth models that rely exclusively on distance rules. While such rules can generate topologies with high clustering and short path lengths, they do not generally yield multiple modules or clusters which are characteristic of most structural brain networks. Multiple modules can be obtained, however, if different parts of the network develop in different time windows (Kaiser and Hilgetag, 2007; Nisbach and Kaiser, 2007). Time windows are introduced by modulating the probability that a connection is generated between two nodes as a function of their distance as well as an intrinsic time parameter that defines a preferred window within which connections are made. This temporal property is inherited by newly generated nodes on the basis of proximity to other already existing nodes. Multiple clusters and a small-world (but not scale-free) topology emerge if the growth process is seeded with "pioneer nodes" that are appropriately positioned. The size and overlap of clusters depends on the width and overlap of time windows for synaptogenesis.

More realistic growth models emulate cellular processes of neural development to create realistic neuron morphologies and connectivity patterns. For example, Arjen van Ooyen and colleagues have developed a model for network growth called NETMORPH that allows the generation of artificial neural networks that are fully embedded in three-dimensional space and incorporate neuronal growth processes such as growth cone extension, neurite outgrowth, branching, and synaptogenesis (Koene et al., 2009; see figure 11.3, plate 14). Neurons created within NETMORPH exhibit characteristic dendritic and axonal morphologies, as well as spatial distributions of synaptic connections. While the resulting network topologies have not yet been comprehensively studied, initial results indicate the presence of small-world attributes (de Ridder

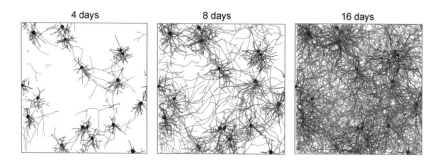

Figure 11.3 (plate 14)
A computational model of network development. Images show simulated neurons and their interconnections within a 400 μm × 400 μm cross-section of space, depicted after the equivalent of 4, 8, and 16 days of development. Neuronal cell bodies are shown as blue circles, dendrites are blue, and axons are green. Note that some cell bodies are located above or below the imaged volume, and some axons and dendrites thus appear as disconnected fragments in the plot. Reproduced from Koene et al. (2009) with permission.

et al., 2009). Another example is the simulation tool CX3D (Zubler and Douglas, 2009) which aims at modeling neurobiological growth processes within a realistic three-dimensional environment that captures mechanical forces as well as chemical diffusion. Simulations carried out with CX3D have reproduced some of the key stages in the formation of multiple layers in cortex.

As these examples show, growth models that account for spatial dimensions and distance-dependent processes can generate networks that match some of the spatial distributions and topological patterns seen in real nervous systems. All of the models discussed so far have focused on distance-dependent processes for the addition of nodes and edges but have not considered the role of neural activity. However, there is abundant evidence that the structure of brain networks is also shaped by ongoing and evoked neural activity. Such activity-dependent processes govern the stability and persistence of neural connections, and they likely continue to do so throughout life.

Symbiotic Relationship between Structural and Functional Connectivity

In cortical networks, structural and functional connectivity mutually influence each other on multiple time scales. On fast as well as slower time scales, structural connections shape the topology of functional networks (see chapter 8). Conversely, functional connectivity can also mold synaptic patterns via a number of activity-dependent mechanisms. Thus, structure shapes neural activity, and activity in turn shapes structure. This mutual or "symbiotic" relationship (Rubinov et al., 2009b) is important in guiding the development of structural and functional brain networks. The mutual interdependency of network topology and dynamics in the brain is an example of what Gross and Blasius (2008) have referred to as "adaptive coevolutionary networks" (see figure 11.4). In these networks, dynamic processes unfolding on a relatively fast time scale shape the topology of the network on a slower time scale. These changes in topology in turn alter the dynamics of the system. Many real-world networks incorporate these interdependencies, which are essential ingredients in their growth and development. For example, a traffic or communication network may experience congestion, a form of dynamic failure, which triggers efforts to construct new links to ease traffic flow (Gross and Blasius, 2008). The brain is a particularly striking example of a network where fast dynamic processes continually shape and are shaped by the topology of structural connections.

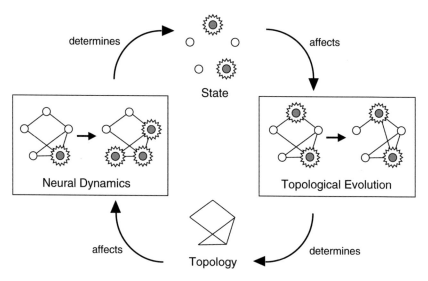

Figure 11.4
Network dynamics and topological evolution. This schematic diagram illustrates the interplay between neural dynamics and the temporal evolution of the connection topology, an
example of an adaptive coevolutionary network. The figure is based on a similar diagram
in Gross and Blasius (2008).

Several network modeling studies have explored the role of neural
dynamics in forming network topology. The interplay between structural
and functional connectivity was investigated in a series of computational
models using an adaptive rewiring rule based on synchrony (Gong and
Van Leeuwen, 2004; Kwok et al., 2007; Rubinov et al., 2009b). Gong and
Van Leeuwen (2004) proposed a network growth model that used an
activity-dependent rewiring rule to guide the time evolution of structural
connectivity. The rewiring rule had Hebbian characteristics, in that connections were established between synchronously active pairs of neurons
and were pruned away between neurons that were asynchronous. Neural
units were modeled as coupled logistic maps with each of the units
exhibiting chaotic dynamics. Starting from an initially random network
topology, connections between units were rewired based on the difference in their instantaneous activation values. Connections were made, or
persisted, between units with similar activation values while units with
dissimilar activation values tended to lose connectivity. Over time, this
adaptive rewiring algorithm produced small-world network topologies
with high clustering and single-scale degree distributions. Kwok et al.
(2007) performed similar studies in randomly coupled networks of neural

oscillators whose coupling structure was rewired based on a pairwise synchrony measure. Again, networks gradually evolved toward small-world connectivity, characterized by high clustering and short path lengths.

A similar model with a synchrony-based adaptive rewiring rule was implemented by Rubinov et al. (2009b). The model tracked the temporal pattern of structural and functional connectivity and their mutual interplay. Over time, random structural connectivity was reshaped by ordered functional connectivity toward a small-world, modular architecture. The relationship between functional connectivity and structural connectivity was particularly strong when functional connections were estimated over longer time scales, consistent with empirical and modeling results (see chapter 8). In agreement with other models (Honey et al., 2007), functional networks were found to exhibit significant fast-time scale fluctuations. These fluctuations were found to be enabled by hub nodes that exhibited high-dimensional "cloud-like" noisy dynamics. The greater variability of hub node dynamics allows these hubs to participate in different configurations with nodes that belong to more local neighborhoods or modules.

Numerous studies have demonstrated that spontaneous neuronal activity plays an important role in shaping connectivity in the developing brain (Katz and Shatz, 1996). For example, neurons in the developing retina and lateral geniculate nucleus exhibit characteristic patterns of spontaneous activity that guide the establishment of synaptic connections within the various stages of the visual pathway. Patterns of spontaneous activity within the visual system are the result of multiple interacting mechanisms, partly driven by external sources of input, for example, waves of activity originating in the retina, and partly produced by endogenous neuronal oscillations within thalamus or cortex (Weliky and Katz, 1999). Silencing spontaneous activity during development can have profound effects on the patterning of functional neuronal circuits. For example, the disruption of spontaneous retinal waves disturbs the retinotopic mapping of geniculate to cortical neurons (Cang et al., 2005). There are multiple potential sources of spontaneous neuronal activity in developing organisms, including those that result in self-generated motor activity. In the developing human fetus, spontaneous movement can generate sensory inputs that drive somatotopically mapped cortical oscillations and aid in the formation of functional circuits in the somatosensory cortex (Milh et al., 2007).

A broad range of cellular mechanisms render synaptic networks sensitive to neural activity and dynamics. Learning-related changes in the nervous system are not limited to changes in synaptic weights of existing connections but include structural plasticity—for example, the remodeling or rewiring of synapses (Butz et al., 2009), and even changes in the structure of cortical white matter linking distant regions in the human brain (Scholz et al., 2009). While synaptic remodeling has been demonstrated in a number of systems, the extent to which structural rewiring occurs either spontaneously or in conjunction with neural activity or learning events is still unknown. Some evidence points to learning-related structural changes in dendritic spines as a basis for long-term memory (Yang et al., 2009). Chklovskii et al. (2004) have argued that synaptic weight and wiring changes must be distinguished and that the capacity to rewire connections could significantly increase the number of functionally distinct circuits available for encoding of information. The close spatial proximity of axonal and dendritic branches within cortical tissue creates many opportunities for the formation of new synapses without the need for significant additional growth of neural processes. The many points of close apposition between dendrites and axons have been called potential synapses (Stepanyants et al., 2002; Stepanyants and Chklovskii, 2005), and their number far exceeds the number of actually realized synaptic junctions. Potential synapses thus theoretically allow for a great number of new structural patterns that "lie in waiting" and could be rapidly configured by synaptic rewiring. Wen et al. (2009) have suggested that the complex branching patterns of neuronal dendrites are arranged such that the local repertoire of potential synapses is maximized while keeping the cost (length, volume) of dendrites low. As cellular mapping and reconstruction techniques (see chapter 5) begin to deliver cellular network topologies, even closer linkages between cell morphology and connectivity will likely be discovered.

Development of Brain Networks across the Human Life Span

The topology of brain networks changes dramatically across the human life span with important consequences for cognitive development. Changes in the number (e.g., Huttenlocher, 1990) and arrangement of structural nodes and edges in the brain influence the effectiveness and spatial pattern of their dynamic interactions at all scales. It is important to emphasize that network growth and plasticity is but one major mechanism that drives cognitive development. Equally important, particularly in the case of humans, is the role of the organism's physical and social environment, the physical growth of its body and motor apparatus, continual self-reference (Körner and Matsumoto, 2002), and embodied interactions with the surrounding world (Thelen and Smith, 1994; Smith and Thelen, 2003). Development depends not only on intrinsic programs that inexorably lead toward a "mature" end state but rather involves dynamic interactions between brain, body, and environment that guide the expression and continued modification of morphology and behavior. The development of brain networks does not involve brain processes alone. For example, neural mechanisms of learning and plasticity allow the developing brain to extract statistical regularities in the environment. These regularities are partly the result of sensorimotor interactions between the learning organism and the surrounding physical and social world (see chapter 14). Development can only be fully understood if the networks of the brain are considered in the context of interactions between brain and environment.

Computational models, particularly connectionist approaches, have yielded many important insights into mechanisms of learning and development (Elman et al., 1996; Marcus, 2001). However, they do not address how network growth and plasticity shape the emergence of neural dynamics supporting cognition. Most connectionist models focus on algorithms for learning that are implemented in simple multilayer neural networks. The arrangement of nodes and edges in connectionist models bears little resemblance to the complex network architecture of the brain. Furthermore, most connectionist models do not possess rich non-linear dynamics, and their development mainly involves adjustments of synaptic weights without including physical growth or network evolution. To be fair, connectionist models focus on different problem domains, and they address a different set of questions about development (Elman, 2005). Their success lies in their ability to capture patterns of change in human behavior, and this success is a continuing challenge to more anatomically and biophysically based models of brain networks. Ultimately, we need realistic models that can show us how we can get from neural dynamics and network evolution all the way to behavior and cognition.

The connectivity patterns and growth mechanisms of such models will be informed by neuroimaging studies of the human brain across different age groups, including mapping of structural and functional connectivity. Such studies have begun to cast light on neural substrates of cognitive development (Casey et al., 2000; 2005; Johnson, 2001) and aging (Grady, 2008). Comprehensive structural network analyses across several developmental stages of the human brain are still lacking. Developmental changes in the myelination of long-range fiber pathways create additional challenges for diffusion imaging and tractography. Diffusion imaging has been employed for noninvasive measurements of white matter maturation indexed by fractional anisotropy and mean diffusivity in 1- to 4-month-old infants (Dubois et al., 2006). The development of specific thalamocortical tracts in the cat brain was investigated with high-resolution DSI (Takahashi et al., 2010). The method allowed for the delineation and three-dimensional imaging of several tracts including corticothalamic and corticocortical pathways across several months of postnatal development. Whole-brain structural networks of the developing human brain have not yet been comprehensively mapped.

An important role in understanding the development of human brain networks is played by observations of endogenous or spontaneous neural activity (see chapter 8). Spontaneous brain activity can be recorded across all developmental stages and during the entire human life span without the need to communicate or specify behavioral or cognitive tasks. Spontaneous neural activity offers an opportunity to observe functional interactions across numerous brain regions and record their developmental time course. Several studies have examined spontaneous brain activity during early development and have found significant changes over time in the way brain regions are functionally connected. Based on studies in the adult brain where structural and functional connectivity have been shown to be correlated it appears likely that changes in functional linkage across developmental time partly reflect the growth and maturation of brain regions and white matter pathways. A large number of studies, many of them involving diffusion MRI, document the importance of the physiological maturation of specific white matter pathways in cognitive development (Paus et al., 2001).

Spontaneous neural activity can be recorded from human infants soon after birth.[7] Five different resting-state networks were identified in the brains of preterm infants scanned at term-equivalent age, with fMRI data acquired during periods of sleep (Fransson et al., 2007). Resting-state networks appeared predominantly to link homologous areas in the two hemispheres, and the adult pattern of the default mode network, particularly the linkage between its anterior and posterior components, was not found. Fransson et al. suggest that the absence of a fully connected default mode network may reflect the relative immaturity of the infant brain's structural organization. Gao et al. (2009; see also Lin et al., 2008) performed resting-state fMRI recordings in healthy pediatric subjects between 2 weeks and 2 years of age. In very young infants, the default mode network was not yet fully represented, and additional components became linked at about 1 year of age. By 2 years of age, all major components of the default mode network appeared to be functionally connected. Throughout this early developmental period, a region comprising the posterior cingulate/precuneus and retrosplenial cortex occupied the most central position and was most strongly linked to other regions within the emerging default network. While Gao et al. (2009) found evidence for a relatively early emergence of the default mode network, results by Fair et al. (2008) argue for a slower developmental time course. Fair et al. (2008) found that the default mode network exhibits significant differences in children (ages 7–9 years) compared to young adults (ages 21–31 years). While interhemispheric connections between homotopic cortical regions were found to be strong in children, other linkages were significantly weaker than those in the adult network (see figure 11.5). Default regions were only sparsely connected, with most connections

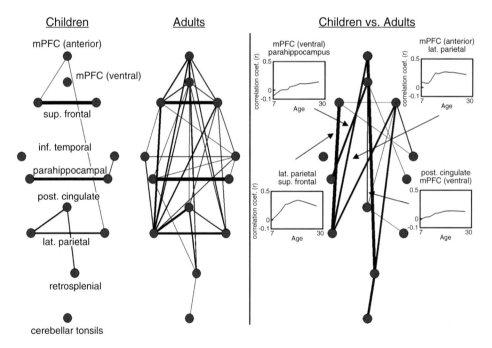

Figure 11.5
Development of the human default mode network. Resting-state functional connectivity between regions of the default network is sparse in children (ages 7–9 years) while the same set of regions is highly connected in young adults (ages 21–31 years). The plot at the right shows statistically significant differences, as well as time courses for several individual functional connections. mPFC, medial prefrontal cortex; sup., superior; inf., inferior; post., posterior; lat., lateral. Modified and reproduced from Fair et al. (2008), with permission.

spanning the brain in the anterior–posterior direction entirely absent. Most functional connections were significantly weaker in children than in adults, an effect that could be due to weaker coupling or to coupling that is more variable across time. The latter explanation is less likely since a separate study using the same subjects and examining other, task-related brain networks (Fair et al., 2007) showed both increases and decreases in the strength of functional connectivity across time.

As discussed in chapters 8 and 9, the use of resting-state fMRI allows for the identification of specialized functional brain networks that become engaged in varying conditions of rest or goal-related cognitive processes. Fair et al. (2009) characterized the development of four previously identified functional networks in subjects ages 7–31 years by using a variety of network measures, most notably community and modularity detection. This study did not find significant trends across developmental time for several network metrics, including modularity and small-world attributes. Children and adults exhibited high clustering and short path lengths, consistent with a small-world organization and overall high efficiency of information flow. Fair et al. found clearly delineated modules or communities of brain regions in both children and adults, but community membership changed significantly over time. Interestingly, Fair et al. found a decrease in the strengths of functional connections linking regions that were close in space (separated by less than 30 mm) while the opposite pattern was seen for long-distance functional connections (exceeding a length of 90 mm). This developmental pattern with a progression from a more local to a more distributed organization (see figure 11.6, plate 15) held across multiple resting-state networks and may reflect the overall tendency of the brain's functional architecture to develop toward more highly integrated and spatially distributed large-scale functional networks. Another comparative study of functional brain networks obtained from a cohort of children (ages 7–9 years) and young adults (ages 19–22 years) confirms several of these findings, including basic similarities in their small-world organization (Supekar et al., 2009). Differences were seen in their hierarchical patterning, with children exhibiting stronger coupling between subcortical and cortical regions while stronger corticocortical coupling was found for the brains of young adults. Furthermore, comparison of functional connectivity with wiring lengths derived from diffusion imaging again revealed a developmental trend toward weakening of short-range and strengthening of long-range functional connections. This trend indicates a rebalancing of functional segregation and functional integration during early development.

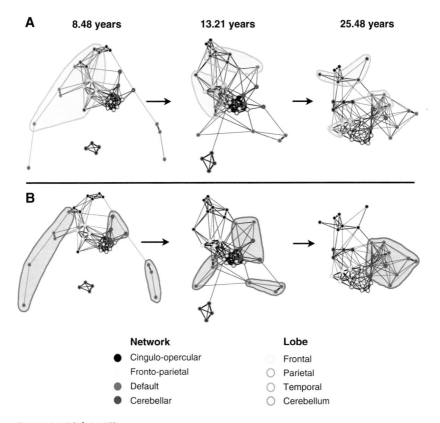

Network
● Cingulo-opercular
  Fronto-parietal
● Default
● Cerebellar

Lobe
○ Frontal
○ Parietal
○ Temporal
○ Cerebellum

Figure 11.6 (plate 15)
Development of default and task-control networks from children to young adults. Individual frames show the development of resting-state functional connectivity measured with functional magnetic resonance imaging at approximate ages of 8, 13, and 25 years. Networks are displayed using a spring-embedding algorithm which places regions that are functionally highly interactive close to each other. The plots in the top row show a coherent cluster of frontal regions (light blue) whose members are anatomically close as well as functionally coupled ("segregation"). The members of this cluster become more widely dispersed across the network later in development. Conversely, member regions of the default network (bottom row, red), which are functionally strongly coupled in the adult ("integration"), are more widely dispersed and uncoupled in children. Development of functional networks appears to progress from a local or segregated to a more distributed or integrated mode of organization. Reproduced from Fair et al. (2009).

Functional brain networks continue to change throughout the adult life span and into senescence. Grady et al. (2006) examined cortical activations with fMRI in the brains of young, middle-aged, and older adults during rest and across a variety of encoding and recognition tasks. Areas that are commonly deactivated during the performance of cognitive tasks exhibited age-related increases in activation while task-related regions decreased with age. These results suggest a progressive decrease in the ability to suspend default mode activity during transitions from rest to task-related processing, which could account for observed age-related cognitive changes. Andrews-Hanna et al. (2007) showed reduced functional connectivity between anterior and posterior components of the default network, specifically the posterior cingulate and the medial frontal cortex, in older subjects (see figure 11.7). Both anterior and posterior components of the default mode network also exhibited reduced activity levels in elderly subjects (Damoiseaux et al., 2008), possibly reflecting a reduction in stimulus-independent mental activity with age. Small-world attributes of brain functional networks were also shown to be affected by age, with a decrease in global efficiency (corresponding

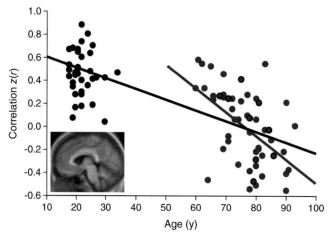

Figure 11.7
Reduced anterior–posterior functional correlations in aging. The plots shows the relationship between the age of participants and the strength of the functional connection between the medial prefrontal cortex and the posterior cingulate/retrosplenial cortex, two of the major components of the default mode network (seed regions are shown in the image on the lower left). Data from young adult participants (black dots) is shown together with data from older adults (gray dots). Modified and reproduced from Andrews-Hanna et al. (2007) with permission.

to an increase in the path length) in older brains (Achard and Bullmore, 2007). The extent to which the topology of structural brain networks changes with aging is still unknown. There are indications that globally measured white matter integrity decreases with age (Damoiseaux et al., 2009), a likely substrate for changes in brain dynamics.

Age-related changes in brain functional networks also involve the grouping of areas into clusters whose members are functionally coupled and the role of individual regions in interlinking these clusters as hubs. Network modularity was studied by Meunier et al. (2009a) in two groups of healthy participants, composed of younger (ages 18–33 years) and older adults (ages 62–76 years), using whole-brain fMRI time series data and a wavelet-based measure of correlation. There were significant differences in the number, relative size, and membership structure of network modules, as well as differences in interlinking hub regions. For example, brains of young adults exhibited fewer but larger modules that were less extensively interconnected. A large module consisting of fronto–cingulo–parietal regions was found to be split into two smaller and more local medial posterior and fronto–striato–thalamic modules in older brains. Intermodular links between regions in the posterior and central cortex were increased in the brains of older subjects while links between frontal and posterior as well as frontal and central modules were significantly decreased. These changes in the composition and linkage of functional linkage in brains of subjects from different age groups strongly suggest that brain networks continue to change throughout adulthood and normal senescence. The relationship of these changes in brain networks to parallel changes in cognition and behavior awaits further empirical study.

In summary, endogenous brain activity results in resting-state functional networks that exhibit characteristic differences between children, young adults, and elderly adults. The topology of functional networks changes throughout development, adulthood, and aging. The first major developmental changes involve the emergence of robust and globally linked resting-state networks by a process that coordinates functional specialization with integration. In children, short-range functional interactions dominate while longer-range interactions appear later in adolescence. Late adulthood and aging are accompanied by a breakup of larger modules into smaller ones that are less well delineated and exhibit greater cross-linkage. Overall, the growing and the aging brain go through gradual rebalancing of functional relationships while preserving large-scale features such as small-world connectivity. Developmental trends in functional segregation and integration are strong candidates for potential neural substrates of cognitive change across the human life span.

Network Development and Self-Organization

The topology of structural and functional brain networks changes profoundly during neural development, adulthood, and senescence, due to a multitude of mechanisms for growth and plasticity, operating on different cellular substrates and time scales. These processes also account for the resilience of brain networks against structural alteration and damage, topics considered in detail in the preceding chapter. As we learn more about the dynamics of connectivity, mounting evidence indicates that most connectional changes are not the outcome of environmental "imprinting," the permanent transfer of useful associations or linkages into the brain's wiring pattern. Instead, the picture is one of self-organization, the complex interplay between the formation of organized topology and ongoing neural dynamics. Nervous systems do not converge onto a final stable pattern of optimal functionality; rather, their connectivity continues to be in flux throughout life. As Turing noted in his paper on morphogenesis, "Most of an organism, most of the time, is developing from one pattern into another, rather than from homogeneity into a pattern" (Turing, 1952, pp. 71–72).

Models of neural development are beginning to provide insight into the fundamental cellular and synaptic mechanisms that drive connectional change. Disturbances of these mechanisms are potential candidates in a variety of neurodevelopmental disorders (see chapter 10), and they highlight the delicate balance that must be maintained for properly organized connectivity to emerge. One of the most puzzling aspects of structural brain networks at the cellular scale is their extraordinary propensity for rewiring and remodeling in the presence or absence of neural activity (Minerbi et al., 2009). Some studies suggest that individual synapses can change shape and even come into and go out of existence on time scales far shorter than those of some forms of memory. Many elements of the brain's "wiring pattern," or structural connectivity graph, at the scale of cells and synapses, appear to be highly dynamic, and the relative instability of individual synapses casts doubt on their reliability as sites of long-term modification and memory. If these observations are further extended and found to generalize across much of the brain, then processes that ensure some degree of stability or "functional homeosta-sis" at the level of the entire system will become of central importance (see chapter 4).

Processes of self-organization also appear to underlie the highly vari-able yet robust nature of brain dynamics. It turns out that mechanisms of plasticity may play an important role in maintaining the networks of the brain in a dynamic regime that ensures high sensitivity to inputs, high information capacity, and high complexity.

A singular, specific cell assembly underlies the emergence and operation of every cognitive act. In other words, the emergence of a cognitive act is a matter of coordination of many different regions allowing for different capacities: perception, memory, motivation, and so on. They must be bound together in specific grouping appropriate to the specifics of the current situation [...] and are thus necessarily transient. [...] A specific CA [cell assembly] is selected through the fast, transient phase locking of activated neurons belonging to sub-threshold competing CAs.[1]
—Francisco Varela, 1995

Francisco Varela advanced a set of ideas that squarely aimed at characterizing mental states on the basis of physical events occurring in brain networks (Varela, 1995; see figure 12.1). He envisioned brain dynamics as the ongoing operation of a "transient coherency-generating process" that unified dispersed neural activity through synchronous relationships. The transience of the process is essential because it allows for "a continual emergence," an ongoing dynamic flow in a cognitive–mental space. According to Varela's theory, coherent patterns are assembled and dissolved depending upon changing conditions of input or task demand, and their configurations corresponded to sequences of mental states experienced at each moment in time. The brain's ability to self-organize and undergo transient state dynamics is crucial for its capability to simultaneously satisfy momentary demands posed by the environment and integrate these exogenous signals with the endogenous activity of brain and body. Integrated brain activity forms the neural basis for the unity of mind and experience.

Why should we care about dynamic diversity? The importance of diverse dynamical states for self-organization and robustness was recognized early in the history of cybernetics. Ashby's "law of requisite variety" (Ashby, 1958) dealt with the impact of environmental perturbations on

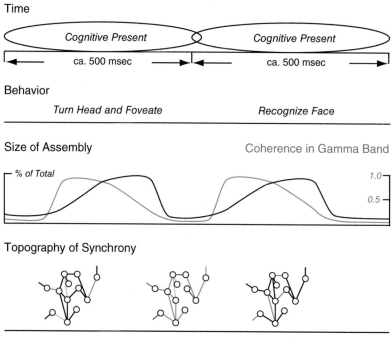

Time

Cognitive Present   Cognitive Present

ca. 500 msec   ca. 500 msec

Behavior

Turn Head and Foveate   *Recognize Face*

Size of Assembly   Coherence in Gamma Band

% of Total   1.0

0.5

Topography of Synchrony

Figure 12.1
Varela's model of synchronous cell assemblies: cognitive states are associated with increased gamma band coherence resulting in binding of cell assemblies. The neural correlate of cognition is a time-varying "synchronous neural hypergraph" illustrated at the bottom of the diagram. Modified and reproduced from Varela (1995).

the stability and homeostasis of a system or organism. The law states that if these environmental perturbations are of great variety, then the system must have a matching variety of responses at its disposal with which to counter them in order to maintain internal stability. Ashby did not explicitly consider the importance of cooperative interactions among system components for maintaining robust responses. Yaneer Bar-Yam arrived at a generalized law of requisite variety by suggesting a trade-off between the variety of responses displayed by system components, analogous to modules, and scales of coordination (Bar-Yam, 2004). Networked systems can respond to challenges and perturbations with responses that range from minute to large-scale and often involve the coordinated action of several components to accomplish an adaptive task. An effective system maintains a variety of coordinated responses at each relevant scale while maintaining a balance between functional coupling and independence. Distributed control enhances this variety while centralized control limits it severely by constraining the variance of the system's response to the variance of the central controller. It has long been recognized that dynamic and hostile environments demand decentralized control (Galbraith, 1973; Anderson, 1999; Axelrod and Cohen, 1999). As we will see in the next chapter, the capacity of a brain-like system to perform a wide range of actions across multiple scales of organization can be quantified as its complexity and degeneracy.

After sketching out links between structural and functional connectivity in earlier chapters (chapters 8–10) we need to reemphasize that structural connections only constrain, but do not rigidly determine, functional interactions in the brain. This is particularly true for the patterns of dynamic coupling and coherence observed over short time scales. Over hundreds of milliseconds, functional coupling of neurons and brain regions exhibits significant variability, even in the course of spontaneous activity. These fluctuations occur despite the fact that the underlying structural anatomy remains fixed over the same time frame. What is the origin of this dynamic diversity, and how does it relate to the variety and flow of cognitive and mental states? Our discussion will lead us back to the idea of a "functional repertoire" of brain states as a potential substrate for higher cognition, and to the possibility that the brain exists in a critical state, delicately poised between random and regular behavior.

Dynamic Processes on Multiscale Network Architectures

Most complex networks are of interest to us because of the dynamic processes they sustain (Barrat et al., 2008). These dynamic processes manifest themselves in the global states and state transitions of cells, brains, ecosystems, power and transportation grids, collective social behavior, the Web, and the economy, to name but a few examples. Each network engages in characteristic types of dynamics, including diffusion, random walks, synchronization, information flow, search, vehicle traffic, energy flux, and the spreading of rumors, cultural innovations, or infectious disease. Each type of dynamics can be described and modeled, often with the goal of predicting the future time evolution of the global states of the system. In nearly all cases, the connection topology of the network plays an important role in the emergence of global or collective dynamic states.

This problem is particularly pressing in modeling and forecasting the local and global spread of infectious diseases.[2] Epidemic models are instructive examples of how information about the interactions and movements of people can inform the prediction of the potentially global impact of an emerging disease. As in the case of the brain, models of epidemics range from models of simple compartments that assume homogeneous mixing of individuals to models that incorporate hetero-geneous transmission rates and connectivity patterns on multiple spatial scales. Homogeneous models assume that all members of a population are perfectly mixed and interact uniformly, and they allow the analytic definition of an "epidemic threshold," determined by the relationship of the rates of disease spreading and recovery. However, the assumption of homogeneous mixing is fundamentally flawed as it fails to take into account social and geographical constraints on the movements and inter-actions of individuals. In addition, transportation networks at multiple scales, from commuting to global air travel, play a major role in determin-ing whether epidemic outbreaks remain local events or become global pandemics (Colizza et al., 2006). The heterogeneity of these networks requires numerical simulations of multiscale and/or agent-based models to improve the accuracy of epidemic forecasting (Colizza et al., 2007; Colizza and Vespignani, 2008; Balcan et al., 2009; Vespignani, 2009).

Heterogeneous coupling and multiscale dynamics are also ubiquitous features of the brain. Brain connectivity is organized on a hierarchy of scales from local circuits of neurons to modules of functional brain systems. Distinct dynamic processes on local and global scales generate multiple levels of segregation and integration and give rise to spatially differentiated patterns of coherence (Nunez, 2000). Neural dynamics at each scale is determined not only by processes at the same scale but also by the dynamics at smaller and larger scales (Breakspear and Stam, 2005). For example, the dynamics of a large neural population depend on the interactions among individual neurons unfolding at a smaller scale, as well as on the collective behavior of large-scale brain systems, and even on brain–body–environment interactions. Multiscale brain dynamics can be modeled through mean-field approaches that bridge neural microstructure and macroscale dynamics (Robinson et al., 2005)—for example, neural mass models (Deco et al., 2008). Mean-field models mainly address dynamic effects at one scale by averaging over the dynamics of components at smaller scales. However, truly multiscale or scale-free dynamics requires the consideration of a nested hierarchy of linear and nonlinear dependencies. One way to achieve a more complete understanding of such hierarchical interactions involves the use of wavelet transforms that explicitly model distinct spatial and temporal scales (Breakspear and Stam, 2005).

Heterogeneous, multiscale patterns of structural connectivity shape the functional interactions of neural units, the spreading of activation and the appearance of synchrony and coherence. Synchronization is thought to be an important mechanism for flexible binding of individual neurons into cell assemblies (see chapters 8 and 9), and thus the role of network topology in neuronal synchronization has been investigated in some detail. A number of studies have focused on the capacity of networks to become globally fully synchronized, a type of dynamics often seen in networks that are composed of uniformly connected, identical or noise-free oscillators. Networks with a completely regular lattice-like connection pattern are difficult to synchronize globally, and the admixture of randomized connections, a key feature of the small-world architecture of Watts and Strogatz (1998), generally facilitates global synchrony (Barahona and Pecora, 2002). This trend toward greater synchronizability in small-world networks has been observed in numerous studies, and it occurs largely independently of the details of the node dynamics that are employed in the model (Nishikawa et al., 2003; Buzsáki et al., 2004; Masuda and Aihara, 2004; Netoff et al., 2004; Roxin et al., 2004). Enhanced synchronizability in these models is mainly attributed to the decrease in path length, or increase in efficiency, induced by the small number of random shortcuts (long-range connections). Networks with fully randomized connectivity tend to exhibit even greater synchronizability but incur high connection cost due to many long axons (Buzsáki et al., 2004; see chapter 7). Disproportional communication load on hub nodes, however, can disrupt synchronization, leading Nishikawa et al. (2003) to suggest that decreases in path length need to be accompanied by balanced node degrees.

A more realistic situation arises when oscillators exhibit heterogeneous or broadened degree distributions, when they exhibit slight variations in their intrinsic parameters, or when they operate under the influence of noise in a weak coupling regime. Under these conditions, networks exhibit more complex synchronization behavior with partial coherence among changing subsets of nodes. Zhou and Kurths (2006) investigated the synchronization behavior of noisy nonidentical oscillators linked in networks with heterogeneous (scale-free) degree distributions and weak coupling. Heterogeneous networks showed hierarchical synchronization with high-degree nodes becoming most strongly synchronized and forming a dynamic "network core" that most closely reflected the global behavior and functional connectivity of the system. Other studies have confirmed that the network's degree distribution can affect the emergence of synchronized patterns. Moreno and Pacheco (2004) studied coupled scale-free networks of simple phase oscillators and found that the onset of synchronization could occur at very low values of a critical parameter related to coupling strength. Gómez-Gardeñes et al. (2007a; 2007b) demonstrated that synchronization in heterogeneous networks is driven by a core of highly connected hub nodes, while networks with homogeneous (Gaussian) degrees allow for the coexistence of several synchronization clusters reflecting structurally highly connected communities that gradually coalesce on the path to global synchrony. Synchronization behavior can be disturbed, resulting in pathological network states, as was demonstrated in a physiologically realistic model of the dentate gyrus (Morgan and Soltesz, 2008). Alterations in neural connectivity due to pathological processes can create highly connected cellular hubs whose presence renders the circuit prone to abnormally high levels of global synchronization corresponding to epileptic network states.

Synchronization models have been applied to study synchrony in large-scale structural connectivity patterns of the mammalian cerebral cortex. Zhou et al. (2006; 2007a; Zemanová et al., 2006) have investigated synchronization behavior of the connection matrix of the cat cortex (Scannell et al., 1999), known to be composed of several clusters of structurally related and linked cortical areas (Hilgetag and Kaiser, 2004; see chapter 6). In the weak coupling regime, synchronization patterns conformed to these structurally defined clusters and exhibited a hierarchically modular arrangement. Areas found to be crucial for intercluster functional linkage largely corresponded to structural hubs. A more detailed analysis of the cat cortex revealed dynamic behavior that is indicative of hierarchical modularity and was strongly shaped by the network's modular connectivity (Müller-Linow et al., 2008).

In addition to synchronization, the spreading of perturbations arising from local events within the nervous system or from external stimuli is directly influenced by the community structure of the multiscale network architecture (Wu et al., 2009). Local perturbations of clustered network architectures result in a repertoire of nonglobal dynamic activation states greater than that of comparable random networks, due to the relative isolation of clustered communities (Kaiser et al., 2007a; see figure 12.2). Hierarchically clustered networks produce limited yet sustained neural activity over a larger parameter range than equivalent single-scale small-world networks. Kaiser and colleagues have suggested that multilevel clustered network architectures naturally promote rich and stable

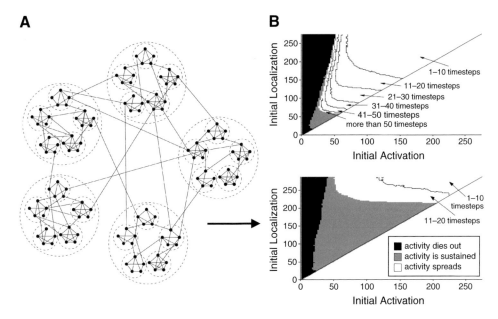

Figure 12.2
Hierarchical modularity and sustained network activation. (A) An example of a network
with hierarchical modularity. The network consists of five modules, which, in turn, can be
divided into five smaller modules each. The network has high clustering and a short path
length. (B) Summary plot of sustained network activity for a (nonmodular) small-world
network (top) and a network with hierarchical modularity (bottom) from Kaiser et al.
(2007a). Networks consist of 1,000 nodes and 12,000 edges and engage in simple spreading
dynamics. Simulation runs involved activating between 1 and 250 seed nodes ("initial
activation"), which were randomly spread out ("initial localization"). Dynamics were
allowed to proceed for 80 time steps, and activity at the end of this time period either had
died out (black region), had spread throughout the network (white region), or was sustained at intermediate levels (gray region). Note that the area of sustained activity is significantly larger for the hierarchical modular as compared to the nonmodular small-world
network. Reproduced from Kaiser et al. (2007a) with permission.

dynamic behavior reminiscent of criticality (see below). In support of
this idea, computational models of hierarchical "fractal" connectivity
were shown to exhibit high dynamic complexity and a great variety of
functional motifs (Sporns, 2006). These dynamic features were tightly
correlated with the appearance of structural small-world attributes in a
fractal connectivity pattern, suggesting that they emerge together.

   A recurrent theme in studies of collective behavior in complex networks, from epidemic to brain models, is its dependence on the network's
multiscale architecture, its nested levels of clustered communities. The
functional significance of the hierarchical nature of the brain's structural
and functional connectivity is still largely unexplored. Computational

studies suggest that nested hierarchies promote structured and diverse dynamics. An additional level of diversity results from activity-dependent plasticity and structural alterations at the level of cells and synapses. Dynamic processes are not only shaped by network topology but also actively participate in the carving of structural connection patterns during development (see chapter 11) and in the continual adjustment of synaptic weights. Hence, dynamic diversity is likely accompanied by an as yet unknown level of diversity in synaptic patterns.

Neural Transients, Metastability, and Coordination Dynamics

Neuronal activity unfolds on multiple time scales from fast synaptic processes in the millisecond range to dynamic states that can persist for several seconds to long-lasting changes in neural interactions due to plasticity. Over time, neural activity and behavior display variability which can be due to a variety of sources. Some of these sources are considered "noise," because they give rise to random fluctuations and do not form "part of a signal" (Faisal et al., 2008), for example, the stochastic openings and closings of ion channels or subthreshold fluctuations in cellular membrane potentials. Much of neuronal variability, however, is not due to noise in molecular or cellular components but is the result of the deterministic behavior of the brain as a coupled system. This variability makes significant contributions to neuronal signals and is ultimately expressed in variable cognitive states and behavioral performance. For example, the ongoing fluctuations of endogenous neural activity that are characteristic of the brain's resting state have been shown to account for a significant part of the trial-to-trial variability of behavioral responses (see chapter 8), and variable dynamics on multiple time scales is readily seen in large-scale computational models (Honey et al., 2007). What is the extent of this variability, how can we characterize it, and what are the network mechanisms by which it is generated?

Brain dynamics is inherently variable and "labile," consisting of sequences of transient spatiotemporal patterns that mediate perception and cognition (Kelso, 1995; Friston, 2000; Rabinovich et al., 2006). These sequences of transients are a hallmark of dynamics that are neither entirely stable nor completely unstable and instead may be called metastable. Metastable dynamics unfolds on an attractor that forms a complex manifold with many mutually joined "pockets" that slow or entrap the system's trajectory and thus create its intermittent, quasi-stable temporal behavior (see figure 12.3). Such a manifold may be visualized as a surface

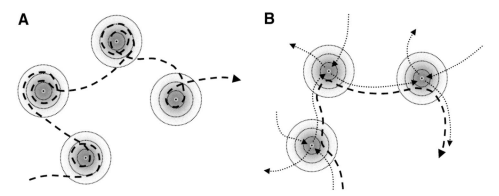

Figure 12.3
Metastability and heteroclinic channels. Both diagrams visualize the time evolution of a
system state in phase space (hatched arrow). In panel (A) the system's attractor manifold
has numerous weakly or marginally stable states. These "pockets" trap the system's motion
temporarily until a small perturbation results in a transition to another nearby pocket. In
panel (B) metastable states are created by linked saddle points in the attractor that channel
the trajectory along a sequence that is determined by the linkage of the heteroclinic skeleton. The system is able to describe reproducible sequences of metastable states and is, at
the same time, sensitive to external perturbations that can result in switching between
channels. Panel (B) modified and redrawn after Rabinovich et al. (2008a).

with numerous shallow indentations or wells. An object that moves along
the surface will fall into a well, where it becomes trapped for a while
before jumping out again. The wells represent metastable states that are
occupied for some time, but not permanently, and that may be visited
repeatedly. The transitions between these metastable states occur in
intervals that are typically much longer than the elementary time constants of any of the system's components. In simulated neural systems,
metastability is associated with sparse extrinsic connections that link
modules or clusters, and its dynamics can be characterized by the entropy
of its spectral density (Friston, 1997).

The concept of metastability is related to "chaotic itinerancy" (Kaneko
and Tsuda, 2003), the itinerant or roaming motion of the trajectory of a
high-dimensional system among varieties of ordered states. Chaotic itinerancy is found in a number of physical systems that are globally coupled,
that are far from equilibrium, or that engage in turbulent flow, for
example, coupled electrochemical oscillators, lasers, and chaotic fluid and
atmospheric dynamics. It has also been observed in brain recordings
(Freeman, 2003) and neural network models (Raffone and van Leeuwen,
2003). Over time, systems exhibiting chaotic itinerancy alternate
between ordered low-dimensional motion within a dynamically unstable

"attractor ruin" and high-dimensional chaotic transitions. System variables are coherently coupled, their dynamics slow down during ordered motion, and they transiently lose coherence as the system trajectory rapidly moves between attractor ruins.

Another way to create metastable and transient dynamics involves configurations of so-called saddle points connected together into chains forming a network within a dynamic manifold (Afraimovich et al., 2004; Rabinovich et al., 2008a; see figure 12.3). Because of the nature of saddle points, a trajectory traversing this space will be both attracted and repelled by these structures and slow down in their immediate vicinity. The trajectory spontaneously transitions between saddle points that are "nearby" in state space and interconnected. These interconnected saddle points form "stable heteroclinic channels" that determine sequences of transient states. The arrangement of metastable states along these channels allows for robust and reliable sequences of neural states following a stimulus-evoked response. Rabinovich et al. (2008a) have investigated neural implementations of heteroclinic channels as a possible model for cognitive processes such as sequential decision making. The existence of heteroclinic channels depends on certain required attributes of structural connectivity, for example, asymmetrical coupling.

Neural computations as unique sequences of transient states triggered by inputs present an alternative to more classical models of computation with fixed-point attractors that cannot easily account for variable brain dynamics (Rabinovich et al., 2008b). Wolfgang Maass proposed the idea of "liquid-state computing" as a model of neural processing based on trajectories in state space instead of fixed points (Maass et al., 2002). The term "liquid state" expresses an analogy with the physical properties of an excitable medium, such as a liquid, that can be transiently perturbed, with each perturbation leaving a characteristic dynamic trace. Liquid-state machines rely on the dynamics of transient perturbations for real-time computing, unlike standard attractor networks, which compute in sequences of discrete states. Applied to the brain, the model is based on the intrinsic and high-dimensional transient dynamics generated by heterogeneous recurrent neural circuits from which information about past and present inputs can be extracted. The model can be implemented in a generic neural microcircuit (Legenstein and Maass, 2007). Haeusler et al. (2009) investigated the computational performance and connectivity structure of two different cortical microcircuit templates and found that despite differences in the connection topology, both circuit models showed similar computational capabilities. A critical feature for achieving high computational performance was the degree distribution of the circuits. These and other models of transient state dynamics offer a plausible set of mechanisms for self-sustained computation in the nervous system (Gros, 2009).

Scott Kelso developed the theoretical framework of "coordination dynamics" to account for the self-organizing nature of both brain and behavior (Kelso, 1995; Bressler and Kelso, 2001). In this framework, coordination, defined as the functional ordering among interacting components, and its dynamics, which combines stability and transformation, are essential elements of brain and cognition. Cognitive dynamics depends upon the coupling and uncoupling of sets of brain regions, patterns of coordination that evolve through time. Bressler and Kelso (2001) describe these processes with the language and tools of dynamic systems. Phase relations between regions capture their temporal ordering and interrelationships and serve as state variables that describe the collective dynamics of the system. The relative, time-varying coordination of brain areas reflects local and global features of the cortical architecture and gives rise to metastable dynamics. Metastability reconciles functional segregation and integration in the brain, by accounting for the tendency of individual system components to express their autonomy, as well as their synergistic behavior (Kelso and Tognoli, 2007). Coordination dynamics places special importance on metastable regimes and interregional phase relationships. Tognoli and Kelso (2009) examined the dynamic signatures of metastability in noninvasive electrophysiological recordings, and they developed new analytic techniques that allow the unambiguous detection of metastable episodes and phase locking in EEG.

Relative phase between local oscillators represents an important collective variable that can characterize the dynamics of both brain and behavior (Kelso, 1995). Collective variables that govern the coordinated behavior of interacting components are important ingredients in coordination dynamics. Their creation effectively involves a reduction in the dimensionality of the system. Integration of system components through coordination eliminates most available degrees of freedom and leaves only a few that are relevant and needed to describe the system's structure and time evolution. Thus, coordination greatly "simplifies" complexity. Several connectional features of brain networks promote dimension reduction. One example is the existence of modules which blend together functional contributions from within their membership and compete with those of other modules. The first process is more consistent with phase synchrony or coherence while the second results in phase dispersion or scattering. Modules define the major axes of a low-dimensional dynamic space or manifold which is traversed by the dynamic trajectory of the system in continual cycles of transience and stability.

Persistent variability raises a number of important issues for our interpretation of dynamic brain networks. Clearly, patterns of coordination are time dependent on fast time scales (hundreds of milliseconds). Functional brain networks engage in fast transitions between metastable states that result from their own intrinsic dynamics and are not necessarily driven by external influences. Each metastable state can be characterized as a set of functional relationships between system elements, described by a functional network. Transitions between these states therefore result in switches between networks and, thus, in fluctuations of network properties of nodes and edges. In the large-scale model of Honey et al. (2007), the attractor dynamics resulted in fast-time scale fluctuations of connectivity and a large repertoire of functional networks that were visited over time. These transitions also caused fluctuations of key functional network measures such as small-world attributes and centrality. Hub nodes expressed their global influence over the network in a time-dependent manner. Whether such temporal modulations of network properties on fast time scales accompany transitions between empirically observed metastable neural states is an interesting but open question.

Can dynamic diversity explain the flexibility of cognition? An important piece of evidence that supports this idea comes from an analysis of brain signal variability across developmental stages from children to adults. McIntosh et al. (2008) found increased variability in the brains of adults as compared to children and a negative correlation of this brain variability with the variability of behavioral performance. As brain and behavior become more mature, more stability in behavioral performance was accompanied by an increase in the variability of neural activity. In this study, greater functional variability and a larger repertoire of metastable functional states are found to be associated with more mature cognitive capacities.

Power Laws and Criticality

Rapid transitions in global patterns of functional correlations have been observed in numerous electrophysiological studies, in both task-evoked and spontaneous neural activity. Spontaneous fluctuations in amplitude and coherence exhibit "heavy-tail" or power-law distributions, scale invariance across multiple frequencies, and transient long-range correlations.[3] One of the first reports of scale-free phenomena in cortical potentials found long-range correlations and power-law scaling of amplitude fluctuations in MEG and EEG recordings (Linkenkaer-Hansen et al., 2001). Walter Freeman reported the occurrence of episodes of intermittent phase locking at scales from millimeters to that of an entire cortical hemisphere in spontaneous human EEG recordings (Freeman, 2003). Gong et al. (2003) recorded episodes of scale-invariant intermittent phase synchrony in human EEG. Stam and de Bruin (2004) detected scale-free distributions of global synchronization time in recordings of spontaneous EEG across several frequencies, ranging from the fast gamma to the slow delta band. Multiple studies have demonstrated the alternating occurrence of periods of phase shift or reset and phase synchrony or stability, with reset occurring typically within less than 100 milliseconds and periods of stability ranging from 100 milliseconds to seconds (Freeman et al., 2006; Rudrauf et al., 2006). Perturbations of ongoing fluctuations modify their scale-free characteristics by reducing the power-law exponent and diminishing long-range temporal correlations (Linkenkaer-Hansen et al., 2004).

What is the origin of power-law fluctuations in cortical potentials? Several authors have attributed power laws in cortical dynamics to the existence of a self-organized critical state. Per Bak and colleagues (Bak et al., 1987) suggested that complex behavior of dynamic and spatially extended systems can emerge spontaneously, as a result of the system's own self-organization. The system's complex behavior is characterized by scale-invariant fractal properties in its spatial patterning as well as scale-free distributions of dynamic events. Bak called this regime "self-organized criticality" (SOC) because systems naturally evolve toward this state and exhibit a fine balance of robust interactions and sensitivity to perturbations. A classic example is a pile of sand. As more and more grains of sand are added to the pile, it will grow and its slope will at first increase, until it reaches a critical value. At this "angle of repose" the addition of more grains of sand cannot increase the angle further. Instead, avalanches will occur that continually restore the critical angle. These avalanches come in all sizes, and their distribution follows a power law. When it occupies this type of dynamical regime, the system is said to display "critical" behavior. Importantly, in the case of the sandpile, the system reaches this critical state on its own, without the need for external tuning or parameter adjustment. The system maintains this critical behavior indefinitely by continually restoring the balance between its internal structure and external perturbations. Other physical systems can be tuned to show critical behavior by setting a single control parameter, such as the temperature in the Ising model of spin magnetization (see figure 12.4).

A critical state is reached when a system evolving from an ordered into a disordered state approaches the "edge of chaos." Chris Langton (1990) studied cellular automata in ordered, critical, and chaotic dynamic regimes, and concluded that the computational capacity of these automata was greatest at the border between order and chaos, in a critical state.[4] Models of interaction networks of cellular proteins (Kauffman, 1993) also exhibited self-organized criticality, as did a number of neuronal network models (see below). The diversity of these models raised the intriguing possibility that SOC could explain the spontaneous emergence and stability of complex modes of organization in a wide variety of systems (Bak, 1996). All of the modeled systems exhibiting SOC shared certain attributes, for example, the existence of scale-free distributions of dynamic events (often called avalanches in keeping with the example of the sandpile), the presence of a phase transition taking the system from an ordered to a disordered regime, and the spontaneous and robust evolution toward criticality without the need to adjust or fine-tune system parameters.

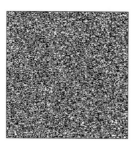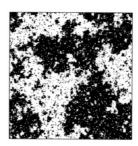

Figure 12.4
The Ising model. Individual elements arranged in a two-dimensional grid have a magnetic moment or spin, pointing up or down (black and white in the figure). Nearest neighbors on the grid interact with each other, and there is a tendency for neighboring spins to become aligned. Pairs of same orientation lower the system's overall potential energy, while pairs of unequal orientation increase it. The model is statistical in nature, and the energy function is temperature dependent. At high temperatures, the system is more disordered, and as the temperature is lowered, the system transitions from a disordered to an ordered state by way of a phase transition at the critical temperature. The figure shows a 200×200 grid of spin configurations obtained at high, critical, and low temperatures (left to right). At or near the critical temperature, fluctuating patterns persist for a long time and occur at all spatial scales.

Dante Chialvo and Per Bak suggested that self-organized criticality was a plausible model for adaptation and dynamic diversity in the brain (Chialvo and Bak, 1999; Bak and Chialvo, 2001). Empirical evidence for SOC in neuronal networks came from the work of John Beggs and Dietmar Plenz, who examined spontaneous patterns of neuronal activity recorded with microelectrode arrays from slices of rat cortex (Beggs and Plenz, 2003; see figure 12.5). Sequences of propagating spikes emitted during spontaneous neural activity form "neuronal avalanches" whose

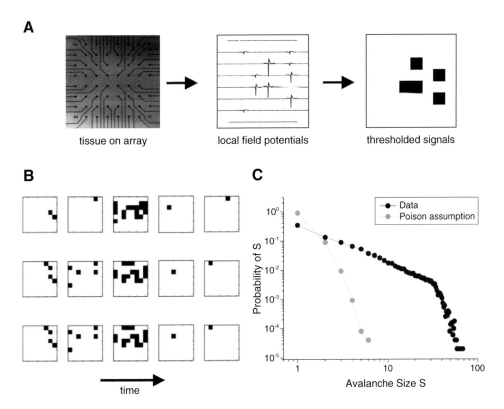

Figure 12.5
Neuronal avalanches. (A) Multielectrode recording array with 60 electrodes, an example of field potential traces and thresholded activity pattern. (B) Three sequences of activity patterns, each forming a neuronal avalanche. These three examples form a family of repeating avalanches, which may recur over time periods of up to several hours. The avalanche size is the total number of active nodes (electrodes) over one instance. (C) The distribution of avalanche sizes follows a power law, with a cutoff near the limit of system size (for another example of a power law, see figure 2.4). Data from larger recording arrays show a more extended range of the scale-free regime. Note that shuffled data (Poisson) do not follow a power law. Images from Beggs (2007), modified and reproduced with permission.

size distribution follows a power law.[5] The continual integration and redistribution of neuronal impulses can be represented as a critical branching process. Beggs and Plenz found that slice preparations of rat cortex operate at or near criticality. In the critical regime, the branching parameter expressing the ratio of descendant spikes from ancestor spikes is near unity, such that a triggering event causes a long sequence of spikes that neither dies out quickly (subcritical) nor grows explosively (supercritical). Neuronal avalanches, while lasting only for a few milliseconds, are often repeated several times over time periods of minutes to hours (Beggs and Plenz, 2004). This repeatability of avalanches suggests that they might play a role in information storage and that they form a stably reproducible repertoire of diverse patterns across multiple spatial scales (Plenz and Thiagarajan, 2007).

The critical dynamic regime has many properties that are highly desirable for neural information-processing systems. Modeling of branching processes demonstrated that criticality is associated with maximal information transfer (Beggs and Plenz, 2003) and thus with high efficiency of neuronal information processing. The critical regime also sustains a maximal number of metastable dynamical states (Haldeman and Beggs, 2005).[6] The parallel existence of many attractor states maximizes the network's capacity to store information. In addition, the critical regime allows neural systems to respond with optimal sensitivity and dynamic range to exogenous perturbations (Kinouchi and Copelli, 2006). "Liquid-state" recurrent neural networks can perform complex computations only at or near the critical boundary separating ordered and chaotic dynamics (Bertschinger and Natschläger, 2004; see figure 12.6). Furthermore, power-law distributions of size and duration of neuronal avalanches are indicative of long-range correlations across all spatial scales in the system. The critical state thus ensures that the system can access a very wide and diverse state space or functional repertoire.

If the critical state is indeed privileged in regard to information processing and dynamic diversity, then how might neural systems reach this state and how might they tune themselves in a self-organized manner to maintain it? Simple models of network growth result in a convergence of the network topology toward characteristic critical values (Bornholdt and Rohlf, 2000; Bornholdt and Röhl, 2003). Other modeling studies suggest that neural plasticity may play an important role in generating and maintaining the critical state. For example, a spiking neural network model with dynamic synapses was found to exhibit robustly self-organized critical behavior (Levina et al., 2007). A form of plasticity that

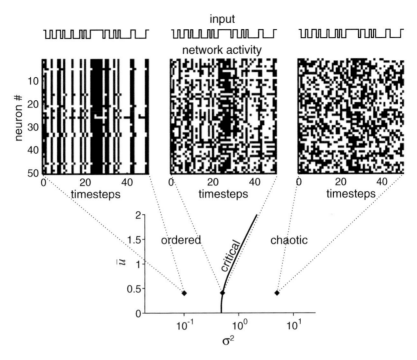

Figure 12.6
Computation at the edge of chaos. The diagram shows examples of the time evolution of a randomly connected network of simple threshold neurons, for three different settings of two parameters. Varying one of these parameters, the variance σ^2 of the network's nonzero connection weights, results in qualitatively different types of network dynamics, taking the system through a phase transition from an ordered to a critical to a chaotic regime (left to right). Corresponding time series for a single fixed input sequence are shown at the top. Note that in the ordered state the system largely follows the current input state while in the chaotic regime even small changes in input result in large variations in response. The ordered system quickly "forgets" about previous states while the chaotic system is extremely sensitive to even small fluctuations in the past. Networks in the critical regime combine memory of the past with sensitivity to current input. Reproduced from Bertschinger and Natschläger (2004) with permission.

is sensitive to the relative timing of presynaptic and postsynaptic responses, called spike-timing-dependent plasticity, can mold the connectivity structure of a globally connected neuronal network into a scale-free small-world network that resides in a critical dynamic regime (Shin and Kim, 2006). Even after the critical state is attained, spontaneous activity results in fluctuations in synaptic weights while global distributions of connection weights remain stable. Hsu and Beggs (2006) designed a neural model that converged on a critical dynamic regime through synaptic plasticity. Plastic changes accrued as a result of a homeostatic mechanism that preserved firing rate, resulting in network behavior that converged onto criticality and was stable against perturbations. Siri et al. (2008) investigated the effect of Hebbian plasticity on the capacity of a random recurrent neural network to learn and retrieve specific patterns. Plasticity results in profound changes of network behavior, leading the network from chaotic to fixed-point dynamics through a series of bifurcations. The sensitivity of the network to input is greatest while it occupies a critical regime "at the edge of chaos." The authors suggest that additional mechanisms of homeostatic plasticity may serve to stabilize the system within this functionally important state.

The relationship between SOC in neuronal networks and their structural connection topology remains largely unresolved. A variety of growth, rewiring, or plasticity rules can give rise to SOC behavior, but it is unclear if SOC can occur regardless of connection topology, or whether some network architectures selectively promote its occurrence. Pajevic and Plenz (2009) have suggested an association between avalanche dynamics and small-world connectivity. Introducing a novel algorithm for the inference of directed functional networks from physiological recordings, they demonstrated that neuronal avalanches in slice cultures of rat cortex form functional networks with a large excess in clustering and a small network diameter, consistent with a small-world topology.

Evidence for the existence of a critical state in large-scale neural systems also comes from EEG/MEG and fMRI recordings of human brain activity. The presence of power-law distributions of coherent states or transients (see above) may be viewed as supporting the existence of a critical state, although it does not necessarily indicate the presence of a phase transition or a critical branching process. In a multiscale analysis of human MEG data during cognitive rest and task-evoked activity, Bassett et al. (2006) found evidence for a fractal self-similar organization of functional brain connectivity. Functional networks exhibited consistent topological characteristics over a broad range of frequencies, from fast (100 Hz) to ultraslow (0.1 Hz), indicative of a fractal organization of network topology across multiple frequency ranges. In addition, an analysis of dynamical properties, particularly the level of synchronizability, strongly suggested that the observed networks operated at or close to the boundary between a subcritical and supercritical regime.

Further evidence for critical dynamics in the human brain comes from MEG and fMRI data obtained during the resting state. Kitzbichler et al. (2009) obtained distributions of pairwise phase-lock intervals and the lability of global synchronization for simple computational models as well as for empirical brain recordings. Phase locking between pairs of units or recording sites showed highly variable interaction lengths and, like global synchronization measures, exhibited power-law scaling in both models and empirical data.[7] This scaling behavior was seen across a broad range of frequencies, from <0.1 Hz to >100 Hz, and in MEG as well as fMRI recordings, indicating that these observations are independent of the frequency range or the nature of the physiological signal. "Broadband criticality" may promote rapid changes in phase synchrony, flexible response to external perturbations, and high capacity for information transmission and storage across multiple frequency bands at once. Fraiman et al. (2009) have compared various statistical properties of networks extracted from a two-dimensional Ising model of magnetic spin coupling near the critical temperature to those obtained from human resting-state fMRI and concluded that these two sets of networks were virtually indistinguishable. The Ising model is a well-studied example of a coupled system undergoing a phase transition and exhibiting critical dynamics, and the observed similarity of this system with brain functional networks is seen to support the existence of critical brain dynamics. Poil et al. (2008) have compared temporal statistics of human MEG recordings with a model of a critical branching process. The model supported a link between the distribution of fluctuating bursts of alpha-frequency activity and sequences of neural transients generated in the model. Interestingly, the model could not account for very long time scale temporal correlations between burst events observed in the empirical data. This indicates that branching models can reproduce some (but not all) temporal characteristics of spontaneous MEG activity.

Taken together, these observations imply that transient patterns of synchrony, like those envisioned in Francisco Varela's theoretical proposal discussed at the beginning of this chapter, are an abundant feature of human brain dynamics. These transient patterns can occur over multiple time scales, with particularly broad distributions during spontaneous neural activity (see also Freeman, 2007). Their scaling behavior and characteristics of the dynamics within which they reside are at least highly suggestive of an underlying self-organized critical regime in the brain, possibly at multiple scales from neurons to systems (Werner, 2007). However, current evidence is still incomplete, and other explanations for power-law scaling have to be considered as well. Power laws can arise in many different living and nonliving systems and as a result of numerous processes of varying degree of "complexity" (Newman, 2005). For example, power laws are a prominent feature of systems that are in a state of turbulence. Initial studies suggest that turbulence is insufficient to explain power-law dynamics as recorded in the brain (Suckling et al., 2008). Other authors have suggested that the appearance of power laws in physiological recordings of brain activity could be the result of "simple" phenomena such as broadband or filtered noise in neural activity (Bédard et al., 2006; Milstein et al., 2009) and is thus not necessarily reflective of critical dynamics. Clearly, much additional work is needed to define the conditions and range of critical behavior in neural systems.

How Essential Is Dynamic Diversity?

The picture of neural dynamics drawn in this chapter is substantially different from that of most "standard" models of neural computation that place much greater emphasis on serial processing, noise-free signal transmission, and reliable encoding and retrieval of information. Such models have been remarkably successful in well-defined problem domains and in the absence of conflicting or competing demands. In contrast, the computational capacity of network models incorporating dynamic transients, coordination dynamics, or criticality is still relatively unexplored. Yet, these phenomena seem to pervade neural dynamics at all scales, from cellular avalanches to large-scale power-law distributions of synchrony and coherence. Initial indications are that the dynamic diversity expressed when a neural system is in the critical state has numerous computational advantages, including high information transmission and storage capacity. Only when operating at or near the critical point can neural systems preserve and transmit information about a stimulus or environmental perturbation over long periods of time since critical networks can sustain long and diverse neural transients (Kinouchi and Copelli, 2006).[8] In contrast, subcritical and supercritical systems possess a much more compressed dynamical range of responses. Criticality may thus be a preferred dynamic regime, especially when considered in relation to an environment that consists of a mixture of randomness and regularity, perhaps residing in its own critical regime.

While some authors have suggested that critical dynamics are favored by certain connection topologies, the relation between structural connection patterns and dynamic diversity is far from understood. In a neural system, its metastable itinerant motion and the linkages in state space between weakly stable or unstable attractors are determined in large part by the pattern of structural connections. These connections effectively constrain and shape the system's trajectory, and its responses to external perturbations. A plausible hypothesis is that clustered and modular connectivity promotes the reduction of the system's dimensionality by contracting the region of the state space it can access. Modular connectivity may thus give rise to a dynamic small world of attractor ruins (or saddle points) linked by bridges or channels that allow for the system to transition between its available metastable states in few steps. Hub regions may be instrumental in triggering transitions of the system between low-dimensional and high-dimensional states and guiding its trajectory from channel to channel.

Power-law scaling is not only found in the brain but is also a pervasive feature of variations in human behavior. Evidence for scaling, coordination, and dimension reduction are found in behavioral activity such as limb movements, locomotion, and speech, as well as cognitive processes such as visual search, mental rotation, and word naming (Kelso, 1995; Kello et al., 2007). Chris Kello and colleagues have argued that power-law scaling of behavioral variables such as fluctuations in the acoustic characteristics of a spoken word are due to metastability and that this metastability reveals the origin of cognition in the organization and reorganization of spatiotemporal patterns of brain, body, and environment (Kello et al., 2008). This attractive hypothesis offers the potential for a deep conceptual linkage between neural dynamics and behavioral/cognitive processes. Yet, the mechanistic basis of power-law scaling in behavior and cognition is still relatively unexplored, and there is much work still to be done before alternative explanations for the appearance of scaling and power laws in terms of stochastic noise, filtering, or physiological artifacts can be ruled out.

Bearing in mind these caveats, there is much converging evidence to suggest that metastability and relative coordination, finely balanced between segregation and integration, is a defining feature of the complexity of brain and behavior. The remaining chapters of this book will bring this essential quality of neural complexity and its manifestation in embodied systems into sharper focus. First, let us try to clarify what it means for a system such as the brain to be complex, and why complexity matters.

13   Neural Complexity

One path to the construction of a nontrivial theory of complex systems is by way of a theory of hierarchy. Empirically a large proportion of the complex systems we observe in nature exhibit hierarchic structure. On theoretical grounds we could expect complex systems to be hierarchies in a world in which complexity had to evolve from simplicity. In their dynamics, hierarchies have a property, near decomposability, that greatly simplifies their behavior.[1]
—Herbert Simon, 1962

Most readers would probably agree with the statement that the brain is extraordinarily complex. However, there is considerably less agreement as to how complexity can be defined or measured in the brain or elsewhere. So far, it has proven difficult to identify a common theoretical foundation for the many manifestations of complexity in systems as diverse as societies, cells, or brains, and the existence of a general theory of complexity is still in question.[2] Nevertheless, it is undeniable that many complex systems have certain common characteristics, one of which is a mode of organization that is reminiscent of "hierarchical modularity" (see chapters 9 and 12). As Herbert Simon noted in 1962, many complex systems are hierarchically organized and composed of interrelated subsystems, which themselves may have hierarchical structure (Simon, 1962), defined by nested clusters of strong or dense interactions. Importantly, interactions within subsystems are stronger than interactions among subsystems, thus rendering the system "nearly decomposable" into independent components. In such nearly decomposable systems, "the short-run behavior of each of the component subsystems is approximately independent of the short-run behavior of the other components," and "in the long run the behavior of any one of the components depends in only an aggregate way on the behavior of the other components" (Simon, 1962, p. 474).

Simon pointed out that in complex systems "the whole is more than the sum of the parts" such that "given the properties of the parts and the laws of their interaction, it is not a trivial matter to infer the properties of the whole" (Simon, 1962, p. 468). All complex systems contain numerous components that engage in organized interactions and give rise to "emergent" phenomena. These phenomena cannot be reduced to properties of the components. Reductionist approaches have only limited success when applied to complex biological systems. For example, a recent review on cellular networks states that "the reductionist approach has successfully identified most of the components and many interactions but, unfortunately, offers no convincing concepts and methods to comprehend how system properties emerge" (Sauer et al., 2007, p. 550). The authors continue to propose that "[…] the pluralism of causes and effects in biological networks is better addressed by observing, through quantitative measures, multiple components simultaneously, and by rigorous data integration with mathematical models," the research program of the emerging discipline of systems biology (Kitano, 2002). The highly interconnected, hierarchical, and dynamic nature of biological systems poses a significant experimental and theoretical challenge, one that is not adequately addressed by the reductionist paradigm. However, what exactly is complexity, and how can it help us to better understand the structure and function of nervous systems? Complexity describes systems that are composed of a large number and a great variety of components. In addition, complexity refers to a mode of organized interaction, a functional coherence that transcends the intrinsic capacities of each individual component. The pervasiveness of complexity in the brain raises the question of whether a better understanding of complexity offers important clues about the nature of brain function (Koch and Laurent, 1999) and whether it can inform us about how nervous systems are structurally and functionally organized.

Here I argue that the union or coexistence of segregation and integration expressed in the multiscale dynamics of brain networks is the origin of neural complexity. Once I have developed an intuitive understanding of complexity, I will attempt to define it more formally on the basis of how information is distributed and organized in the brain. While this definition of complexity depends mostly on statistical aspects of neural interactions, one may ask if there are specific patterns or motifs in structural connectivity that favor or enable the emergence of highly complex dynamic patterns. I will identify some candidates for such structural patterns and compare them to our current knowledge of how brains are anatomically organized. Finally, I will examine the relationship of neural complexity to consciousness and will explore the potential evolutionary origins of complexity in the brain.

What Is Complexity?

While there is much ongoing discussion about how complexity should be mathematically defined and measured in real systems, there is some agreement across different problem domains and fields of science about the ingredients that are shared by most, if not all, complex systems. First, as discussed by Herbert Simon, most complex systems can be decomposed into components and interactions, possibly on several hierarchical levels. Second, complexity is a mixture of order and disorder, or regularity and randomness, which together account for the nontrivial, non-repeating nature of complex structures and their diverse dynamics (see chapter 12).

The components of complex systems are structural elements that have some autonomy and are capable of generating local behavior mostly determined by their intrinsic processes. If these components can be further subdivided into smaller elements, they give rise to multiple hierarchical levels. For a system composed of such elements to be capable of complex behavior, the behavior of individual components must partly depend on that of other elements in the system, that is, the system must be "nearly decomposable" with "weak links" between components that can serve as the basis for system-wide coordination and emergence. The brain is a good example of a system that consists of components nested across multiple hierarchical levels, including neurocognitive networks, individual brain regions, specialized neural populations, and single neurons.[3]

Interactions between components integrate or bind together their individual activities into an organized whole. They create dependencies between components, and they also affect the component's individual actions and behaviors. Interactions are often shaped by structured communication paths or connections. These connections can vary in their sparseness and strength, and their specific pattern has an important role in determining the collective behavior of the system. Different network topologies can give rise to qualitatively different global system states. In the brain, interactions are relayed by structural connections, and they can be further modulated intrinsically by diffuse chemical signals or extrinsically by statistical relationships in environmental stimuli.

The interactions of components in a nearly, but not fully, decomposable system generate phenomena that cannot be reduced to or predicted from the properties of the individual components considered in isolation. Sequences of amino acids in peptide chains give rise to three-dimensional folding patterns of proteins that determine their functional properties. Predation and competition among species control their survival and reproduction within ecosystems. Geographic dispersion, specialization of skills, and social stratification of individual humans shape their societal and economic organization. These emergent phenomena cannot be fully explained by dissecting the system into components, nor can their full functionality be revealed by an examination of isolated components or interactions alone. In many cases, different levels of scale interact. Local coupling shapes emergent global states of the system, which in turn can modify the internal structure of components or reconfigure their interactions.[4]

While there is general agreement that complex systems contain numerous components whose structured interactions generate emergent phenomena, their empirical observation poses many challenges. Systematic observation of complex systems requires that the system be sensibly partitioned into components and interactions whose states can be tracked over time. Defining components and interactions, or nodes and edges in the language of complex networks, requires a number of choices about relevant spatial and temporal scales, resolution, or empirical recording methods, all of which can influence the nature of the reconstructed observed dynamics (see chapter 3). This subtle but important point is often neglected. Unlike idealized systems such as cellular automata or spin glasses, where the elementary components and their interactions are exactly defined, most real-world systems contain components that blend into each other, form nested hierarchies, come into or go out of existence, and engage in dynamics on multiple time scales. In such systems, choices about how components are defined and observed must be carefully justified, because they can impact the computation and interpretation of network or complexity measures.

Measuring Complexity: Randomness and Organization

Despite broad agreement on some of the defining features of complexity, there is currently no general way to measure or estimate the complexity of an empirically observed system. Numerous complexity measures have been defined, usually within the context of a specific application or problem domain (Lloyd, 2001; Sporns, 2007; Mitchell, 2009). This heterogeneity reflects the nascent state of the field of complexity theory, as well as real differences in the way complexity is conceptualized in physical, biological, or social systems. Measures of complexity define a common metric that allows different systems or different instantiations of the same system at different points in time to be compared to one another. Such comparisons make sense only for systems that are structurally or functionally related. For example, a comparison of the complexity of two nervous systems in different states of endogenous or evoked activity may reveal meaningful differences in their dynamic organization while it makes little sense to quantitatively compare the complexity of a cell phone network with that of a network of interacting proteins.

There are two main categories of complexity measures. Measures in one category measure complexity by how difficult it is to describe or build a given system. Within this category, measures of complexity based on description length generally quantify the degree of randomness, and while they have had significant applications in physics and computation, they are less interesting in a biological and neural context. One of these measures, algorithmic information content, defines complexity as the amount of information contained in a string of symbols (Chaitin, 1977). This information can be measured by the length of the shortest computer program that generates the string. Symbol strings that are regular or periodic can be computed by short programs and thus contain little information (low complexity) while random strings can only be generated by a program that is as long as the string itself and are, thus, maximally complex. Other measures of complexity such as logical depth (Bennett, 1988) or thermodynamic depth (Lloyd and Pagels, 1988) are related to algorithmic information content in that they become maximal for systems that are "hard to build" or whose future state is difficult to predict. Thus, these measures evaluate the length or cost of a system's generative process rather than its actual dynamics or its responses to perturbations.

A second category of complexity measures captures the degree to which a system is organized or the "amount of interesting structure" it contains, and these measures are highly relevant in the context of biological and neural systems. Several different measures exist within this category, and most of them have in common that they place complexity somewhere in between order and disorder (see figure 13.1; Huberman and Hogg, 1986). In other words, complex systems combine some degree of randomness and disorganized behavior with some degree of order and

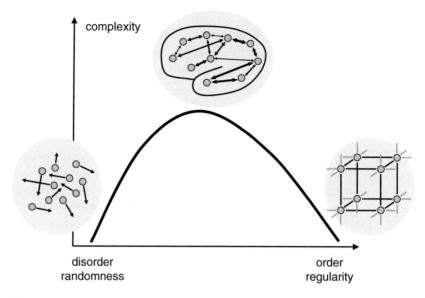

Figure 13.1
Complexity as a mixture of order and disorder. This schematic diagram illustrates different levels of complexity present in highly disordered systems ("gas"), highly ordered systems ("crystal"), and systems that combine elements of order and disorder ("brain").

regularity. Complexity is high when order and disorder coexist, and low when one or the other prevails. How do order and disorder manifest themselves in a neural context? One way to create a neural system that is highly disordered is to isolate its components from one another so that each of them acts independently. In such a system, all components only express their own response preferences and are maximally specialized (segregated). A neural system that is highly ordered might be one where all components are strongly coupled to one another to the point where the system becomes fully synchronized and integrated. In this case, the interactions have overwhelmed any local specialization and the system acts as if it were composed of only one independent component. Clearly, neither of these extreme cases of order and disorder corresponds to the type of organization seen in any real nervous system. Instead, a mixture of order and disorder, of randomness and regularity, segregation and integration, prevails in brain structure and function.

Order and disorder are closely related to the concepts of information and entropy, and it is therefore no surprise that many measures of complexity that quantify the degree of organization, regardless of where they are applied, use information as their basic building block. A foundational measure of information theory is entropy, whose origins trace back to thermodynamics. In Boltzmann's formulation, entropy links the macrostate of a system (e.g., its temperature) to a probability distribution of its microstates (e.g., the kinetic energy of gas molecules). In the context of Shannon's information theory (Shannon, 1948), the entropy of a system is high if it occupies many states in its available state space with equal probability. In that case, an observation of the state of the system provides a high amount of information because the outcome of the observation is highly uncertain. If the system visits only very few states, then its entropy is low and its observation delivers little information.

Several measures of complexity as organization have been proposed, including effective complexity (Gell-Mann, 1995) and physical complexity (Adami and Cerf, 2000). Effective complexity measures the minimum description length of a system's regularities and attempts to distinguish features of the system that are regular or random. As such, it is a formal measure of the system's information content resulting from its intrinsic regularities, but it cannot easily be obtained from empirical observations. Physical complexity specifically addresses the complexity of biological systems. Chris Adami has argued that the complexity of a biological organism must depend crucially on the environment within which it functions (Adami et al., 2000; Adami, 2002). Therefore, the physical complexity of a biological system can be understood as the mutual information between gene sequences (genomes) and the ecological environment within which they are expressed. The physical complexity of a given genetic sequence is the amount of information it encodes about the environment to which the organism is adapting. Physical complexity of an organism therefore depends on the ecological context within which the organism has evolved. An application of this measure of complexity to the nervous system has not yet been attempted, but it might involve an estimation of how much structured information about an environment is captured in regularities of brain structure or function.

While all of these measures of complexity highlight interesting aspects of various physical and biological systems, none seem particularly well suited for quantifying the amount of organization or complexity encountered in neural systems. What are the key markers of complexity in the brain? Network analyses have consistently pointed to the importance of segregation and integration in the structural and functional organization of the brain. Structurally, segregation and integration are enabled by the small-world modular architecture of brain networks (see chapter 6). Functionally, the interplay of specialized and integrated information is what enables the variety and flexibility of cognition (see chapter 9). Segregation and integration are essential organizational features of brain networks. As I will argue in the next section, they can be quantified with information-theoretic approaches, and the coexistence of segregation and integration is a major determinant of neural complexity.

Neural Complexity and the Balance of Segregation and Integration

From an information-theoretic perspective, nervous systems need to cope with two major challenges. First, their neural elements need to capture statistical regularities present in their input space by creating specialized, or segregated, information. Second, to generate coherent behavioral responses and cognitive states, these specialized resources need to become functionally integrated. Segregation requires that neural responses remain encapsulated and distinct from one another in order to preserve their specialized response profiles. Integration requires that neural responses be coordinated through interneuronal interactions, which inevitably results in a partial loss of specialization. Thus, segregation and integration place seemingly irreconcilable demands on neural processing, yet they must be realized within a single architecture. These informational challenges can be met by a connectivity that combines segregation and integration in a "nearly decomposable," modular small-world network.

Segregation and integration in the dynamic patterns of functional and effective brain connectivity can be defined in terms of statistical dependencies between distinct neural units forming nodes in a network (see chapter 3). Statistical dependencies can be expressed as information, and functional and effective connectivity essentially quantify how information is distributed, shared, and integrated within a network. Let us consider a system that is composed of a set of neural units representing individual neurons or brain regions, which generates observable dynamics that can be analyzed with the methods of information theory. Can we characterize how information is distributed within the system?

A first step is to look at pairwise interactions and characterize them in terms of information and entropy.[5] The information shared by two elements, their mutual information, expresses their statistical dependence, that is, how much information the observation of one element can provide about the state of the other element. It is defined as the difference between the sum of the two individual entropies and the joint entropy. If no statistical dependence exists between the two elements, then observing the state of one element provides no information about the state of the other, and the mutual information is zero. Unlike correlation, which is a linear measure of association between variables, mutual information captures linear and nonlinear relationships. Importantly, mutual information does not describe causal effects or directed dependencies between variables.

A multivariate extension of mutual information, the integration of the system, measures the total amount of statistical dependence among an arbitrarily large number of elements (Tononi et al., 1994).[6] Integration is mathematically defined as the difference between the sum of the entropies of the individual units and their joint entropy. Like mutual information, integration always takes on positive values or is equal to zero. Zero integration is obtained for a system whose elements behave independently. In such a system, knowledge of the state of any of its elements provides no information about the states of any of the other elements, and the joint entropy of the system is therefore exactly equal to the sum of the individual entropies. If there is any degree of statistical dependence between any of the elements, then the joint entropy of the system will be smaller than the sum of all individual entropies, resulting in a positive value for integration.

This formalism for integration signals why we are interested in applying it to functional brain networks. Dynamic coupling is usually defined as a statistical dependence (linear or nonlinear), and a measure of integration should be able to quantify such dependencies between arbitrary numbers of neural units. Furthermore, integration seems well suited to serve as a building block for assessing the balance between segregation (statistical independence) and integration (statistical dependence). The modular and hierarchical nature of brain networks requires a formalism that is sensitive to segregation and integration at multiple scales. To that end, we consider the integration of subsets of elements of a given system across all scales, ranging from subsets of sizes 2, 3, and so on up to the size of the full system. Statistical dependencies that reside at one or several spatial scales can thus be captured in a single measure which we called neural complexity (Tononi et al., 1994; 1998). The hierarchical nature of neural complexity is inherently well suited for a system such as the brain, which exhibits modularity at several different levels. Neural complexity captures the amount of structure or organization present within the system across all spatial scales. It takes on low values for systems whose elements behave independently from one another. These systems are characterized by high segregation (each element is informationally encapsulated) but very low integration (absence of dynamic coupling). Neural complexity also takes on low values for systems whose elements are fully coupled. These systems contain very little segregation (all elements are behaving identically) but are highly integrated because of strong global coupling. Only systems that combine segregation and integration generate high complexity.

A closer analysis reveals that the measure can be identically formulated in terms of the distribution of mutual information across all bipartitions of the system, where "bipartitions" refers to a way of dividing the system into two complementary parts (see figure 13.2). Expressed in these terms, the neural complexity of a system is high when, on average, the mutual information between any subset of the system and its complement is high. High mutual information between many possible subsets of a system indicates a diverse set of statistical dependencies between the different portions of an integrated system. Thus, complexity emerges when rich and dynamic contextual influences prevail, and complexity is low when such influences are either completely absent (as in systems that engage in random activity) or completely homogeneous (as in systems that are highly regular).

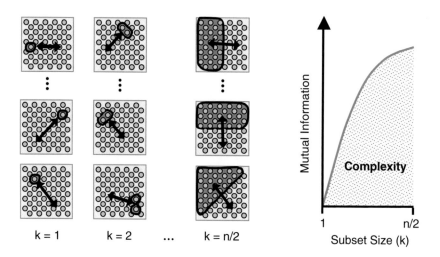

Figure 13.2
Neural complexity as mutual information on multiple spatial scales. Plots on the left illustrate the sampling of subsets of the system, ranging from single units (k = 1) to the maximal subset size of k = n/2. For each subset, the mutual information between the subset and its complement (the rest of the system) is determined, and averages for each subset size are plotted on the right. The sum of the average mutual information across all subset sizes gives the neural complexity. Redrawn after Tononi et al. (1998).

Extensions of neural complexity that take into account the external inputs and outputs of a system have been proposed (Tononi et al., 1996; 1999). To capture the effects of inputs on dynamics, we considered that one of the effects of an external perturbation consists of changing the pattern of intrinsic correlations. Stimuli that are discordant with the intrinsic dynamic organization of the system will have little effect, because they do not "integrate well" with the system's spontaneous activity. Other stimuli may enhance a distinct set of statistical relationships within the system. In the former case, the intrinsic complexity of the system, as defined by its internal statistical structure, remains unchanged, while in the latter case, it is selectively increased. A statistical measure called matching complexity (Tononi et al., 1996) quantifies the effect of a stimulus on the distribution of segregated and integrated information in a complex network. The measure explicitly evaluates the informational gain resulting from a sensory perturbation of an endogenously active network (see chapter 8, figure 8.11). Network outputs are considered in the context of degeneracy, a key ingredient of network robustness, which was discussed earlier in chapter 10.

The analytic foundations of the measure of neural complexity have been further studied by Jürgen Jost and colleagues. Olbrich et al. (2008) noted a close relationship of neural complexity with another statistical measure of complexity based on the idea of excess entropy (Crutchfield and Feldman, 2003), defined as the amount of uncertainty about the state of a subsystem that remains after the state of the remainder of the system is known. Olbrich et al. also suggested that neural complexity be normalized by the number of elements of the system in order to avoid counterintuitive increases in complexity due to the addition of independent elements or systems. A related approach to neural complexity examined the distribution of information in networked systems on the basis of a decomposition of the system's integration (or multi-information) into "connected information" (Schneidman et al., 2003).

Networks for Complexity

Structural networks determine which neural units can communicate and thus shape the statistics of neural firing patterns. Dynamic processes unfolding on complex networks depend critically on the connection topology (see chapter 12) in addition to the response characteristics of the individual nodes. Some topologies are more suitable for the creation of stable attractors, others for global synchronization, and still others for dynamic transients and critical behavior. Which network topologies promote high neural complexity, and do these patterns have anything in common with those of empirical cellular or large-scale brain networks? The question can be addressed by varying topological patterns and examining how these variations affect global dynamics and measures of complexity. However, a complete inspection of all connection topologies is impractical because they occupy a vast space of possible configurations.[7]

A computational approach similar to an evolutionary algorithm allows the systematic exploration of the relationship between structural topology and dynamics.[8] First, structural variants of a system are created, their dynamics are evaluated under a cost function, and the variant whose performance most closely matches the desired goal is selected.[9] This variant is copied forward into the next generation together with a set of nearly identical copies ("offspring") that incorporate random structural variations. Once again, their dynamics are compared to the cost function and selection ensues. The cycle of variation and selection continues until no further improvement occurs or the goal defined by the cost function is attained. Effectively, the procedure searches for systems that optimally satisfy the cost function within a high-dimensional parameter space. In our context, the parameters correspond to wiring patterns and the cost function is given by a global measure of network dynamics, such as integration or complexity. What kinds of structural connectivity patterns are associated with high values for these dynamic cost functions?

A crucial ingredient in this approach is the type of neural dynamics that is used to derive covariance patterns (functional connectivity) from the pattern of structural connections. Even given an identical pattern of structural connectivity, different choices of dynamics can result in very different functional connectivity. The systematic exploration of how connection topology shapes realistic nonlinear neural dynamics requires the simulation of very large numbers of network variants and is therefore computationally quite costly. Linear systems are better suited for such an analysis because the system's covariance structure can be derived analytically from the structural connectivity matrix (Tononi et al., 1994; Galán, 2008) under the assumption that the basic statistics of the dynamics remain stationary over time. The covariance matrix can then be used to compute entropies (Cover and Thomas, 1991) and thus estimate multivariate information-theoretic measures such as integration and complexity. Linear systems are a poor model for the highly nonlinear and nonstationary dynamics of single neurons but capture at least some of the characteristic behavior of very large neuronal populations. Thus, they may serve as a proxy for neural dynamics that remains close to the assumptions of linearity and stationarity. The covariance structure of linear systems tends to reflect the patterning of the underlying structural connectivity, reminiscent of the close structure–function relationship seen in large-scale brain networks during spontaneous activity (see chapter 8).

A series of computational studies explored the link between connection topology and neural dynamics for a simple variant of linear systems.[10] Consistently, networks optimized for high entropy, integration, and complexity displayed characteristic network topologies (see figure 13.3). Only networks that are optimized for high complexity show patterns that resemble those observed in real cortical connection matrices (Sporns et al., 2000a; 2000b; Sporns and Tononi, 2002). Specifically, such networks exhibit an abundance of reciprocal (reentrant) connections and a strong

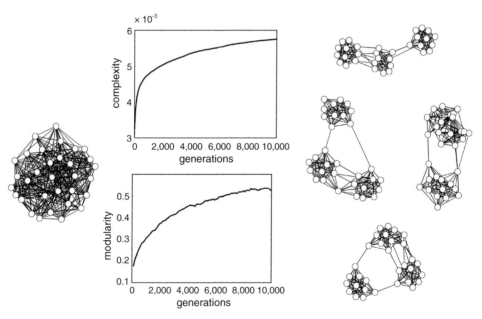

Figure 13.3
Optimizing neural complexity. Plots show graph selection for high neural complexity, shown for graphs composed of 32 nodes and 160 edges, and using a model for linear neural dynamics (Galán, 2008). Starting from a population of random networks (an example is shown on the left), neural complexity increases nearly twofold as edges are rewired. The resulting graph topologies resemble modular small-world networks (examples shown on the right). Note that modularity increases in parallel with neural complexity.

tendency to form modules interlinked by hub nodes. The rise in complexity during network optimization is paralleled by the appearance of high clustering and short path lengths, arranged in a modular small-world architecture (Sporns et al., 2000a; Sporns and Tononi, 2002; see figure 13.3). The resulting connection topologies can be wired efficiently when the network nodes are embedded in three-dimensional space (see chapter 7). Hierarchical modularity and self-similar "fractal" connection patterns also promote high complexity (Sporns, 2006; see figure 13.4), a result that further supports the idea that hierarchical networks are associated with complex critical dynamics (see chapter 12).

While more realistic nonlinear dynamics have not yet been systematically employed in the context of optimizing connectivity for complexity, the comparison of specific instances of networks with various connection topologies supports the idea that high dynamic complexity is indeed associated with structural patterns that are similar to those found in empirical brain networks. The influence of structural connections on endogenous modes of neuronal dynamics has been studied in computational models of cortical and corticothalamic systems. For example, nonlinear models of patchy connections between functionally segregated neuronal groups (Tononi et al., 1994; Sporns, 2004) as well as an example of an optimization of nonlinear networks (Sporns and Tononi, 2002) yield results that are consistent with a strong link between dynamic complexity and modular small-world network architectures (see figure 13.5).

Nonlinear models exhibit additional dynamic features associated with complexity. Varying the spatial pattern of corticocortical connections produced differences in dynamics such as varying degrees of local and global synchronization (Tononi et al., 1994; Sporns, 2004). Connectivity composed of a mixture of short-range and long-range connections gives rise to spontaneous activity patterns with variable correlation structure, characterized by a waxing and waning of functional coupling that generates a rich repertoire of cortical states and high neural complexity (see chapters 8 and 12). Rich spatial and temporal patterning depends on the presence of small-world network topology. For example, random rewiring of a large-scale model of the macaque cortex not only degrades its structural small-world attributes but also reduces dynamic correlations within and between functional clusters (Honey et al., 2007). Rich dynamics are also promoted by heterogeneous connection topologies (Jirsa and Kelso, 2000; Jirsa 2004), as well as conduction delays (Ghosh et al., 2008a,b). In virtually all cases where dynamic complexity has been

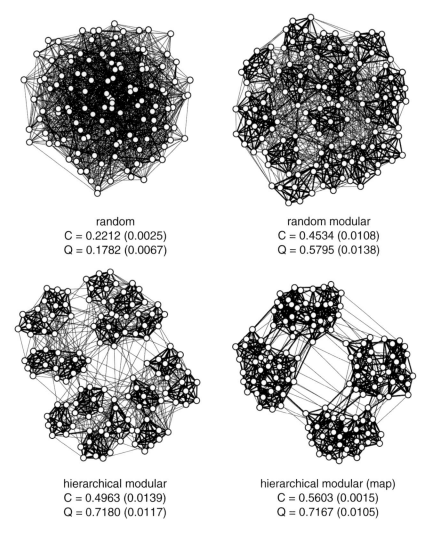

random
C = 0.2212 (0.0025)
Q = 0.1782 (0.0067)

random modular
C = 0.4534 (0.0108)
Q = 0.5795 (0.0138)

hierarchical modular
C = 0.4963 (0.0139)
Q = 0.7180 (0.0117)

hierarchical modular (map)
C = 0.5603 (0.0015)
Q = 0.7167 (0.0105)

Figure 13.4
Complexity and hierarchical modularity. Graph plots show networks composed of 128 nodes and approximately 10,000 edges. Values for C and Q give mean and standard deviation of neural complexity (based on a linear model as in figure 13.3) and modularity, respectively, averaged over 10 instantiations of each network type. Top left: Random graph. Top right: Modular graph consisting of 16 randomly linked modules. Bottom left: Modular graph consisting of 16 modules that are linked by hierarchically arranged random connections. Bottom right: Modular graph consisting of 16 modules linked by topographically mapped hierarchical connections. Note that neural complexity is highest for networks with hierarchical modularity (see figure 12.2). Connection matrices were constructed as described in Sporns (2006).

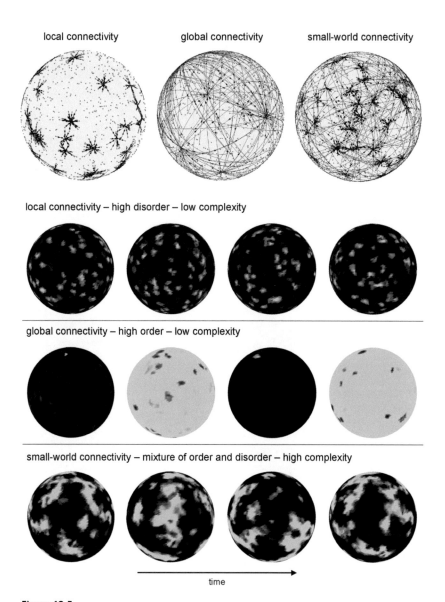

Figure 13.5
Variations of connectivity patterns and their associated neural dynamics. Images show structural connectivity (top) and dynamics (bottom) obtained from a demonstration model consisting of 1,600 spontaneously active Wilson–Cowan neural mass units randomly arranged on a sphere and coupled by excitatory connections. Structural connectivity plots only depict connections for 2 percent of all excitatory nodes. Three cases are shown: local connectivity (only short-distance connections), global connectivity (only long-range connections), and small-world connectivity (a mixture of short- and long-distance connections). Neural complexity (Tononi et al., 1994; Sporns et al., 2000a; 2000b) is highest for dynamics unfolding on the small-world network. A movie showing all three cases is referenced in Sporns (2007).

examined, it has been found to be associated with structural network properties also encountered in the nervous system. These computational studies suggest that only specific classes of connectivity patterns that are structurally similar to cortical networks simultaneously support short wiring, small-world attributes, hierarchical modular architectures (all structural features), and high complexity (a global index of functional connectivity).

Complex Networks and the Origin of Consciousness

A science of the brain that does not account for subjective experience and conscious mental states is incomplete. Consciousness, long the domain of philosophers and psychologists, has finally become a legitimate topic of neuroscientific discourse and investigation. The search for "neural correlates of consciousness" has delivered a plethora of observations about the neural basis of the phenomenon (Crick and Koch, 1998b; Rees et al., 2002; Tononi and Koch, 2008). We know that certain brain regions, notably the cerebral cortex, are more important for consciousness than others and that the presence of neural activity alone is insufficient to create it since we lose consciousness every time we sleep. Yet, no amount of empirical data alone can answer fundamental questions about why and how certain physical processes occurring in neural tissue can generate subjective experience. As Giulio Tononi has argued, empirical studies must be complemented by a theoretical framework (Tononi, 2008).

William James famously referred to consciousness as a continuous process or stream: "Consciousness [...] does not appear to itself chopped up in bits. Such words as 'chain' or 'train' do not describe it fitly as it presents itself in the first instance. It is nothing jointed; it flows. A 'river' or a 'stream' are the metaphors by which it is most naturally described" (James, 1890, p. 239).[11] The phenomenology of consciousness highlights several of its key properties, the integration of the many facets of subjective experience into a unified mental state, the high level of differentiation of each of these states seemingly drawn from an inexhaustible repertoire of possible mental configurations, and the dynamic flow of highly integrated and differentiable states on a fast time scale. Tononi and Edelman (1998) have argued that these dynamic and integrative aspects of consciousness require a unified neural process—specifically, reentrant interactions between distributed regions of the thalamocortical system. The dynamic reciprocal coupling of neural activity provides the neural substrate for rapid and flexible integration (see chapter 9) while at the same time maintaining differentiated neural states drawn from a large repertoire. The coexistence of high integration and high differentiation can be formally expressed using measures of statistical information, for example, the measure of neural complexity defined earlier. High complexity in a neural system is attained if the system allows for a large number of differentiable states and at the same time achieves their functional integration by creating statistical dependencies that bind together its various individual components. Dynamically bound neural elements that evolve through a rich state space form a functional cluster or "dynamic core" (Tononi and Edelman, 1998; Edelman and Tononi, 2000). The boundaries of the core define the extent of the neural substrate encompassing a particular conscious experience. Neural elements outside of the core cannot contribute to it as they are not functionally integrated.

An essential aspect of the dynamic core is that it must be able to select, based on its intrinsic interactions, its own causal flow, the series of transitions between states within a large repertoire of possibilities. A core capable of selecting from among only a handful of states does not generate consciousness. The core must possess high complexity, that is, the interactions of its elements must create high amounts of information. As discussed earlier, a major (but not the only) factor promoting high complexity is the arrangement of structural connections that shape the statistics of neural dynamics. However, a single instance of a structural network can transition from high to low complexity and from high to low consciousness, as in the transition from waking to sleep, deep anesthesia, or epilepsy. These transitions can be caused by over- or underactivity of individual brain regions or the actions of neuromodulatory systems.

Giulio Tononi developed an extended theoretical framework for addressing the two main problems of consciousness, dealing with the quantity or level of consciousness expressed in a given system and with its quality or content (Tononi, 2004). The central proposal of the theory is that consciousness corresponds to the capacity of a system to integrate information. This capacity is determined by the coexistence of differentiation (a large number of possible states forming a dynamic repertoire) and integration (accounting for the unity of experience). The capacity for information integration can be measured as the amount of causally effective information that can be integrated across a minimal bipartition, called Φ (Tononi and Sporns, 2003). The value of Φ depends in large part on the topology of the system's structural connectivity (see figure 13.6). A system that can be divided into two completely separate modules would, as a whole, have zero capacity to integrate information. In turn, a system with high effective information across all its bipartitions will have high Φ. What kinds of structural connection patterns emerge if networks are optimized for high Φ? Optimization of Φ resulted in networks composed of a heterogeneous arrangement of structural connections such that each network element had a unique connectional fingerprint (indicative of functional specialization or segregation; see chapter 4) and was highly interactive with all other elements in the network (high functional integration). Tononi's information integration theory predicts that consciousness depends solely on the capacity of a

A Corticothalamic system

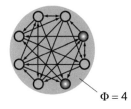

$\Phi = 4$

B Cerebellar system

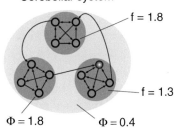

f = 1.8

f = 1.3

$\Phi = 1.8$ $\Phi = 0.4$

C Afferent pathways

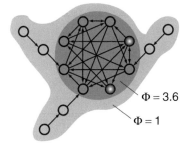

$\Phi = 3.6$

$\Phi = 1$

D Cortical-subcortical loops

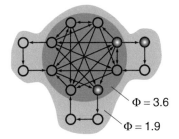

$\Phi = 3.6$

$\Phi = 1.9$

Figure 13.6
Integrated information and patterns of structural connectivity. Panels (A) to (D) show examples of networks that differ in their structural connectivity and in their capacity to integrate information, Φ. (A) A network that is both functionally integrated and specialized ("corticothalamic system") generates high Φ. The network shown was generated by optimizing Φ (Tononi and Sporns, 2003). It is fully connected, it has a short path length (functional integration), and each node maintains a unique pattern of connections (functional specialization). (B, C, D) Architectures that are modeled on the cerebellum, or include afferent pathways or loops, are associated with lower values of Φ. Reproduced from Tononi (2008), with permission from the Marine Biological Laboratory, Woods Hole, Massachusetts.

physical system to integrate information and that it is independent of other properties that are often associated with consciousness, such as language, emotion, a sense of self, or immersion in an environment. However, the theory recognizes that in order for neural circuits capable of high Φ to arise, a physical system may have to go through individual development and learn about regularities in its sensory inputs through experience-dependent plasticity and embodiment.[12]

Information integration as captured by Φ relies on a measure of effective information which, unlike mutual information, reflects causal interactions. Causal interactivity can also be estimated from actual neural dynamics, for example, with Granger causality or transfer entropy (see chapter 3). Anil Seth has suggested a measure called causal density, which is computed as the ratio of the total number of significant causal interactions out of all possible ones (Seth, 2005; 2008). The measure can capture both functional segregation and integration since it is sensitive to the level of global coordination within a system (the degree to which its elements can affect each other) as well as its dynamic heterogeneity. Since it considers temporal precedence cues to compute the strengths of causal (directed) influences, causal density can detect interactions that are "smeared over time" and not necessarily instantaneous. The relationship of causal density and network topology is still relatively unexplored. An initial study indicates that high values for causal density may be associated with small-world networks (Shanahan, 2008).

The idea that a "dynamic core" of causally interacting neural elements is associated with consciousness is also reflected in several related theoretical proposals (Shanahan, 2010). For example, Bernard Baars global work space theory (Baars, 2005) posits that consciousness depends on the existence of a central resource (the global work space) that enables the distribution of signals among specialized processors that by themselves are functionally independent from each other and informationally encapsulated (cognitive modules). Mental content is determined by which of these modules gain access to the global work space. Within the global work space, sequences of serially organized integrated states occur and correspond to sequences of conscious mental events. A dynamic approach related to global work space theory has pointed to potential neural substrates (see figure 13.7), for example, a "neuronal global work space" where sensory stimuli can trigger global and large-scale patterns of integrated neural activity (Dehaene et al., 2003; 2006). A sensory stimulus gains access to consciousness if it succeeds in activating a set of central work space neurons, thought to be preferentially localized to the

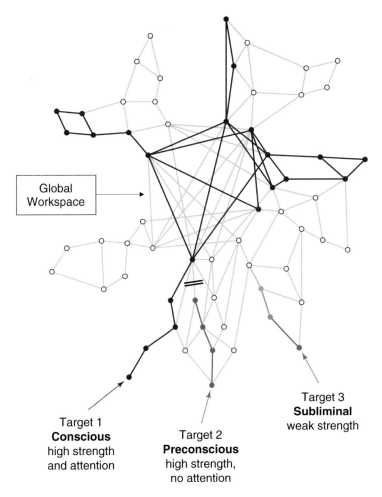

Global
Workspace

Target 1
Conscious
high strength
and attention

Target 2
Preconscious
high strength,
no attention

Target 3
Subliminal
weak strength

Figure 13.7
Schematic representation of the global neuronal work space model. A strong and attended
target stimulus ("Target 1") activates a set of "central work space" neurons and is con-
sciously accessed. A second strong stimulus ("Target 2") loses the competition for attention
and central access and does not gain access to the central work space. A weak stimulus
presented near threshold ("Target 3") remains subliminal. Central work space neurons are
thought to be particularly dense in parietal, prefrontal, and cingulate cortices. Redrawn
and modified after Dehaene et al. (2006).

prefrontal and cingulate cortex. The strength of a sensory stimulus, as well as the presence of "top-down" attentional modulation, contributes to its conscious perception.

A detailed comparison of these different theoretical approaches to consciousness is beyond the scope of this chapter. A common theme is that all of them are based, in one form or another, on network interactions, on patterns of functional or effective connectivity that are constrained by anatomy. For consciousness to arise, these interactions have to be properly configured. Several of these proposed theories stress the importance of both integration and differentiation (or segregation) in the process. Key attributes of structural and functional brain networks— for example, the existence of modules interlinked by hub regions and the prevalence of recurrent connections—are associated with several of the proposed measures or models for consciousness. The link between consciousness and patterns of brain connectivity naturally argues for the graded nature of consciousness across the animal kingdom and may shed light on its natural history.

Consciousness emerges from complex brain networks as the outcome of a special kind of neural dynamics. Whether consciousness is an adaptation and has been selected for during evolution remains an open question, particularly when we consider this issue in the context of the biological evolution of brain networks (see chapter 7). It is possible, then, that consciousness arose as a result of evolving patterns of neural connections that were shaped by competing needs for economy in design, for efficiency in neural processing, and for diverse and complex neural dynamics. Consciousness, as we currently find it in the natural world, requires a physical substrate (a network) to generate and integrate information, but it may not depend on the specific biological substrate of the brain. Can consciousness be created artificially or at least emulated in systems that use neither neurons nor synapses? Is it possible to create machine consciousness, perhaps capable of reaching levels that cannot be attained by biological organisms? If consciousness does indeed emerge as a collective property of a complex network, then these questions must be answered affirmatively. Machine consciousness may be within our reach (Koch and Tononi, 2008).

Evolution of Complexity

Does complexity itself evolve? Does evolution drive organisms and their nervous systems toward greater complexity? Does a progressive increase in complexity, should it actually occur, signify purpose and necessity behind the evolutionary process? These are charged questions that have been answered in different ways by different authors, and not always entirely on the basis of empirical facts.[13] There is little doubt that the complexity of living forms, their morphology and behavior, has on average increased over time, but is this increase the manifestation of purpose and direction in evolution or the result of an accidental history? An eloquent proponent of the latter view, Stephen J. Gould, attributed the observed trend toward an increase in biological complexity to the existence of a lower limit, below which viable organisms cannot exist, combined with an increase in variation (Gould, 1996). According to Gould, the combination of these two factors makes systems diverge away from the lower limit, thus leading to an average increase in complexity. Others have taken the opposite view, attributing observed trends toward greater complexity to increased adaptation and natural selection (e.g., Bonner, 1988; Dawkins, 1996; Adami, 2002).

Even when leaving aside the teleological aspects of the questions posed above, we are still left with the difficult problem of explaining how something as complex as the mammalian or human brain evolved from the much simpler nervous systems of creatures alive hundreds of millions of years ago. In chapter 7, I tried to shed light on the evolution of complex brain networks, and I concluded that not all properties of such networks are adaptations but that some architectural features likely have simpler explanations such as physical growth processes and allometric scaling. The answer to the question of how complexity has evolved may not be revealed entirely by the neural substrate itself but also depend on the interactions between organism and environment. In chapter 12, I surveyed the many sources of diverse and variable neural dynamics and discussed the potential benefits of this dynamic diversity for creating a large repertoire of internal states and a rich capacity to react to external perturbations. Hence, the dynamic diversity of nervous systems makes a fundamental contribution to the organism's adaptive success. The observed trend toward an increase in the complexity of a nervous system, expressed in its structural and functional connectivity, may partly be the result of an increase in the complexity of the organism's environment, which is composed of a mixture of statistical regularities and randomness. Neural complexity confers an adaptive advantage because it enables a greater range of response and a greater capacity for generating and integrating information about the external world as accessed through the senses.

The link between brain and environment becomes even more intricate when one considers that the environment of an organism cannot be objectively defined in terms of physical properties alone. In the words of Richard Lewontin, "The organism and the environment are not actually separately determined. [...] The environment is not an autonomous process but a reflection of the biology of the species" (Lewontin, 1983, pp. 75–76). The biological form, its morphology and behavior, creates its own environment by virtue of its complement of sensors and effectors and by actively shaping the statistics of its sensory input (see chapter 14). Abstract models of brain/environment interactions support the idea that neural complexity reaches higher values when the statistical structure of environmental stimuli contains a mixture of order and disorder, that is, high complexity. The informational gain produced within a complex network resulting from a sensory input can be quantified with matching complexity, a measure of the transient gain in network complexity due to a perturbation by a stimulus (Tononi et al., 1996). Optimizing matching complexity in simple networks strongly favors increased complexity of spontaneous neural activity (Sporns et al., 2000a, 2000b). Repeated encounters with structured inputs reorganize intrinsic connections in a way that endogenously recapitulates salient stimulus features (see chapter 8). More complex stimulation thus naturally leads to more complex intrinsic dynamics. In a related study, Seth and Edelman (2004) evolved neural controllers for gaze control in a simulated head/eye system under varying conditions of environmental and phenotypic complexity. Adaptation in environments that contained visual targets capable of more variable motions and with a phenotype allowing for a greater range of head/eye movements resulted in greater neural complexity than simpler environmental or phenotypic conditions. These results are consistent with the idea that increases in neural complexity may be driven by a greater repertoire of behavioral actions and sensory stimuli. The rudimentary nature of behavior and environment in these simple models raises questions about the generality of these conclusions. A more complete exploration of the origin of neural complexity requires the use of sophisticated software platforms capable of simulating more realistic forms of artificial evolution.

Larry Yaeger's Polyworld (see figure 13.8) is a model of a computational ecology in which evolutionary processes act upon encoded descriptions of autonomous agents equipped with sensors, effectors, and nervous systems that control the agent's behaviors (Yaeger, 1994). Energy is consumed by all agent activities, including neural processing, and must

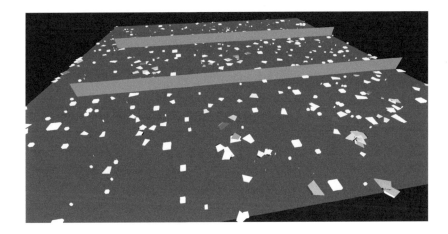

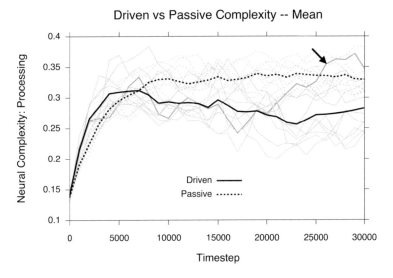

Figure 13.8
Polyworld. The plot at the top shows a view of the Polyworld environment. Trapezoid
shapes are agents, bright squares are food objects, and elongated barriers are walls that
restrict the movement of agents. Agents can navigate along the surface of the environment
and sense their surroundings with visual sensors. The plot at the bottom shows neural
complexity as a function of time in a set of "driven" runs, in which natural selection operates normally, and a set of "passive" runs, in which agents perform a random walk in gene
space. Light lines are individual runs, and dark lines are averages of 10 runs each. Note
that individual driven runs can outperform passive runs in the long term (arrow). Image
at the top courtesy of Larry Yaeger (Indiana University), plot at the bottom redrawn from
data reported in Yaeger et al. (2008).

be replenished by the activities of the agents—by either foraging for food or killing and eating other agents. Reproduction is accomplished when two agents come into contact and express their mating behavior, and a successful mating applies crossover and mutation to the parents' haploid genetic material to produce their offspring. Food grows in patches that may be static or dynamic. Barriers can isolate populations entirely, partially, or not at all and may also be dynamic. These ecological challenges generate selection pressure on agents, particularly on their network architectures, which are the primary subject of evolution in Polyworld. Over evolution, individual network structures arise that are highly varied, due to a stochastic, generative model of network design partly specified in the agents' genomes, in terms of clusters of excitatory and inhibitory neurons and their connection densities and topologies, and partly the result of neural development. Once neural architectures are specified and built, the agent's neural activations over its entire "lifetime," as well as its behavioral activity, are recorded and can be analyzed offline. Importantly, Polyworld can run in a "natural selection" mode, without a user-specified fitness function, with evolutionary changes that accrue due to selection based on the survival and reproduction of competing agents within a particular set of ecological conditions. Observed evolutionary trends due to natural selection can be compared to control runs that simulate genetic drift or that make use of standard fitness functions to directly maximize specific traits or behaviors.

Does natural selection in Polyworld favor the emergence of nervous systems with higher complexity or with specific connectional features? Agents within Polyworld exhibit consistent evolutionary trends that shape their structural connection patterns and promote the emergence of increasing levels of neural complexity (Yaeger and Sporns, 2006; Yaeger et al., 2008; Yaeger, 2009). Agents evolve toward greater connection densities while maintaining a dynamic balance between excitation and inhibition, as well as greatly increasing levels of synaptic plasticity. Concomitant with these trends in network architecture, the neural activity of evolving agents displays increasing levels of neural complexity. Graph-theoretical analysis of evolved connection patterns show that these increases in neural complexity are associated with the appearance of small-world attributes such as high clustering and short path lengths (Lizier et al., 2009). Importantly, these trends emerge without an explicit cost function that directly selects for complexity or small-world architectures. Instead, the observed increases in neural complexity are the result of natural selection in a computational ecology. In Polyworld, the evolution of neural complexity appears linked to the ecological demands of the environment within which evolution occurs.

This last point is underscored by a comparison (see figure 13.8) between the evolution of complexity in Polyworld under conditions of natural selection ("driven"), random genetic drift ("passive"), and direct optimization for complexity. Starting from a simple uniform seed population of agents, natural selection clearly favored the emergence of nervous systems with higher levels of neural complexity, but only up to a point, until a solution that is "good enough" under the constraints of the model's ecology has arisen. At that point complexity leveled off although individual simulations continued to exhibit innovations, reminiscent of speciation events that yield even higher complexity. Random genetic drift, akin to Gould's random walk away from an immutable lower boundary, also resulted in increased complexity, reaching levels that exceeded those of driven runs. Direct optimization for complexity generated organisms whose complexity far exceeded both driven and passive conditions, but their behavior evolved in a direction that would be maladaptive if natural selection would prevail. These simulation results obtained within the computational ecology of Polyworld suggest that neural complexity will emerge in the course of natural selection if it is of evolutionary advantage, but it is not optimized in any simple-minded sense of the word. Instead, once the neural complexity of a population of agents is sufficient to support their continued survival, it remains stable, until further evolutionary change takes place. Further increases in complexity then depend on increases in the complexity of the environment, resulting in an expansion of the world's ecospace (Knoll and Bambach, 2000).

Why Complexity Matters

There are patterns within the complexity of the brain. The brain's complexity does not derive from the "complicatedness" of trillions of seemingly independent and variable components. The brain's complexity is about patterns, structural and functional organization, cooperative processes, dynamic diversity, and the relationship between brain and environment. The brain's complexity is no accident—instead, complexity is one of its central "design features" and essential to its flexible and robust operation. Complexity, and with it the capacity to respond and act differently under different circumstances, is the brain's answer to the persistent challenges of a variable and only partly predictable environment. The fact that the complex organization of neural systems is bound up with recognizable patterns in structural and functional brain networks means that its origins can be traced and its defining features discerned and enumerated. The measures and approaches sketched out in this chapter are only the beginning of what must ultimately be a much more sustained and comprehensive inquiry. A focus on networks appears to be a promising avenue in this endeavor as networks naturally tie the functioning of nerve cells to the emergence of behavior and the mental life of the organism.

The story of brain connectivity now must take one last turn that places the brain back into its natural context of body and world. The networks of the brain are shaped by this context in ways that are both fundamentally important and rarely appreciated. Cognition is generally thought to involve neural activity and its continual propagation and transformation *within* the brain—patterns of neural activity causing other patterns of neural activity through networked interactions that underlie information processing. However, neural patterns can cause other neural patterns also by way of bodily actions and movements, for example, those that select and structure sensory inputs. Hence, functional brain networks are powerfully reconfigured as a result of sensory events in the real world that are the outcome of brain activity manifested as environmental change. The networks of the brain extend outwards, to the sensors and effectors of the body and into the physical world.

14   Brain and Body

The anatomist may be excused for thinking that communication between part and part in the brain can take place only through some anatomically or histologically demonstrable tract or fibres. The student of function will, however, be aware that channels are also possible through the environment. An elementary example occurs when the brain monitors the acts of the vocal cords by a feedback that passes, partly at least, through the air before reaching the brain. [...] *coordination between parts can take place through the environment; communication within the nervous system is not always necessary.*[1]
—W. Ross Ashby, 1960

When we think of brain networks, we think of neurons that are connected to other neurons and of the patterned flow of neural activity among cell populations and brain regions that underlies neural information processing. However, structural connections are not the only means by which neurons can causally affect the activity of other neurons. Another way in which neural states can cause other neural states is through the environment, as a result of bodily movement that causes changes in sensory inputs. Historically, this point formed a key rationale for the cybernetic approach to brain function. Norbert Wiener noted that cybernetics must take into account the "circular processes, emerging from the nervous system into the muscles, and re-entering the nervous system through the sense organs" (Wiener, 1948, p. 8) and thus cannot view the brain as "self-contained." W. Ross Ashby emphasized that organism and environment must be treated as a single system, and that "the dividing line [...] becomes partly conceptual, and to that extent arbitrary" (Ashby, 1960, p. 40). Humberto Maturana and Francisco Varela extended the idea in a different direction, describing the brain as a "closed system in which neuronal activity always leads to neuronal activity," either through a network of interacting neurons or through linkages between sensors and effectors that extend through the environment

(Maturana and Varela, 1980, p. 127).[2] By acting on the environment, the brain generates perturbations that lead to new inputs and transitions between network states. Environmental interactions thus further expand the available repertoire of functional brain networks.

Much of this book has been devoted to the link between the topology of structural brain networks and the dynamic patterns of functional and effective connectivity they generate. To give a full account of these structure–function linkages, it does not suffice to focus only on the structure and physiology of the nervous system. The physiology of the organism as a whole profoundly affects brain structure and function. Examples for physiological links between brain and body are the metabolic coupling of neural tissue with surrounding glial cells and the cerebral vasculature, the circadian regulation of brain and behavior, and the actions of hormones on neural circuits.[3] The primacy of biological regulation for guiding behavior and the importance of sensing the physiological state of the body for emotion and "higher" cognition (Damasio, 1994) are only beginning to be recognized. In addition to these powerful physiological couplings between brain and body, the important roles of body and environment in shaping the statistics of neural events cannot be ignored. Nervous systems function, develop, and evolve while connected to the body's sensors and effectors. Sensors relay information about exogenous signals that perturb network states of the brain, and network activity triggers effectors, resulting in bodily movement and the repositioning of sensors. Hence, the body forms a dynamic interface between brain and environment, enabling neural activity to generate actions that in turn lead to new sensory inputs.[4] As a result of this interaction, patterns of functional connectivity in the brain are shaped not only by internal dynamics and processing but also by sensorimotor activity that occurs as a result of brain–body–environment interactions (Chiel and Beer, 1997; Chiel et al., 2009; see figure 14.1).

In this final chapter, I will argue that brain–body–environment interactions can have profound effects on brain networks on both slow and fast time scales. These interactions are essential for natural sensing and multimodal perception, and they are integral components of cognitive and social development. Brain–body–environment interactions can be conceptualized as an extension of functional connectivity beyond the boundaries of the physical nervous system. The influence of these extended dynamic relationships modulates neural interactions by generating perturbations that add to the diversity of the brain's functional repertoire. Approaches from dynamical system and information theory provide a

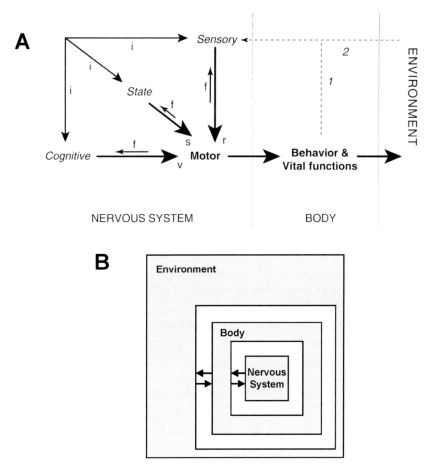

Figure 14.1
Dynamic coupling between brain, body, and environment. (A) A "four systems model of
the basic plan of the nervous system," illustrating the interactions between nervous system,
body, and environment. The brain is divided into several components primarily concerned
with sensory, cognitive, and motor function, as well as information related to the internal
state of the organism. Motor outputs result in sensory inputs via body and environment. i,
interconnections between sensory, behavioral state, and cognitive systems; f, feedback
signals provided by the motor system; r, direct sensory inputs to the motor system mediating reflex behaviors; v, inputs from the cognitive system mediating voluntary behavior; s,
inputs mediating state control influences; 1 and 2, sensory feedback signals to the nervous
system due to behavioral influences on the internal and external environment, respectively.
From Swanson (2003), reproduced with permission. (B) A schematic diagram of dynamic
interactions between brain, body, and environment, from the work of Beer (2000).

common framework for describing and analyzing the extended networks of brain, body, and environment.

Embodiment, Intelligence, and Morphology

Complex behavior can arise from even the simplest of processing mechanisms, provided these mechanisms are expressed in relation to an external environment. Herbert Simon illustrated this idea with the following example (Simon, 1969). Suppose we watch an ant making its way across a sandy beach. Moving, turning and pausing, avoiding pebbles and seaweed, traveling over and across uneven surfaces, its path is anything but straight. Instead, its path appears to be geometrically complex and difficult to describe. However, this complexity is not a result of complex internal processing on the part of the ant. Rather, the complexity emerges from the interaction of the ant with its environment, the irregularities of the terrain and the abundance of obstacles. As Simon put it, "The ant, viewed as a behaving system, is quite simple. The apparent complexity of its behavior over time is largely a reflection of the complexity of the environment in which it finds itself." (Simon, 1969; quoted after Simon, 1996, p. 52).[5] A related point was made by Valentino Braitenberg, who envisioned the construction of a series of synthetic autonomous agents, equipped with sensors and motors (Braitenberg, 1984; see figure 14.2). While the agents are extremely simple in their internal construction, once they are put into a "natural environment," often surprising patterns of behavior can arise. Differences in the internal wiring of Braitenberg's vehicles, for example, in the connections between sensors and motors, result not only in differences in behavior but also in radical changes in the composition of the vehicle's sensory world.

Simon's "ant on the beach" and Braitenberg's "vehicles" illustrate the inseparability of brain, body, and environment. Complex behavior is the result of their interaction, not the end product or readout of centralized control. The coupling between brain, body, and environment has become a cornerstone of the theoretical framework of "embodied cognition." The rise of embodied cognition acts as a counterweight to more traditional approaches to artificial intelligence (AI), first developed in the 1950s, that emphasized symbolic representations and computation.[6] According to embodied cognition, cognitive function is not based on symbolic computation but rather is shaped by the structure of our bodies, the morphology of muscles and bones, hands and arms, eyes and brains (Varela et al., 1991; Thelen and Smith, 1994; Clark, 1997; Lakoff and Johnson, 1999).

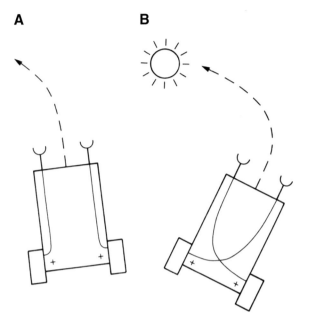

Figure 14.2
Braitenberg's vehicles. In both examples shown here a single sensor is connected to a single motor (driving a wheel), but the arrangement of the connections differs. In one case the vehicle will turn away from a light source while in the other it will approach it. From Braitenberg (1984), reproduced with permission.

Most theories of embodied cognition incorporate the notion that coherent, coordinated, or intelligent behavior results from the dynamic interactions between brain, body, and environment (Chiel and Beer, 1997; Pfeifer and Scheier, 1999; Iida et al., 2004; Pfeifer and Bongard, 2007). Cognition does not occur all in the head—instead it stretches beyond the boundaries of the nervous system. Andy Clark has made a compelling argument that the minds of highly evolved cognitive agents extend into their environments and include tools, symbols, and other artifacts that serve as external substrates for representing, structuring, and performing mental operations (Clark, 2008). If this view of cognition as extending into body and world is correct, then cognition is not "brain bound" but depends on a web of interactions involving both neural and nonneural elements. The networks of the brain fundamentally build on this extended web that binds together perception and action and that grounds internal neural states in the external physical world.

The failure of traditional AI to solve unconstrained real-world problems spurred the development of new approaches to robotics that explicitly addressed interactions between a robot, its control architecture, and a dynamic environment. Turning away from the prevailing paradigm of centralized control, Rodney Brooks argued that "coherent intelligence can emerge from independent subprocesses interacting in the world" (Brooks, 1991, p. 1228). Hence, the design of intelligent systems requires working with "complete agents," fully embodied systems that are autonomous in their actions and are situated and embedded in an environment. Brooks envisioned a modular rather than serial organization for the internal control architecture, in which each module has access to sensory input and motor output, and where coordinated behavior emerges from the interaction of these modules mediated by both brain and body, situated in the real world. Variations of decentralized control have been successfully implemented in robot models of various types of movement and locomotion (walking, running, crawling, etc.), manipulation of objects, and recognition and categorization, as well as models of imitation and social interaction. Many of the robot models employed in this work were directly inspired by specific biological systems (Pfeifer et al., 2007), for example, cricket phonotaxis (Webb, 1995), landmark-based homing behavior of ants and bees (Möller, 2000), insect walking (Gallagher et al., 1996; Cruse et al., 2007), and amphibious movements of the salamander (Ijspeert et al., 2007). Other models attempted to emulate complex cognitive abilities. One such model involved the construction of a humanoid robot equipped with sensors and effectors for real-world sensorimotor activity, and a modular control system for vision and sound, balance and posture, recognition and motor control (Brooks et al., 1999). What all these models and robots have in common is that they act autonomously *in the real world*. Building such systems is extraordinarily revealing about the relations between neural control and bodily action, the role of material properties and movements of sensors in delivering useful information, and the dependency of cognitive processes on sensorimotor interactions.[7]

Rolf Pfeifer and colleagues formulated a set of principles that underlie the operation of complete embodied agents (e.g., Pfeifer and Bongard, 2007). All such agents share a number of properties. They are subject to physical laws that govern the function of their control architectures as well as their bodies. They act on their environment and, through their actions, generate sensory inputs. Their brains and bodies form a single dynamical system with attractor states that are configured partly through interactions with the environment. Finally, their body joins in the task of information processing by performing functions that otherwise would have to be performed by the brain. This last property, which Pfeifer refers to as "morphological computation," is illustrated in figure 14.3. Consider locomotion or walking. A robot built according to traditional AI applies complex control algorithms to maintain posture and stability. As a result, its movements appear sluggish, stiff, and unbiological, and its algorithms are slow to adapt to changes in terrain, surface properties, physical load, or energy supply. In contrast, animals exploit not only neural control but also the physical and material properties of their bodies to achieve stable and adaptive motion. The compliant "hardware" of arms and legs, their sensor-rich muscles, tendons, and joints, participate in the dynamics of movement and promote stability and flexibility. This aspect of morphological computation can also be exploited by mechanical agents or robots that incorporate elastic joints, flexible materials, and a control architecture that models body and brain as an integrated dynamical system. To achieve flexible control, such a system naturally exploits the processing capacities of brain networks (and thus of brain morphology) as well as the material properties of the body and its coupling to the physical world.

As Rolf Pfeifer has argued, intelligence is not only a function of neural processing or, more generally, of a set of clever control algorithms. Rather, intelligence is distributed throughout brain and body. This view

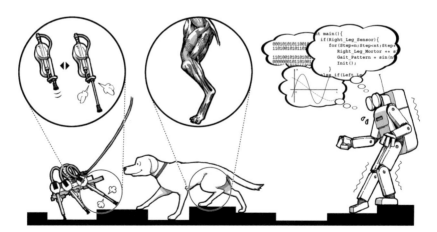

Figure 14.3
Morphological computation. (Left) A robot with pneumatic actuators moves over uneven terrain, without the need for centralized control or internal representation of the environment. (Middle) An animal uses a combination of neural control and the elasticity of its musculoskeletal system for locomotion. (Right) A robot built from servomotors and stiff materials must use complex algorithms to control its own body. Courtesy of Shun Iwasawa (Studio Ghibli, Inc.), reproduced from Pfeifer and Bongard (2007) with permission.

has important consequences not only for the efficient design of intelligent machines but also for biological questions such as the evolutionary origin of intelligence. Intelligence depends not only on the architecture of the brain but on the architecture of brain and body—brain and body evolve together. Embodiment greatly expands the space of possibilities by which evolution can achieve an increased capacity of organisms to process information, by partly offloading computation to the morphology and material properties of the organism's body. Recall that morphological considerations, not of the body but of the brain itself, were a major focus of an earlier chapter (chapter 7). It was noted that the three-dimensional structure of the brain and the spatiotemporal continuity of physical processes occurring during development, from axonal outgrowth to tension-based folding of the brain's surface, play important roles in shaping the organization of structural brain networks. Here, I merely extend this idea to include the rest of the body and its behavior. Evolutionary changes to the development and morphology of an organism's body, for example, the placement or capabilities of its sensory surfaces, the articulation or muscular control of its motor appendages, or its weight or size, necessitate concomitant changes in the nervous system.

Not only is the physical structure of the brain inseparable from that of the body and its sensorimotor repertoire, its dynamics and functional networks are continually modulated by interactions with the environment. Before we turn to an emerging theoretical framework for body–brain interactions that builds on information theory and complex networks, let us examine how some of the neural mechanisms that underlie sensory processes, multimodal perception, cognitive development, and social interactions relate to embodied cognition.

From Natural Sensing to Social Interactions

Sensation and perception result from motion and action within the physical world.[8] Organisms are not passive recipients of information. Instead, they actively explore their environments, and their motor activity *generates* and *selects* sensory inputs (Ahissar and Arieli, 2001; Kleinfeld et al., 2006; Chiel et al., 2009). Active movement of receptor arrays in visual, auditory, and tactile systems creates variations in spatiotemporal patterns of stimulus energy, enhances spatial and temporal detail, and prevents receptor adaptation. Among animal species, examples for active sensing abound. Echolocation in bats and dolphins requires body movement as well as active probing of the surrounding space. Rodents detect, localize, and categorize objects by rapidly scanning their surfaces with their vibrissae. Lobsters and crabs live in a turbulent underwater environment and rely on olfactory cues to locate food by actively moving antennules studded with chemosensors across odor plumes. These examples suggest that the full capacity of biological sensory systems is only revealed in their natural environment and with ecologically meaningful sensory inputs. Unfortunately, the complex interaction between sensing and moving can be difficult to control in a laboratory experiment, and thus sensory physiology generally employs idealized stimuli in immobilized or anesthetized animal preparations.[9] Increasingly, however, physiological studies involve natural stimulation and allow organisms to produce motor activity, with results that document the complexity of natural sensory stimulation and the close interaction of sensing and moving.

Most natural sensory environments are rich and complex, and sensory networks must effectively respond to a virtually infinite range of possible inputs. Sensory responses to natural and behaviorally significant stimuli often differ from those to highly simplified "trigger" stimuli (Braun, 2003; Kayser et al., 2003). Neural responses in visual cortex depend not only on visual features present in the neuron's classical receptive field but also on the composition of the visual background and on the context of the entire visual scene. Simple "nonnatural" stimuli such as single oriented contours presented on a blank background result in stronger neural responses than similar stimuli that are part of a natural scene (Gallant et al., 1998). Natural visual stimulation tends to decorrelate neuronal responses in V1 (Vinje and Gallant, 2000) and increases the efficiency of information transmission (Vinje and Gallant, 2002), thus improving the capacity of visual cortex to encode the sparsely distributed information present in typical real-world environments. These context-dependent effects on neuronal responses in visual cortex are likely the result of network interactions mediated by recurrent horizontal and feedback connections.

Sensory responses of visual neurons throughout all levels of the visual hierarchy are modulated by eye movements—for example, microsaccades used to direct attention and gaze in the visual environment (Melloni et al., 2009). Saccades are an extremely frequent behavior about which we experience very little.[10] Effects of abrupt and frequent shifts in the visual field due to saccadic motion are largely suppressed to ensure perceptual stability of the visual scene. The alternation of saccadic motion and stable fixation structures the timing of visual information flow and directs visual processing and thus cognitive resources to specific locations in the environment. Active exploration has physiological effects on neural responses. For example, whether a stimulus is presented passively or enters a neuron's receptive field as a result of a saccadic eye movement matters to the temporal response pattern of orientation-selective neurons in primate V1 (MacEvoy et al., 2008). Furthermore, human eye movements select locations in the visual environment that are relevant for particular perceptual or cognitive tasks.[11] The selection of fixation points in a visual scene is determined by image content and the saliency of local visual features, as well as exploratory movements, and together these factors shape the statistics of visual inputs (Parkhurst and Niebur, 2003; Betsch et al., 2004) and direct the deployment of cognitive resources. Outputs influence inputs, and by directing fixation and visual gaze, motor neurons guiding eye, head, and body movements profoundly influence patterns of functional connectivity in the visual brain.

The value of movement in sensory processing was recognized two decades ago by researchers in machine vision who struggled with the difficult problem of object recognition. At the time, the traditional approach to machine vision started from the premise that the purpose of vision is to generate an accurate and comprehensive internal representation of the surrounding three-dimensional world by extracting information from two-dimensional images. In this view, movement merely implements the outcome of perceptual decision making, but it does not participate in visual information processing. An alternative strategy, called active vision, postulated that vision is best understood in the context of visual behaviors and that motor activity can improve the quality of visual input and thus support visual computation (Bajcsy, 1988; Ballard, 1991). For example, visuomotor behaviors greatly facilitate efficient sampling of sensory environments, and invariant pattern recognition benefits from sensorimotor activity such as foveation which reduces variance across multiple views of the same object. In addition, visual agents can utilize and continually reference objects in the outside world during the generation of behavior, instead of relying exclusively on internal models and representations to guide action.

The role of active vision strategies for shaping visual processing has been explored in a number of robot models of visual development. Almassy et al. (1998) studied the development of invariant visual recognition in a mobile robot that freely explored its environment. The natural flow of sensorimotor activity created temporal continuity in visual inputs that enabled the development of neural units with invariant receptive field properties similar to those found in the mammalian visual cortex. When active exploration was disabled and inputs were presented in a discontinuous manner, these receptive fields did not arise. Floreano et al. (2005; Suzuki and Floreano, 2008) created more abstract network models of similar visual processes and again found that active vision strategies promote efficient visual development. Behavior, expressed as specific patterns of brain–body–environment interactions, modulated learning through altering the statistical structure of sensory inputs. Other robot models have documented the role of behavior in perceptual learning (Verschure et al., 2003), reward conditioning (Alexander and Sporns, 2002), and visual binding (Seth et al., 2004). A compelling example for the role of active manipulation in visual perception came from work carried out with the upper-torso humanoid robot Cog (Metta and Fitzpatrick, 2003; see figure 14.4). Cog's ability to swipe at objects and thus displace them relative to their background generated new information about object boundaries. This information allowed the robot's visual system to learn about scene segmentation, a process that is as important in machine vision as it is in human visual development (Fitzpatrick et al., 2008).[12]

Active manipulation of stimulus objects also supports the development of human visual object recognition. When people are handed a three-dimensional object and given the opportunity to freely explore it

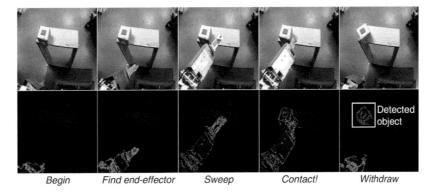

Begin   Find end-effector   Sweep   Contact!   Withdraw

Figure 14.4
Better vision through manipulation. These images are taken through a head-mounted camera attached to the upper-torso humanoid robot Cog (Brooks et al., 1999). The images show an object (a wooden cube) placed on a table top in front of the robot. Cog's exploratory arm movements result in a collision and in contact with the object. The lateral displacement of the object generates coherent motion and thus new sensory information. Reproduced from Metta and Fitzpatrick (2003) with permission.

by rotating it in front of their eyes, they dwell on specific orientations of the object and rarely inspect intermediate views (Harman et al., 1999; James et al., 2001). This active control of visual input not only shapes the statistics of sensory inputs but also results in object recognition that is more efficient compared to passive viewing. Manipulation of objects allows the selection of viewing angles that are most informative about object identity or that present frequently encountered patterns and features to which sensors are most attuned. By reducing the dimensionality of sensory inputs, active manipulation and exploration support visual recognition, including its developmental origin (Pereira and Smith, 2009).

Object manipulation naturally gives rise to multimodal sensory input, through simultaneous stimulation of the haptic and visual system. Different sensory modalities continually sample signals that are temporally correlated because they relate to the same physical object or event in the environment. Given the pervasiveness of such correlations and given the recurrent connectivity of cortical networks (see chapter 9), it is perhaps not surprising that much of the cortex devoted to sensory processing may be considered multimodal (Ghazanfar and Schroeder, 2006). Classical multisensory areas such as the superior temporal sulcus (STS) are regions where signals from multiple sensory systems converge and are integrated. For example, the primate STS is activated by stimuli indicating biological motion of body or face (Puce and Perrett, 2003) and plays an important role in social perception (Allison et al., 2000). Moreover, the STS responds to combinations of visual and auditory stimuli, accompanying vocalization, human walking, or the tearing of paper (Barraclough et al., 2005). Visual responses to these stimuli are either augmented or attenuated by the simultaneous presentation of corresponding sounds, indicative of a nonlinear integrative process. Multimodal responses are essential for speech recognition and can greatly facilitate detection and discrimination of stimuli in the presence of ambient noise. Nonhuman primates recognize the correspondence of facial and vocal signals and the activity of neurons in superior temporal cortex as well as "unimodal" auditory cortex (Ghazanfar et al., 2005) are modulated by a combination of visual and auditory signals. Monkeys observing vocalizing conspecifics preferentially fixated on the mouth during the onset of mouth movements (Ghazanfar et al., 2006), an effect also seen in humans (Vatikiotis-Bateson et al., 1998). These studies indicate that active sensing strategies are deployed to selectively gather multimodal information in speech perception. Thus, stimulus integration of a brain region such as STS does not depend solely on convergent neural connectivity and intrinsic flow of information (see chapter 9); integration can be greatly enhanced by coordinated movement of the body.

Embodiment naturally generates correlations and redundancies across multiple sensory modalities. Such multimodal correlations help to disambiguate sensory inputs and reduce the effective dimensionality of the sensory space, thus supporting concept formation, categorization, and other cognitive processes (Thelen and Smith, 1994). Additionally, normal development, especially in humans, is accompanied by coordinated social interactions—"development takes place among conspecifics with *similar internal systems and similar external bodies*" (Smith and Breazeal, 2007, p. 63, italics theirs). The observation of bodily behaviors of others provides information about their internal state, and one's own bodily behaviors provide information about one's own internal state to others. These bodily and environmental linkages create dynamic couplings between otherwise distinct cognitive systems, and they become the means by which the behavior of others can become part of the internal model of each agent, an essential component of social development.

The immersion of humans in a social environment and the embodied nature of human cognition are increasingly recognized as important determinants of social cognition (Hari and Kujala, 2009). An emphasis on social interactions and the concurrent recruitment of shared brain systems for perception and action among individuals has been proposed as a core ingredient of a "new science of learning" (Meltzoff et al., 2009). Emerging evidence from social neuroscience suggests that social interactions can modulate neural activations and functional connectivity within the brains of interacting individuals. In a set of experiments combining simultaneous behavioral and neural recordings, Emmanuelle Tognoli and colleagues have studied social coordination in pairs of interacting individuals (Tognoli et al., 2007). Pairs of participants performed repetitive finger movements at their own preferred frequency, either in the presence or absence of visual contact. When the relative phase between the movement of each individual participant was examined, several different classes of social coordination could be distinguished, among them "social neglect" (an absence of phase coupling), as well as transient (metastable) and sustained phase locking (see figure 14.5). Simultaneous recording of brain activity with a dual-EEG system revealed the presence of specific rhythms during times of visual contact. Rhythmic activity in the 10–12 Hz frequency range near right centroparietal electrodes, termed the "φ-complex" by Tognoli et al. (2007), varied systematically

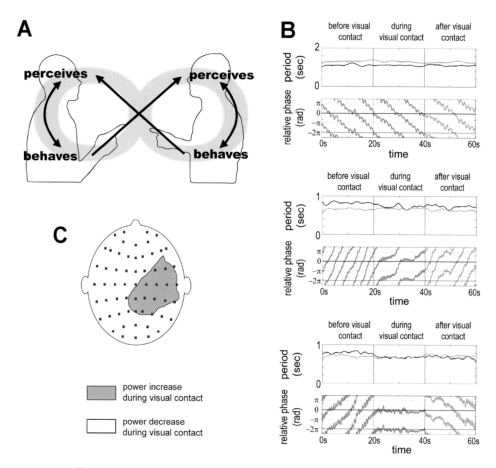

Figure 14.5
Social coordination. (A) Coupling of perception and action in two interacting individuals. (B) Examples of behavioral patterns observed before, during, and after periods of visual contact in pairs of participants. Plots illustrate relative phase difference of finger movements in trials where movements were uncoupled (top) and during transient (middle) as well as sustained phase locking (bottom). (C) Centroparietal EEG electrodes exhibited significant increase in power around 10–12 Hz during visual contact. Different frequency components were selectively engaged during coordinated and uncoordinated interactions. Reproduced from Tognoli (2008) with permission.

with the degree of social coordination during times of potential interaction. Two distinct spectral components showed increases during coordinated and uncoordinated behavior, respectively. These results indicate that the presence or absence of coordinated behavior *between* participants has a neural correlate *within* their individual nervous systems. An open question concerns the degree of mutual synchronization or coupling between brains of socially engaged individuals.[13]

Social interactions that modulate the activation and coactivation of neural elements in brain networks are a special instance of brain–body–environment interactions. Their prevalence in human behavior reminds us of the essential role of social interactions in shaping brain connectivity. As mentioned many times in this book, social interactions also give rise to networks among people. The dynamic coupling of the brains and bodies of interacting individuals blends into the complex networks that pervade social structures and organizations. Hence, social networks and brain networks are fundamentally interwoven, adjacent levels of a multi-scale architecture, possibly with some of the same network principles at play.

Is there a common theoretical framework that can capture processes occurring within brain networks, as well as those processes by which brain networks extend their influence into the real world? Can we quantify and measure the impact of brain–body–environment interactions on how information is structured and processed within an organism's or agent's control architecture? A promising candidate for such a framework results from extensions of dynamical systems and information theory, and the next section examines how this prospective framework can help in defining the role of embodiment in neural information processing.

Information Flow in Brain, Body, and Environment

The operation of brain networks depends on a combination of endogenous patterns of neural activity (see chapter 8) and exogenous perturbations such as those generated by stimuli or tasks (see chapter 9). For organisms situated and embodied in their natural environments, the nature and timing of these perturbations are strongly determined by bodily actions and behavior. By generating sequences of perturbations, embodiment generates sequences of network states and, thus, information in the brain. Hence, the activity of an organism in its environment contributes to neural processing and information flow within the nervous system. This raises the possibility that measures of information (see chapter 13) can be productively applied to estimate the degree to which embodiment modulates the interactions of elements of the nervous system.

The embodied nature of cognition is captured by dynamical systems theory, which describes neural, behavioral, and environmental processes within a common formalism (Beer, 2000). Randy Beer has created several examples of simple cognitive agents whose behavior can be modeled and analyzed with the tools of dynamical systems theory. In these agents, traditional cognitive concepts like discrete representation, symbols, or computation are replaced by formulations of system dynamics, modeled as continuous processes that unfold along trajectories in phase space, influenced by intrinsic and extrinsic forces and subject to perturbation. There is an important conceptual link between continuous dynamic models of cognitive processes and models of neural dynamics, particularly at the large scale. Earlier chapters have dealt extensively with complex neural dynamics and its dependence on spontaneous activity, perturbations, network structure, and plasticity. One of the compelling advantages of dynamic approaches to cognition is that they naturally integrate among internal (network-driven) and external (embodiment-driven) forces.

Another approach, fully compatible with a dynamical framework, is provided by modern extensions of information theory. In chapters 12 and 13, I discussed the importance of specialized and integrated information for defining diverse and complex neural dynamics and how complexity can be captured with measures that quantify functional segregation and integration in terms of statistical information. The confluence of dynamic systems approaches and information theory may offer a common theoretical framework for understanding the operation, development, and evolution of complete agents.

The role of embodied interactions in actively structuring sensory inputs has provided a test bed for developing and evaluating such a framework, for example, by examining computational models or robotic implementations of embodied agents (Pfeifer et al., 2008; Ay et al., 2008). Using an active vision robotic platform, Max Lungarella and colleagues (Lungarella et al., 2005; Lungarella and Sporns, 2006) showed that coordinated and dynamically coupled sensorimotor activity can induce quantifiable changes in sensory information. Simple visual behaviors such as foveation and visual tracking resulted in significant gains in structured sensory information, as measured by decreased entropy, increased mutual information, integration, and complexity within specific regions of sensory space (see figure 14.6). The role of sensorimotor coupling for generating this information was documented by comparing two different conditions. In one condition, sensorimotor coupling was intact and unperturbed, resulting in coordinated behavior. In the other condition, the link between sensory inputs and motor outputs was disabled, effectively decoupling motor outputs from their sensory consequences. When

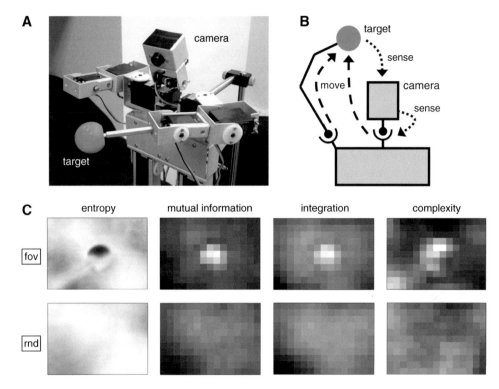

Figure 14.6

Embodiment and structured information. (A) Humanoid robot, consisting of an upper torso, a movable head with a single camera, and a right arm with movable shoulder, elbow, and wrist joints. A visual target is affixed to the tip of the arm, and self-generated arm movements will displace the target in front of the camera (B). (C) During coordinated behavior (condition "fov"), the target is both moved and tracked by the robot. Coordination results in a decrease in entropy and an increase in mutual information, integration, and complexity in the central part of the visual field. Uncoordinated movement of target and camera (condition "rnd") result in loss of information. Modified from Lungarella and Sporns (2006).

these two conditions were compared, intact sensorimotor coupling generated greater amounts of structured information. This additional information was not contained in the stimulus itself; it was created by the sensorimotor interaction. A gain in information has potential benefits for the operation of brain networks, as it promotes both functional specialization and integration. Lungarella and Sporns (2006) suggested that active structuring of sensory information is a fundamental principle of embodied systems and supports a broad range of psychological processes such as perceptual categorization, multimodal sensory integration, and sensorimotor coordination.

The notion of brain–body–environment interaction implicitly (or explicitly) refers to causal effects. Defined somewhat simplistically, a minimally but effectively embodied system is one in which sensory inputs causally affect motor outputs, and these motor outputs, in turn, causally affect sensory inputs. As many proponents of embodied cognition have argued, dynamic "perception–action loops" are fundamental building blocks for learning and development. As dynamic structures, we would expect such loops to be transient, as they are created and dissolved in the course of behavior and involve changing subsets of neural, sensory, and motor elements. Thus, mapping causal relations between sensory and motor states is likely to uncover a temporal progression of perception–action networks that reciprocally link specific subsets of sensory and motor units.

Lungarella and Sporns (2006) used information-theoretic measures to extract patterns of directed information flow between brain, body, and environment. The study mapped noncausal (undirected) as well as causal (directed) relationships between a variety of neural, sensory, and motor variables sampled by two morphologically different robotic platforms, a stationary humanoid and a mobile quadruped. Directed interactions between neural elements, sensors, and effectors were estimated using "model-free" methods based on time series analysis and temporal precedence cues (see chapter 3). Once extracted, these "causal networks" mapped the time-dependent pattern and strength of embodied interactions. In addition, the study demonstrated a relationship between information and body morphology. Different arrangements of sensors, for example, variations in the spatial arrangement and density of photoreceptors on a simulated retina, resulted in different patterns and quantities of information flow. Thus, information processing within the control architecture (e.g., the brain) depended not only on a combination of intrinsic connectivity and sensorimotor interactions but also on body morphology—for example, the physical arrangement of sensory surfaces and motor structures. Once again, the morphology of an agent or organism and the processing capabilities of its neural networks are found to be intricately linked.

If sensorimotor interactions and embodiment contribute to the generation of information, does the optimization of measures of information, in turn, promote the emergence of coordinated behavior? Or put differently, is a general drive toward "better" or "more" information compatible with at least some forms of organized behavioral activity?

The question can be addressed in simple computational models of embodied agents that undergo modification as part of an evolutionary algorithm. Cost or "fitness" functions used for optimizing system performance that are based on behavioral success or on the amount of information available to the agent's control architecture produced virtually identical outcomes (Sporns and Lungarella, 2006). Agents that maximized the complexity of information present in their sensors "evolved" to perform coordinated behavior that was indistinguishable from that of agents that were selected on the basis of their behavioral performance. For example, selecting agents for complexity of sensory inputs yielded organized behavior such as visual tracking, reaching, and tactile exploration (Sporns and Lungarella, 2006), without the need to specify a behavioral task or goal. In the previous chapter (chapter 13), optimization of complexity was found to be associated with modular small-world architectures of brain networks and their capacity to combine segregation and integration. In an embodied setting, information and complexity shape the joint evolution of brain architecture, body morphology, and behavior.

Several candidates for a formal framework of agent–environment systems based on information theory have been proposed. Klyubin et al. (2008) developed an information-based measure, termed "empowerment," which is designed to capture the capacity of an organism to create information in its environment by way of its effectors that can, in turn, be captured by its sensors. The perception–action cycle is viewed as an extension of information processing and information flow and as a means by which organisms increase the information-processing capabilities of their brain networks. Empowerment is a measure of potential rather than actual information flow in an embodied system, quantified as the maximum information flow from a set of actions to future states of sensory variables. As such, empowerment depends on the way the organism is physically coupled to the environment, including the materials and dynamics of its muscles and actuators, as well as the position and functioning of its sensors. Empowerment explicitly relies on the causal nature of the perception–action loop. In a related effort, Jürgen Jost and colleagues have introduced an informational measure of "autonomy" that also addresses the mutual interactions between an agent and its environment (Bertschinger et al., 2008). The measure starts from the intuition that an autonomous system should not be completely determined by its environment and instead should be able to set its own goals. Again, the causal structure of information flow between agent and environment is critical to determine whether observed mutual dependency is the result of the agent acting on the environment or vice versa.

For now, formal models of artificial life or robotic implementation have served as test beds to investigate the role of information in brain–body–environment interactions. The application of such formal models to empirical studies of embodied cognition is a goal for the future. Initial exploratory studies suggest that a combined theoretical framework of dynamical systems and information theory has considerable promise for revealing the interconnectedness of brain and body and for identifying influences of brain–body–environment interactions on the activity of brain networks. Information, generally regarded as an important concept for understanding neural processing within the brain, may also be the key for charting and quantifying mechanisms by which brain states cause other brain states through causal effects on body and environment (Polani, 2009).

It's Networks All the Way Down

Our exploration of brain networks, which has led us from neuroanatomy to neural dynamics, disease, development, and the nature of complexity, is drawing to a close with this brief discussion of the many connections between brain and body. That brain and body share a common evolutionary and developmental history, and that their dynamic linkage is essential for most aspects of behavior and cognition, may, on the surface, seem almost trivial. And yet, the bond between brain and body is at the heart of what it means to be an autonomous organism. The essence of autonomy is self-determination—the actions of an organism within a physical and social environment continually perturb the rich web of dynamic interactions that make up brain and mind. The empirical studies, agent/robot models, and theoretical explorations surveyed in this chapter suggest that the application of network thinking to brain–body–environment interactions promises to reveal principles that enable autonomy and intelligence. These principles do not reside within some clever control algorithm or result from the computations of "higher" brain regions, nor are they deeply embedded within the brain's "blueprint" or wiring diagram. Rather, they draw heavily on ideas of information and dynamics within networks, as well as on embodiment and extended cognition.

It appears unlikely that the extraordinary capacity and flexibility of the human mind can be traced to any single morphological or genetic feature, the appearance of a privileged brain region or pathway or of a specific neural cell type or protein.[14] By itself, even the complete wiring diagram of the brain will not reveal what makes us human, no more so than the complete map of genetic material. The latter point is driven home by the human genome project, which, so far, has fallen short of its original promise of providing "the ultimate answers to the chemical underpinnings of human existence" (Watson, 1990, p. 44) but succeeded in paving the way for new systems-based approaches to understanding how genes turn into phenotypes. Simplistic notions of genetic determinism encounter severe limitations when one is attempting to uncover the biological bases of uniquely human phenotypic traits (Varki et al., 2008). Instead, genome–environment interactions and new concepts in systems biology that build on quantitative methods for network analysis appear to be much more promising. In addition to the identification of specific genetic changes, the complementary study of gene and protein networks provides a new basis for exploring the relationship between genotype and phenotype, including one of the most complex phenotypes, human cognition.

This book has been a single long argument for a similar shift toward networks and complex systems approaches in neuroscience. The study of brain networks defines a new and promising direction for uncovering the mechanisms by which the collective action of large numbers of nerve cells gives rise to the complexity of the human mind. Network approaches are well suited for bridging levels of organization in the nervous system because they place elementary units and processes in a wider functional context. I have argued throughout the book for the considerable power of applying network science and network thinking to neural systems. From the dynamics of social groups to the behavior of single cognitive agents, from the structural and functional connectivity of their neural systems to the morphology and metabolism of individual neurons, and the interactions of their component biomolecules—to modify a popular phrase, it's networks all the way down. Mapping these networks, their extensive sets of elements and interactions, and recording their complex and multiscale dynamics are key steps toward a more complete understanding of how the brain functions as an integrated system, steps toward network neuroscience.

Network Glossary

The following terms are frequently encountered in the network literature and used throughout the book.

Adjacency matrix   The most basic representation of a graph or network in matrix format. In a binary graph, the entries of the matrix record the presence or absence of a connection between node pairs. In a weighted graph, the entries of the matrix equal the weight of the connection (if present). In undirected graphs the matrix is symmetrical along the main diagonal. The adjacency matrix is also referred to as the connection matrix.

Assortativity   The correlation between the degrees of connected node pairs. Positive assortativity indicates that edges tend to link nodes with matching degrees.

Centrality   In general, a measure of how central or influential a node is relative to the rest of the network. There are different measures of centrality. The node degree gives a first indication of centrality, especially in networks with a broad or scale-free degree distribution. Another measure, betweenness centrality, expresses the fraction of short paths between nodes of the network that pass through a given node.

Characteristic path length   The average of all finite distances in a network. A short path length implies the existence of many short paths between node pairs.

Clustering coefficient   The fraction of connections (out of all possible) that connect the neighbors of a given node, thus capturing the degree to which a node's neighbors are also neighbors of each other (i.e., the "cliquishness" of a network neighborhood).

Connectivity   In the book, the term refers to a set of connections among nodes, forming a network of either structural or functional relationships.

Connector hub   Hubs that link nodes across different network modules or communities.

Core   A network core is a set of nodes that are highly and mutually interconnected. A core can be mapped by using a recursive procedure that prunes away weakly connected nodes (i.e., nodes with low degree).

Cycle   A path that returns to its origin, and thus links a node to itself. Cycles are also referred to as loops.

Degree   The number of connections (incoming and outgoing) that are attached to a given node. Across the whole network, all node degrees are often summarized in a degree distribution.

Diameter   The maximum finite distance between any pair of nodes.

Directed graph   A graph that contains directed edges, also referred to as a digraph. Directed edges link a source node to a target node, and the direction of the edge defines the direction of information flow. In the brain, chemical synaptic connections form directed edges between neurons.

Distance   The distance between a pair of nodes is equal to the length of the shortest path between them. If no path exists, the distance is infinite.

Distance matrix   The entries of the distance matrix contain the distances (the lengths of the shortest paths) between all pairs of nodes. The entries are "Inf" if no path exists.

Edge   Pairs of nodes are linked by edges. These edges can be directed or undirected and they can be binary or weighted. In simple graphs, each pair of nodes is linked by, at most, a single undirected edge, or two directed edges (in opposite directions). Edges are also called links, connections, or arcs.

Effective connectivity   The pattern of causal effects of one neural element over another. Effective connectivity may be computed on the basis of temporal precedence cues (Granger causality, transfer entropy) or on the basis of a causal model (e.g., dynamic causal modeling).

Functional connectivity   The pattern of statistical dependencies between distributed and neural elements. Functional connectivity is often expressed as a cross-correlation between neural time series. Other measures of functional connectivity are mutual information or coherence.

Graph   Graphs are abstract descriptions of relationships between the elements of a system. Put differently, a graph is a set of nodes (elements) and edges (relations) which together form a network. Edges can be binary or weighted. In a binary graph, edges between two nodes are either present or absent (one or zero). In a weighted graph edges can take on fractional values.

Hub   Hubs may be identified on the basis of several network measures, including high degree, short average path length, or high betweenness centrality.

Module   Modules or communities may be structurally defined as nodes that are highly interconnected and that overlap in their external connection patterns. Modules may also be functionally defined on the basis of the pattern of functional or effective connections. A given network can be decomposed into a set of non-overlapping, overlapping, or hierarchically arranged modules.

Motif   A small subset of network nodes and edges, forming a subgraph. Any given network can be uniquely decomposed into motifs that each belongs to a specific motif class. For example, for directed networks there are exactly 13 possible connected 3-node motifs.

Neighbors   A node's neighbors are all nodes that are connected to it with either directed or undirected connections.

Node   A network element which may represent a neuron, a neuronal population, a brain region, a brain voxel, or a recording electrode. Nodes are also referred to as vertices.

Path   A series of unique edges that link a pair of nodes. In directed graphs, paths consist of sets of directed edges that connect a source node to a target node. In many cases, a given pair of nodes can be connected by numerous paths.

Path Length   In a binary graph the path length is equal to the path's number of edges. In weighted graphs, the length of the path is the sum of the edge lengths, which can be derived by transforming the edge weights.

Provincial hub   Hubs that belong to a single module or community where they link many of its constituent nodes to each other.

Random network   A network where edges between nodes are randomly assigned with fixed probability. This class of random network is also known as an Erdös-Renyi graph.

Reachability matrix   The binary entries of the reachability matrix record if a path (of any length) exists between a pair of nodes.

Scale-free network   The degree distribution of a scale-free network follows a power law. High-degree nodes are may be network hubs.

Small-world network   A network that combines high clustering with a short characteristic path length. More precisely, compared to a population of random networks composed of the same number of nodes and connections and with equal node degrees, the network's average clustering coefficient is greatly increased, and its characteristic path length is about the same.

Strength   The sum of the connection weights (incoming and outgoing) for all connections attached to a given node.

Structural connectivity   The pattern of physical connections between neural elements. Structural connections can be individual synapses between single neurons, or axonal projections or fiber pathways between neural populations or brain regions. Structural connectivity corresponds to the "wiring diagram" of the brain.

Undirected graph   A graph composed entirely of undirected edges. In functional connectivity, undirected edges often express symmetric statistical relationships. In structural connectivity, undirected edges indicate reciprocal anatomical coupling. Current diffusion imaging techniques generate structural networks of undirected edges.

Notes

Chapter 1

1. The role of networks in linking multiple scales of organization in social systems was recognized decades ago by the sociologist Mark Granovetter in a classic paper entitled "The Strength of Weak Ties" (Granovetter, 1973). Granovetter argued that "the analysis of processes in interpersonal networks provides the most fruitful micro/macro bridge. In one way or another, it is through these networks that small-scale interaction becomes translated into large-scale patterns, and that these, in turn, feed back into small groups" (Granovetter, 1973, p. 1360).

Chapter 2

1. Quoted from the translation of Euler's original paper (Euler, 1736) in Biggs et al. (1976, p. 3).

2. The historical context of Euler's paper is described in Alexanderson (2006).

3. The term "graph" was originally derived from the common use of "graphical notation" to represent the structure of molecules and was introduced by the mathematician James Joseph Sylvester while applying graphical approaches to problems in chemistry in the 1870s (Bonchev and Rouvray, 1990).

4. Several popular books have documented the rise of network science in the natural and social sciences (Barabási, 2002; Buchanan, 2002; Watts, 2003). A collection of key historical and modern papers on network science is also available (Newman et al., 2006).

5. In this book, the term "network" generally refers to both the real-world system and its graph description. Other graph theoretical terms are often used interchangeably. For example, nodes can also be referred to as vertices, and edges are often called links or connections. The "Network Glossary" notes some of these terminological equivalencies.

6. Connections with negative weights are frequently encountered in social networks, where they represent negative affect or dislike, and in cellular signaling and metabolic circuits, which contain an abundance of inhibitory control loops. In both of these fields, graph theory methods that account for negative links have been devised and applied. This is a reminder that the simple graph-based techniques discussed in this book comprise only a minimal tool set and that the arsenal of graph methods in neuroscience is likely to increase in the future.

7. Connectivity-based community detection in networks depends on several factors including the density of connections and the size distribution of modules. Small modules can be difficult to resolve and thus modularity detection algorithms require careful assessment of accuracy and robustness (Fortunato and Barthélemy, 2007).

8. Google's "PageRank" algorithm, used in Google Web searches, employs a variant of eigenvector centrality to establish the authority and importance of Web pages.

9. With the arrival of online services such as MySpace, Facebook, and Twitter, social networking has become a multibillion-dollar economic enterprise as well as an essential part of the social lives of millions of users. At the time of writing, Facebook has hundreds of millions of active users, and the average user is connected to more than 100 "friends."

10. That the actual discovery of a short path in a small-world network may indeed be difficult, however, was demonstrated by the failed attempt in 1999 of the German weekly newspaper *Die Zeit* to find a path with six links or less between the Berlin resident and falafel vendor Salah ben Ghaly and one of his favorite movie actors, Marlon Brando.

11. Highly skewed ("fat-tailed") distributions had been described much earlier. The nineteenth-century economist Vilfredo Pareto observed that economic variables such as land ownership, income, and wealth were distributed according to an 80:20 rule, akin to a power-law relationship. Models of their origin, resembling preferential attachment, were designed by Udny Yule and Herbert Simon more than 50 years ago. Power-law relationships were also described long ago for word frequencies and city sizes by George Zipf. Zipf's law states that the frequency of words is inversely proportional to their rank in usage, and the relationship holds for many human languages.

12. The issue of how power laws are best detected in empirical data sets was recently reexamined by Clauset et al. (2009). Regression analysis of linear relationships in logarithmically transformed data, often used to establish the existence of a power law, may be inapplicable or uninformative. Closer analysis of a number of purported power-law relationships confirms some of them but also reveals that others are more closely approximated by exponential or log-normal distributions. Another issue arises when networks are constructed by sampling from a larger population of nodes. Subsets of nodes may not accurately reflect the topology of the entire network from which they were sampled (Stumpf et al., 2005).

13. The network data set and all software used to compute network measures are freely available at http://www.brain-connectivity-toolbox.net.

14. Note that there is a difference between an Erdös–Rényi random network and a randomly constructed "null hypothesis" random network with fixed degrees. Erdös–Reényi graphs have Poissonian degree distributions, while "null hypothesis" graphs can be constructed for an arbitrary degree distribution.

15. Examples are the "Brain Connectivity Toolbox" maintained by Mika Rubinov and myself (http://www.brain-connectivity-toolbox.net), Katy Börner's "Network Workbench" (http://nwb.slis.indiana.edu), David Gleich's "MatlabBGL" (http://www.stanford.edu/~dgleich/programs/matlab_bgl/), and Pajek (http://vlado.fmf.uni-lj.si/pub/networks/pajek/; Bagatelj and Mrvar, 1998).

Chapter 3

1. Quoted after Shepard (1991, p. 265).

2. A century after Golgi and Cajal shared the Nobel Prize, the neuron doctrine was critically reexamined by Bullock et al. (2005) and Glickstein (2006), who affirmed its continued significance but also pointed to its limitations.

3. Electrocorticography is a more direct method for recording electrical potentials that uses electrodes placed on the exposed surface of the brain. As such, it is an invasive recording method which is usually performed only in patients during or after brain surgery.

4. The spatial resolution of fMRI recordings is largely limited by the voxel size, generally ranging from 2 to 4 millimeters. Specialized application of high-field fMRI can reveal submillimeter-scale structures such as orientation columns (Yacoub et al., 2008).

5. The BOLD response is a complex function of changes in cerebral blood volume, cerebral blood flow, and oxygen consumption, all partially coupled to neural activity. BOLD signals best reflect synaptic inputs to a given region but correlate less well with modulatory inputs or with the neural output of the region (Logothetis and Wandell, 2004). The complex physiology of the BOLD response is rarely considered in the cognitive interpretation of functional imaging data.

6. Karl Friston once remarked on the challenges facing neuroimaging research. He wrote as follows: "Imagine that we took you to a forest and told you, 'Tell us how this forest works […].' You accept the challenge, and, to make things interesting, we place two restrictions on you. First, you can only measure one thing. Second, although you can make measurements anywhere, you can only take them at weekly intervals" (Friston, 1998a, p. 796).

7. A reductionist approach fails to adequately describe complex systems of nonlinearly interacting elements. For instance, the complex patterns of human social activity unfold on multiple scales and, despite the rise of agent-based model in economics and epidemiology, cannot be fully reduced to actions of individuals. Global indicators of economic systems (inflation, economic growth, trade imbalances, consumer confidence, currency pegs, and unemployment) cannot be reduced to the activities of individual shoppers in a supermarket. Instead, these global indicators might well influence the activities of these shoppers, thus further underscoring their independent validity and causal efficacy.

8. If a threshold is necessary to estimate graph measures, it should be varied over a plausible range to generate networks with varying connection density. Networks measures should then be computed across the entire range and compared to appropriate null distributions.

9. Alternative proposals have suggested that neuronal populations are the functional units of the nervous systems—for example, minicolumns or neuronal groups in neocortex (Mountcastle, 1978; Edelman, 1978).

10. Centuries of philosophical debate have left the nature of causality unresolved, leading William James to remark that "we have no definite ideas of what we mean by cause, or of what causality consists in. […] The word 'cause' is, in short, an altar to an unknown god; an empty pedestal still marking the place of a hoped-for statue" (James, 1890, p. 671).

11. The targeted use of perturbations—for example, neuronal microstimulation or transcranial magnetic stimulation (TMS)—can reveal specific dynamic (or cognitive/behavioral) effects. For instance, the combination of TMS with functional neuroimaging allows the quantification of effects of localized perturbations on extended brain networks engaged in the performance of specific tasks (Paus, 1999; Pascual-Leone et al., 2000). Using a combination of TMS and high-density electroencephalography, Massimini et al. (2005) reported a striking reduction in the extent of cortical effective connectivity during non-REM sleep compared to waking.

12. Several other methods for deriving directed interactions on the basis of temporal precedence have been proposed. A computational comparison shows that they differ in their sensitivity and ability to retrieve "true" causal interactions mediated by structural connections (Lungarella et al., 2007).

13. For that reason, some authors argue that time-series-based methods for inferring directed interactions reveal functional, not effective, connectivity (e.g., Friston, 2009a).

14. The skepticism of most empirical neuroscientists with regard to theory was expressed by Santiago Ramon y Cajal in his "Advice for a Young Investigator." Theorists, he writes, combine "a facility for exposition, a creative and restless imagination, an aversion to the laboratory, and an indomitable dislike for concrete science […]. Basically, the theorist is a lazy person masquerading as a diligent one" (Cajal, 1999, pp. 84–85). Of course, Cajal himself was not only a keen observer and brilliant laboratory scientist but also a formidable theoretician (see, e.g., chapter 7).

15. Norbert Wiener was among the first to envision the application of computer models to complex systems "and in particular to the very complicated study of the nervous system which is itself a sort of cerebral meteorology" (Wiener, 1956, p. 260).

16. Eugene Izhikevich carried out a simulation of one hundred billion spiking neurons connected by almost one quadrillion synapses, a neural simulation roughly of the size of the human brain. In late 2005, simulating one second of real time took 50 days on a 27-processor computer cluster. Just storing the weights of the structural connection matrix would take around 10,000 terabytes. Izhikevich has suggested that assuming Moore's law (an assertion that computational power doubles approximately every two years) remains

in effect, real-time simulation of the human brain at the level of single neurons and synapses may become possible as soon as 2016. Near real-time simulations approaching the size of a mouse or cat brain have already been carried out (Djurfeldt et al., 2008; Ananthanarayanan et al., 2009).

Chapter 4

1. Quoted after von Bonin (1960, p. 57).

2. An early critique of this view noted that anatomical localization and physiological specialization are related concepts (John and Schwartz, 1978).

3. Pierre Flourens credits Gall with firmly establishing the proposition that the brain is the exclusive seat of the mind: "The merit of Gall, and it is by no means a slender merit, consists in his having understood better than any of his predecessors the whole of its importance, and in having devoted himself to its demonstration" (Flourens, 1846, p. 28). Indeed, Gall's physiological approach was based on the notion that the organization of the brain caused mental processes and their disturbances: "A few drops of blood extravasated in the cavities of the brain, a few grains of opium, are enough to demonstrate to us, that, in this life, volition and thought are inseparable from cerebral organization" (Gall, 1835, p. 45). Gall's contributions to psychology and neuroscience are reviewed in Zola-Morgan (1995).

4. The American psychologist Shepard Franz sharply criticized the histological studies of Campbell and Brodmann as sophisticated but futile attempts to revive phrenology (Franz, 1912), despite Brodmann's rather explicit disavowal of the concept (see the following note). Phrenology continues to be invoked in critiques of cerebral localization and modular accounts of mental function. For example, the psychologist William Uttal labeled the use of neuroimaging technology to localize functions of the brain as "the new phrenology" (Uttal, 2001). Fodor's views on "modularity of mind," which are generally sympathetic to the old phrenological framework of localized mental faculties, will be discussed further in chapter 9.

5. Brodmann's views on the physiological basis of higher brain function occasionally have a decidedly antilocalizationist ring to them: "In reality there is only one psychic centre: the brain as a whole with all its organs activated for every complex psychic event, either all together or most at the same time, and so widespread over the different parts of the cortical surface that one can never justify any separate specially differentiated 'psychic' centres within this whole" (Brodmann, 1909; quoted after Garey, 1994, p. 255). Brodmann roundly rejected theories "which, like phrenology, attempt to localize complex mental activity [...] to circumscribed cortical zones" (ibid., p. 254), which is all the more remarkable since cytoarchitectonic specialization is often cited in support of such theories.

6. A project to assemble a human brain atlas for gene expression patterns is currently underway at the Allen Institute for Brain Science (Jones et al., 2009). A similar effort resulted in a complete gene expression atlas of the adult mouse brain (Lein et al., 2007). An exciting prospect is the registration of these atlases with whole-brain anatomical connectivity maps (see chapter 5).

7. Novel approaches to noninvasive imaging of anatomical fine structure in both gray and white matter may eventually allow the charting of cytoarchitectonic boundaries in vivo (Duyn et al., 2007).

8. Comparing his own cytoarchitectonic map to the myeloarchitectonic map derived by O. Vogt, Brodmann observed that "in man the fibre architecture of the cortex is often more finely differentiated than the cell architecture" thus making it possible "to subdivide larger cytoarchitectonic zones into smaller fields of specific fibre structure" (Brodmann, 1909; quoted after Garey, 1994, p. 5).

9. Subsequent cluster analyses of regional connectivity obtained with diffusion MRI and tractography have resulted in parcellations of human parietal cortex (Rushworth et al., 2006), lateral premotor cortex (Tomassini et al., 2007), and cingulate cortex (Beckmann et al., 2009).

10. The idea of a distinctive "fingerprint" of each cortical area's inputs and outputs was already noted in Felleman and Van Essen (1991). More recently, Marcel Mesulam underscored the close relationship between connectivity and function: "Nothing defines the function of a neuron more faithfully than the nature of its inputs and outputs" (Mesulam, 2005, p. 6).

11. Karl Lashley was among the first to express the view that inherited variations in brain structure could account for much of individual variability in behavior. He noted that "the brain is extremely variable in every character that has been subjected to measurement. Its diversities of structure within the species are of the same general character as are the differences between related species or even between orders of animals [...]. Individuals start life with brains differing enormously in structure; unlike in number, size, and arrangement of neurons as well as in grosser features. The variation in cells and tracts must have functional significance" (Lashley, 1947, p. 333). Lashley ascribed much of this variability to genetic causes. Genetic influences on brain structure are indeed significant (Thompson et al., 2001) and contribute to structural variation, in addition to epigenetic mechanisms.

12. All cellular components, including all proteins involved in cell structure, signaling, metabolism, and electrophysiology, are continually replaced, on time scales of minutes, hours, and days. Francis Crick noted that this rapid turnover of molecular components poses significant problems for the maintenance of long-term memory (Crick, 1984).

13. Unorganized connectivity refined by learning was a central design feature of most connectionist networks. While connectionist models have significantly added to our understanding of the distributed nature of cognitive processes, their idealized architectures have little to say about how these processes emerge from the networks of the brain.

14. In his book *Perceptual Neuroscience*, Vernon Mountcastle acknowledged the tremendous advances in our understanding of the brain brought about by modern neuroanatomy, but he also states that "in and of itself knowledge of structure provides no direct understanding of dynamic function. *Where is not how*" (Mountcastle, 1998, p. 366, italics his).

Chapter 5

1. Quoted after Steno (1965, p. 121).

2. Steno's contributions to geology are more widely known and recognized. His work on the origin of fossils directly challenged the orthodox Biblical account of the age of the earth. Nevertheless, in his later life Steno turned to religion and became a Catholic priest. He was beatified by Pope John Paul II in 1988.

3. An excellent review of the history of cerebral white matter is provided in an article by Schmahmann and Pandya (2007).

4. In one of his short stories, entitled "On Exactitude in Science," Jorge Luis Borges describes the "Art of Cartography" and how its application leads to "[...] a Map of the Empire whose size was that of the Empire, and which coincided point for point with it. The following Generations, who were not so fond of the Study of Cartography as their Forebears had been, saw that that vast Map was Useless, and not without some Pitilessness was it, that they delivered it up to the Inclemencies of Sun and Winters. In the Deserts of the West, still today, there are Tattered Ruins of that Map, inhabited by Animals and Beggars; in all the Land there is no other Relic of the Disciplines of Geography" (Borges, 2000, p. 181). Might a map of the brain whose size is that of the brain meet a similar fate?

5. "Whole brain emulation," involving the scanning of a brain in fine structural detail and then running an accurate software model that reproduces the brain's functional activity, is one of the central goals of the transhumanist agenda (e.g., Sandberg and Bostrom, 2008).

6. Evidently, not everyone thinks that "connectomics" is a compelling idea worth pursuing. In an interview with the journal *Nature*, Nobel laureate Sydney Brenner referred to connectomics as "a ludicrous term" (Brenner, 2008, p. 9) while also projecting, rather optimistically, that "we may be able to compute behaviour from the wiring diagram of *Caenorhabditis elegans* (with 300 neurons) in the next few years."

7. The program to map the human genome was discussed and eventually endorsed at a meeting sponsored by the Office of Health and Environmental Research of the U.S. Department of Energy, held in Santa Fe in 1986 (DeLisi, 2008). The first map of the human genome was published 15 years later, in 2001.

8. Notably, this number of genes exceeds that for *Drosophila* and is about equal to the current best estimate for the number of genes in the human genome (Pennisi, 2007).

9. The seminal paper by White et al. (1986) opens by noting that "The functional properties of a nervous system are largely determined by the characteristics of its component neurons and the pattern of synaptic connections between them" (p. 2). This simple statement still stands as one of the major rationales for compiling whole-brain maps of structural connectivity.

10. Preceding the reconstruction of the *C. elegans* nervous system, early applications of serial EM sectioning and reconstruction technology yielded complete 3D models of individual neurons in the nervous system of the small crustacean *Daphnia magna* (Macagno et al., 1979).

11. For example, high-resolution serial reconstruction of one cubic millimeter of mammalian brain may generate on the order of 1,000 terabytes of data, with a complete reconstruction of a human brain exceeding one million petabytes (Kasthuri and Lichtman, 2007).

12. A "Committee on a National Neural Circuitry Database" was convened in 1989 by the Institute of Medicine to review the feasibility and potential applications of computer technology in the basic and clinical neurosciences (Pechura and Martin, 1991). The committee report led to the initiation of the Human Brain Project in 1993, funded by five U.S. agencies and led by the National Institute of Mental Health. One of the goals of the Human Brain Project was the creation of a neuroinformatics infrastructure that would support the collection and sharing of neuroscience data sets (Huerta and Koslow, 1996).

13. Bohland et al. estimate that the mouse project "can be completed in five years at a total cost of less than US$20 million" (Bohland et al., 2009, p. 6).

14. Other major disadvantages are sampling biases, the lack of data on cognitive and behavioral performance, and the inability to probe the brain of a deceased person for functional activation patterns.

Chapter 6

1. Quoted after Lorente de Nó (1938, p. 207).

2. Lorente de Nó was a professor at The Rockefeller Institute for Medical Research in New York City. His 1938 review of cortical connectivity was published around the same time as some of the first papers on sociometrics (e.g., Moreno and Jennings, 1938), or social networks, written by Jacob Moreno, who at the time lived only 40 miles away near the town of Beacon, New York.

3. Lorente de Nó's idea of "synaptic chains" was formulated before the role of inhibition in the central nervous system was fully grasped. His emphasis on reciprocal anatomical circuits as a prominent feature of cortical anatomy apparently met with disapproval from his teacher and mentor Cajal (Fairén, 2007).

4. Reentry as a structural and dynamic principle for the interaction of local as well as distant cell populations forms one of the cornerstones of Edelman's theory of neural Darwinism (Edelman, 1987) and is discussed more extensively in chapter 9. The existence of reciprocal connections between brain regions does not necessarily imply that individual neurons are mutually coupled. Long-range axonal projections exhibit characteristic laminar profiles in axonal origin and termination patterns arranged such that direct excitatory feedback loops do not occur. Crick and Koch (1998a) formulated a "no-strong-loops" hypothesis, arguing that these connectivity patterns could lead to dynamic instability and were therefore selected against.

5. White goes on to remark that the abundance of highly connected three-node motifs may reflect a mixture of local and global connectivity: "One of the most striking features of the

circuitry may therefore simply be a consequence of the arrangement of processes into restricted yet highly connected neighborhoods" (White, 1985, p. 281). This prescient statement encapsulates one of the essential elements of what is now called a small-world network.

6. Functional motifs were first described by W. Ross Ashby in his book *Design for a Brain* (Ashby, 1960). Ashby noted that "complex systems may have many interlacing circuits" (Ashby, 1960, p. 53) and that the number of potential subcircuits would increase with the density of interconnections. Later in the book (p. 166), Ashby introduced the notion of "immediate" and "ultimate effects," which resembles the distinction between structural and functional connectivity. A static pattern of immediate effects (structural linkages) can produce "a remarkable variety" of functional patterns, depending on the state of individual network elements.

7. A cautionary point was raised by Ingram et al. (2006), who found that even a simple structural motif exhibits a wide range of dynamic behaviors, depending upon the settings of kinetic (or, in the case of neural systems, biophysical) parameters. Motif decomposition of a complex network therefore is only a first step toward characterizing the network's computational or functional competence. Weighted motifs provide a way to incorporate dynamic parameters as edge weights into the analysis (Onnela et al., 2005).

8. Spandrels were introduced into evolutionary theory by Gould and Lewontin's much-discussed critique of adaptationism, the idea that all or most phenotypic traits are adaptations that have been optimized by natural selection (Gould and Lewontin, 1979). Spandrels are architectural surfaces that arise when arches meet rectangular shapes, as by-products of the building's geometric plan, but without a clearly defined or optimized functional role. Gould and Lewontin argued that many phenotypic traits were spandrels, by-products of evolution instead of adaptations.

9. The first demonstrations of the brain's small-world architecture had to rely on sparse data sets that comprised no more than a hundred nodes and a few hundred connections. These data sets are minuscule in comparison to the large networks routinely studied by computer and social scientists. As Duncan Watts has pointed out (Watts, 1999), one of the prerequisites for small-world architectures is that the system under study has a great number of nodes and edges, that is, is "numerically large." As more highly resolved structural connectivity patterns will become available in the near future, small-world analyses will likely add significantly more detail to the present picture.

10. Optimization algorithms that maximize modularity (Newman and Girvan, 2004) may not actually deliver optimal partitions, as the problem of finding an optimal partition is NP-complete and thus becomes intractable for large graphs or networks (Brandes et al., 2008). A number of other modularity algorithms have been proposed (Danon et al., 2005).

11. Years ago, Marc Raichle and colleagues nicknamed the area "medial mystery parietal area" because of its consistent and yet unexplained involvement in task-related and resting-state fMRI (Raichle and Snyder, 2007).

12. Antonio Damasio described patients with bilateral medial parietal damage as "awake in the usual sense of the term: their eyes can be open, and their muscles have proper tone; they can sit or even walk with assistance; but they will not look at you or at any object with any semblance of intention; and their eyes may stare vacantly or orient towards objects with no discernable motive" (Damasio, 1999, p. 263).

Chapter 7

1. Quoted after Cajal (1995, pp. 115–116).

2. This point was made by Striedter (2005), and it was driven home by Nelson and Bower (1990): "In the nervous system, [...] constraints are [...] likely to be imposed by the large numbers of connections between neurons and the rather strict limitations on cranial capacity. A simple 'back of the envelope' calculation serves to demonstrate the potential severity of this constraint: if the brain's estimated 10^{11} neurons were placed on the surface of a sphere and fully interconnected by individual axons 0.1 μm in radius, the sphere would

have to have a diameter of more than 20 km to accommodate the connections!" (Nelson and Bower, 1990, p. 408).

3. Cajal acknowledged that "histogenesis may clearly reveal how a particular feature assumes its mature form" (Cajal, 1995, p. 125), but he insisted that development alone could not explain the "utilitarian and teleological" reasons behind cell and connectional morphology, which are provided by his proposed laws of conservation.

4. Detailed anatomical reconstructions of axonal arborizations in mammalian neuromuscular circuitry have demonstrated suboptimality for the wiring length of individual axons by as much as 25 percent (Lu et al., 2009). This suggests that factors other than wiring length—for example, circuit functionality or activity-dependent growth mechanisms—play a role in shaping neuromuscular axonal arbors.

5. The idea that cortical folding reduces wiring length has been around for some time. In a discussion of cortical folding patterns, Carl Wernicke referred to the idea that the folding is arranged such that space is optimally conserved as an "old opinion" (Wernicke, 1876, p. 298). Norbert Wiener reflected on the allometric scaling of the brain's gray and white matter and on cortical folding as a way to reduce wiring length as early as 1948.

6. Variations in brain size scale with numerous other morphological variables, including cortical surface area, volume, and convolution, all of which also affect connection topology. Im et al. (2008) suggest that systematic differences in brain size between males and females may account for sex differences in cortical structure.

7. One of the more surprising scaling relations is that between the sizes of the brain and gut in primates. Aiello and Wheeler (1995) suggested that since both tissues are metabolically expensive, increased brain size may have required a reduction in the size of the gut. A secondary consequence of reducing gut size is a shift toward a higher quality diet, including the need for animal protein. Metabolic constraints resulting from increased encephalization may thus be responsible for profound changes in behavior.

8. However, the status of the concept of adaptation in modern evolutionary theory is far from resolved. The renowned evolutionist George C. Williams had this to say about the concept of adaptation: "This biological principle should be used only as a last resort. It should not be invoked when less onerous principles, such as those of physics and chemistry or that of unspecific cause and effect, are sufficient for a complete explanation" (Williams, 1966, p. 11).

9. The recent struggles and controversies among leading evolutionary theorists, concerning in part the role of adaptations in the evolutionary process, are documented in a recent book by Richard Morris (Morris, 2001).

Chapter 8

1. Quoted after Hebb (1949, pp. 6–7).

2. As Valentino Braitenberg pointed out, internal traffic of the cortex exceeds external traffic by a factor of 100 to 1,000 (Braitenberg, 1974). While the number of thalamocortical inputs is small compared to intracortical synapses, their physiological effect may be amplified by greater physiological strength and reliability or by the combined efficacy of multiple synchronous inputs (Bruno and Sakmann, 2006). Physiological recordings can more directly determine the degree to which cortex is autonomously active or driven by sensory input (see, e.g., MacLean et al., 2005).

3. Feedforward models of neural processing are quite successful in capturing some of the neural and cognitive data on object recognition (Riesenhuber and Poggio, 1999; 2000). The idea of a "visual hierarchy" consisting of specialized neurons whose response properties become increasingly sophisticated and invariant undoubtedly captures an important characteristic of the visual cortex. The challenge is to create models that can reconcile the different sets of physiological observations supporting the feedforward and reentrant aspects of visual recognition. A promising framework proposes that information is encoded in the temporal evolution of neural trajectories (see chapter 12) and that neural responses are determined by inputs as well as intrinsic network states (Buonomano and Maass, 2009).

4. The autonomy of the brain leads Llinás to suggest that "the waking state is a dreamlike state [...] guided and shaped by the senses" (Llinás, 2001, p. 94). The mounting evidence for coordinated spontaneous activity in the brain lends support to this surprising notion. The main function of the brain, according to Llinás, is prediction, a consequence of the need to anticipate the effects of motor activity in the environment—we will return to this idea when we discuss the embodied brain in chapter 14.

5. Slow alterations between synchronized UP and DOWN states are encountered mostly during slow-wave sleep. How these UP/DOWN states may be related to cortical activation during wakefulness is an open question.

6. Optical recordings of neuronal activity in hippocampal slices has revealed the presence of highly connected and highly influential "hub neurons" (Bonifazi et al., 2009). These neurons, representing a subpopulation of inhibitory interneurons, maintain a large number of functional connections and, when perturbed, have a large effect on network dynamics.

7. Spontaneous activity occurs at different levels in different areas of the brain. While there are many reports of ongoing neural activity throughout the central nervous system, there is also evidence that suggests that many neurons fire only rarely and are therefore difficult to observe directly, perhaps constituting the brain's "dark matter" (Shoham et al., 2006).

8. High-dimensional models of coupled nonlinear differential equations present significant computational challenges, especially when stochastic noise or conduction delays are taken into account.

9. These dynamic transients reflect spontaneous synchronization and desynchronization events, resulting in a power-law distribution for the lengths of synchronized epochs (Honey et al., 2007). Such power laws can be an indication that the system is in a critical state, associated with high dynamic complexity (see chapter 12).

10. Another modeling study attempted to reconstruct dynamic patterns in cortical activity with a large-scale computational model. Izhikevich and Edelman (2008) created a simulation that was based on DTI-derived structural connectivity combined with an efficiently constructed spiking neuron model. The model incorporated mechanisms for neural plasticity and included both cortical and thalamic regions. Model dynamics displayed organized patterns of spontaneous activity, waves, and rhythms.

11. The authors refer to this data set as functional connectivity. However, their experimental method involves a local perturbation of the excitation/inhibition within a single cortical region and the monitoring of its spread across the brain. The actual data matrix (Stephan et al., 2000) forms a directed graph. Hence, by the definition adopted in chapter 3, this technique reveals effective connectivity, rather than functional connectivity.

12. Interestingly, He et al. demonstrated that network topologies and measures of individual modules showed significant variations and differed from those of the global network, indicating that each module had its own internal pattern of organization.

13. Wang et al. (2009a) performed network analyses of functional connectivity using two different parcellations of the cortical surface into 70 and 90 regions. Both networks exhibited robust small-world attributes and efficient connectivity, but the values of these network measures showed parcellation-dependent differences. This underscores the importance of node definition for any quantitative network analysis (see chapter 3).

14. Regardless of its role in cognition, the resting state offers a unique window on brain connectivity that can be applied in circumstances where data on task-evoked neural activations are difficult, if not impossible, to obtain, including imaging of the brains of very young children, in patients who have suffered traumatic brain injury, or across a wide range of neuropsychiatric disorders (see chapters 10 and 11).

15. Just as spontaneous neural activity reveals rich spatial and temporal structure, the spontaneous behavioral activity of an animal may reveal the same (Maye et al., 2007). Spontaneous turning in flight behavior of *Drosophila* does not appear to be stochastic but displays fractal temporal order indicative of a nonlinear neural generator capable of operating in the absence of any overt sensory input. Thus, spontaneous behavior appears to be an irreducible manifestation of spontaneous neural activity.

Chapter 9

1. Quoted after James (1890, pp. 81–82).

2. The "platform independence" of cognitive functionalism is often seen as a considerable strength as it reduces mental processes to their essential, computational core. This functionalist position so prevalent among cognitive scientists is difficult to reconcile with basic facts of biology, and it seems impoverished when compared to the rich phenomenology of brain networks and their complex evolutionary and developmental origin.

3. For the most part, this chapter will leave aside the embodied aspect of cognition, a topic to which we turn in chapter 14.

4. Karl Lashley wrote in 1931 that the concept of cerebral localization was of limited value, because of "its failure to provide any answer to the question of how the specialized parts of the cortex interact to produce the integration evident in thought and behavior. The problem here is one of the dynamic relations of the diverse parts of the cortex, whether they be cells or cortical fields" (Lashley, 1931, p. 246).

5. Semir Zeki describes the duality of segregation and integration, the "paradox of vision," as he calls it, with unmatched eloquence: "The picture that one obtains from studying the visual cortex is one of multiple areas and of parallel pathways leading to them. It is a picture that shows a deep division of labour [...]. Yet the common, daily experience of the normal brain stands forever opposed to the notion of a division of labour and of functional segregation. For that experience is one of wholeness, of a unitary visual image, in which all the visual attributes take their correct place [...] Nothing in that integrated visual image suggests that different visual attributes are processed in physically separate parts of our cortex" (Zeki, 1993, p. 295).

6. Convergence and phase synchrony map onto single-cell physiology. Cortical neurons can operate in two distinct modes of operation, as "integrators" or as "coincidence detectors," depending on the time scale of synaptic summation (König et al., 1996).

7. The idea of creating specialized neurons for complex stimuli or tasks goes back at least to Sherrington who famously invoked the "ultimate pontifical nerve cell [...] the climax of the whole system of integration [...] receiving all and dispensing all as unitary arbiter of a totalitarian State." Sherrington immediately dismissed this model of centralized integration: "Where it is a question of 'mind' the nervous system does not integrate itself by centralization upon one pontifical cell. Rather it elaborates a million-fold democracy whose each unit is a cell" (Sherrington, 1940, p. 277).

8. Gamma-band synchronization was considered a potential neural correlate of consciousness, although more recent evidence suggests that this idea may have been overly simplistic (Vanderwolf, 2000).

9. The tangled nature of the way in which levels appear to be arranged in the anatomy of the cerebral cortex brings to mind Doug Hofstadter's concept of a "strange loop," a logical structure where one's apparent progress in a given direction is suddenly interrupted by the realization that one has returned to the origin (Hofstadter, 2007). Many neural signals may well travel in such strange loops formed by the pervasive recurrent connectivity of the cortex.

10. The concept of heterarchy originated in a short paper by McCulloch (1945) in which he demonstrated that the existence of "diallels" (circular connections, or "interlocking circularities of preference") in nerve nets yields nontransitive relations that do not fit on any hierarchical scale.

11. In some cases, connection patterns in visual cortex could be directly linked to Gestalt laws of visual perception, for example, the laws of good continuation, similarity, and common fate (Sporns et al., 1991).

12. The creation of computational models of entire mammalian nervous systems (for example, those of a mouse or human), perhaps interfaced with robotic systems, is likely to become a reality in the near future (see chapters 3 and 14).

13. A preferred term nowadays is "reverse engineering." However, reverse engineering requires a theoretical foundation to provide a definition of the essential anatomical and physiological ingredients. Principles of connectivity, informed by a theoretical understanding of brain networks, are of central importance in this endeavor.

Chapter 10

1. Quoted after Wiener (1948, p. 147).

2. Norbert Wiener personally encountered mental illness (Conway and Siegelman, 2005). His younger brother Fritz suffered from schizophrenia over much of his life, and Wiener worried greatly that he himself might one day develop the disorder. Throughout much of his life, Wiener appears to have been prone to periods of manic excitability followed by severe depression and even thoughts of suicide. In the 1950s, Wiener became closely acquainted with the young mathematician John Nash, and they remained in contact during Nash's struggle with schizophrenia.

3. The global economic crisis of 2008 is widely regarded as a failure of distributed financial and regulatory networks. The crisis caught most governments and individuals by surprise, with serious and lasting consequences for global markets. The failure of economic theory and modeling to predict these events has led to a call for a new theoretical foundation that takes into account network dynamics of the global economy. "To develop a proper perspective on systemic phenomena, economics as a science should take stock of the experience of the natural sciences in handling complex systems with strong interactions. A partial reorientation in modelling principles and more methodological flexibility would enable us to tackle more directly those problems that seem to be most vital in our large, globalized economic systems" (Lux and Westerhoff, 2009, p. 3).

4. In some cases, graph analysis is used to identify points of vulnerability in order to deliberately disrupt the functional integrity of networks—for example, those of criminal or terrorist organizations (Krebs, 2002).

5. Based on data and modeling results of protein networks, Siegal et al. (2007) caution that simple network measures such as node degree are insufficient to predict functional properties of a node or the functional impact of its removal from the network. Siegal et al. suggest that more complex measures that are sensitive to the local and global pattern of connectivity such as clustering coefficients or betweenness centrality are more predictive and that the link between network topology and network dynamics urgently requires further exploration.

6. The idea that network biology might help in a mechanistic understanding of a disease state was expressed in a landmark review article by two cancer biologists: "Having fully charted the wiring diagrams of every cellular signaling pathway, it will be possible to lay out the complete 'integrated circuit of the cell' […]. We will then be able to apply the tools of mathematical modeling to explain how specific genetic lesions serve to reprogram this integrated circuit in each of the constituent cell types so as to manifest cancer" (Hanahan and Weinberg, 2000, p. 67).

7. The full extent of the lesion was unknown to Paul Broca since he did not dissect the brains of these two patients after their deaths. Instead, he decided to preserve these brains intact for future study, a fortuitous choice that now enables a careful reanalysis with modern noninvasive imaging technology.

8. The historical roots and different interpretations of the idea of "disconnection" as a major cause of disrupted brain function are reviewed in Catani and ffytche (2005) and Catani and Mesulam (2008).

9. Nonlocal dynamic effects following a focal brain lesion have a counterpart in the emerging idea that local plasticity—for example, within the hippocampus—can have effects on communication patterns elsewhere in the brain. Canals et al. (2009) presented evidence for nonlocal reorganization of limbic and neocortical circuits following hippocampal synaptic modifications, suggesting that even highly localized neural plasticity may have global effects on brain networks.

10. It would be especially intriguing if the molecular basis for amyloid- and tau-induced neuropathologies were to be found in changed interactions among proteins within a cellular network. This would constitute a case of network anomalies at one level of organization (molecules) causing the disruption of another network (neurons, brain regions) at another level within the same biological system. Going a step further, the cognitive manifestations of the disease have serious social ramifications, for the patient as well as the patient's social group, thus perturbing a social network as well.

11. The idea that psychosis is due to disruptions of structural brain connectivity can be traced to Carl Wernicke, who termed these disruptions "sejunctions" whose specific location determined the nature of the pathology.

12. Stephan et al. (2006) adopted the term "dysconnection" to indicate that schizophrenia manifests itself in a disordered pattern of connectivity that may include increases and decreases in the numbers of individual links. In contrast, the older term "disconnection" primarily implies the loss of connectivity.

13. Lichtman et al. (2008) have coined the term "connectopathy" for disorders of the nervous system that are expressed in quantitative or qualitative defects in neural circuitry.

14. In most cases, structural networks are likely the primary target of disruption, with disturbances of functional connectivity a secondary consequence.

Chapter 11

1. Alan Turing in a letter to J. Z. Young, written in 1951 and quoted after Hodges (1983, p. 437).

2. J. Z. Young had just delivered the Ferrier Lecture of the Royal Society on "Growth and Plasticity in the Nervous System" (Young, 1951), where he laid out the then-available evidence for activity-dependent modifications of neuronal structure. At about the same time, Turing was exploring the possibility of creating computing machines from simple, neuron-like elements (Turing, 1948). Turing speculated that by "appropriate inference, mimicking education" an initially unorganized machine could be trained to perform a wide range of functions, an idea that would resurface as "connectionism" many years later.

3. According to the "Official Google Blog," the number of Web pages with unique addresses reached 1 trillion in 2008 and grows by several billion pages per day (http://googleblog.blogspot.com/2008/07/we-knew-web-was-big.html). Thus, the number of nodes in the World Wide Web now far exceeds the number of neurons in the human brain.

4. Modifications of the rules by which edges (or nodes) are added to a growing network can lead to even more abrupt discontinuities, so-called discontinuous or "explosive" phase transitions (Achlioptas et al., 2009).

5. Power-law distributions are found in very many systems (see chapter 2), and various models for how they might be generated have been proposed. One of the most well-known power laws governs the distribution of word frequencies in texts, also called Zipf's law. Zipf's law is universal across all known languages (even random letter strings). More than 50 years ago, Herbert Simon proposed a mechanism for the generation of Zipf's law (Simon, 1955), similar to preferential attachment, and a "cumulative advantage" model accounting for a wide range of stochastic growth processes giving rise to power laws. We will encounter power laws in the brain's dynamic behavior in chapter 12.

6. The validity of purely statistical models for describing real-world networks such as the Internet's router-level topology has been questioned. Willinger et al. (2009) suggested that adequate descriptions of network functions require the inclusion of additional domain-specific knowledge that takes into account the engineering, design constraints, and growth dynamics of the system at hand.

7. The estimation of functional connectivity across brains of different ages is made difficult by changes in the hemodynamic response of maturing and aging brain regions (D'Esposito et al., 2003).

Chapter 12

1. Quoted after Varela (1995, p. 82).

2. The case for the increased and more sophisticated use of modeling tools to predict and, if possible, prevent global pandemics was made in an opinion article by Epstein (2009), published in the summer of 2009, after the initial outbreak of the H1N1 "swine flu."

3. In any real-world system, power-law distributions can only cover a limited range of scales, and exponential fall-offs often exist at the high end of the scale due to resource, energy, or space limitations (Amaral et al., 2000). Physical structures or events cannot grow to infinity.

4. Langton's results and interpretation were later challenged by Mitchell et al. (1993). The controversy surrounding the concept of "edge of chaos" is mostly about whether real-world systems actually reside within this dynamic regime and how they get there. Later work on self-organized criticality attempted to address this question.

5. Cajal observed that the convergence and divergence of neuronal projections has implications for the conduction of excitatory impulses in the nervous system. A stimulus "spreads like a fan to involve increasingly more neurons […]. It advances like an avalanche, gaining mass in proportion to the distance that it falls" (Cajal, 1995, p. 114). Cajal used his concept of "avalanche conduction" to illustrate the macroscopic effects that can result from the stimulation of a single photoreceptor in the retina or a single sound receptor in the inner ear.

6. This point is concordant with the maximal diversity of connected components at the critical point of the Erdös-Rényi phase transition (see figure 11.2).

7. For example, power-law distributions of synchronization lengths were seen in large-scale computational models of the cerebral cortex (Honey et al., 2007).

8. The ongoing accumulation of synaptic changes may require that brain networks are continually tuned and adjusted to remain close to or within the critical regime. Pearlmutter and Houghton (2009) have suggested that the functional role of sleep is to allow the brain to reestablish a "margin of safety" in network parameter space, preventing a spontaneous and highly maladaptive transition from near-critical to supercritical dynamics.

Chapter 13

1. Quoted after Simon (1962, pp. 481–482).

2. John Horgan's scathing critique of complexity theory argued that the grand goal of a unified theory of complexity is unrealistic and that complexity is nothing more than a murky concept, existing "in the eye of the beholder" (Horgan, 1995). While there continues to be disagreement about complexity, modern approaches to complex networks have brought us a step closer to a unified theoretical framework. Albert-László Barabási suggested that universal principles of network topology and a yet to be formulated theory of network dynamics may form essential building blocks of a future unified theory of complexity (Barabási, 2009).

3. This hierarchy can be further extended upward or downward to include individual organisms and their ecologies or societies, or subcellular components and molecular complexes.

4. The action of global emergent properties on local components, the supervenient power of "higher" over "lower" levels of organization in a complex system, is sometimes referred to as "downward causation." Roger Sperry developed a framework for thinking about micro- and macrodetermination in the brain that allows for emergent dynamic processes to act on their mechanistic substrates: "When it comes to brains, remember that the simpler electric, atomic, molecular, and cellular forces and laws, though still present and operating, have been superseded by the configurational forces of higher-level mechanisms. At the top, in the human brain, these include the powers of perception, cognition, reason, judgment,

and the like, the operational, causal effects and forces of which are equally or more potent in brain dynamics than are the outclassed inner chemical forces" (Sperry, 1964).

5. The estimation of entropy for a given neural data set (consisting of spike trains, voltage time series, or BOLD signals) poses numerous challenges that are only beginning to be addressed (e.g., Paninski, 2003).

6. This measure was previously defined by McGill (1954) and was called the multi-information, as it expresses the total information shared by at least two or more elements. Integration (multi-information) differs from another multivariate informational measure called the co-information (Bell, 2003), which captures only the information shared by all elements.

7. Even a very small set of a few dozen nodes and connections can be configured into trillions of distinct networks.

8. Evolutionary algorithms have been applied to select and optimize graphs for specific properties. These optimizations can involve specific structural measures or global functional measures of a dynamic process implemented in the graph. Real-world applications are traffic flow in transportation or information technology networks or susceptibility of networked systems to cascading failures (Motter and Toroczkai, 2007).

9. Evolutionary algorithms are not meant to be exact models of biological evolution, but they incorporate some of its principles, such as variation and selection. The description in the text only refers to a specific example—many other versions of evolutionary algorithms have been proposed.

10. Barnett and colleagues (2009) reexamined the measure of neural complexity applying a formulation of linear system dynamics similar to the approach taken by Galán (2008). Barnett et al. developed a novel approximation for neural complexity and despite differences in the linear model broadly confirmed the conclusions drawn by Tononi et al. (1994). Figures 13.3 and 13.4 were generated with a version of the linear model as formulated by Galán (2008).

11. A dynamic basis for consciousness does not necessarily exclude that it depends on the appearance of a novel cell type, brain region, or neurotransmitter. These structural innovations can alter patterns of brain connectivity and thus promote the emergence of the type of dynamic process underlying consciousness.

12. The theory has been significantly extended to address information integration dependent upon the dynamic state of a system (Balduzzi and Tononi, 2008).

13. Evolutionary ideas, on many occasions, have been used to further ideological goals. The ostensible goal directedness of evolutionary processes underpins the popular notion that evolution is fundamentally a manifestation of progress, inexorably leading to beneficial increases in biological organization.

Chapter 14

1. Quoted after Ashby (1960, pp. 220, 222).

2. Indeed, from the perspective of a single nerve cell, it does not matter whether a change in the statistics of its synaptic inputs is caused by events that are intrinsic to the brain or additionally involve the body. The recurrence of neural connectivity and the reentrant nature of cortical processing make it difficult to attribute specific causes to neural events, whether these causes are intrinsic or extrinsic in nature.

3. Stressful emotional or physiological challenges in our environment can lead to a bodily response and trigger plasticity in the brain (McEwen, 2007). Chronic stress results in significant changes in the morphology of neurons and their circuitry—for example, retraction and remodeling of dendrites in the hippocampus. The chemical basis of the phenomenon is complex and likely involves endogenous adrenal steroids released in response to stressful stimuli, as well as multiple neurotransmitter systems and cell surface molecules involved in cell adhesion. Stress-induced structural plasticity occurs in the hippocampus, amygdala, and prefrontal cortex and results in altered physiological and behavioral responses.

4. As Hughlings Jackson once put it, "A man, physically regarded, is a sensori-motor mechanism" (Hughlings Jackson, 1884, p. 703).

5. Clearly, ants are complex organisms with complex nervous systems. Simon's example was not intended to deny the intrinsic complexity of the ant; rather, in keeping with his idea of complex systems as hierarchical and "nearly decomposable" (see chapter 13), the "microscopic details of the inner environment may be largely irrelevant to the ant's behavior in relation to the outer environment" (Simon, 1969; quoted after Simon, 1996, pp. 52–53).

6. AI, with its emphasis on digital thinking and technology and its reliance on theories of computing and information, was an intellectual antipode to the more dynamic and analog approaches of classical cybernetics. AI's rapid rise in the 1950s temporarily eclipsed cybernetic thought in mainstream science and technology.

7. Edelman et al. (1992) referred to this type of approach as "synthetic neural modeling," explicitly targeting the interactions between nervous system, phenotype (body), and the environment by placing an embodied system controlled by a large-scale neural simulation into a real-world setting. According to Pfeifer, one of the chief aims of the approach is "understanding by building," the discovery of often surprising system properties that are difficult to predict from knowledge of the components alone.

8. The idea was clearly expressed by the philosopher Maurice Merleau-Ponty: "One can, if one wishes, readily treat behavior as an effect of the milieu. But in the same way, since all the stimulations that the organism receives have in turn been possible only by its preceding movements [...] one could also say that behavior is the first cause of all the stimulations" (Merleau-Ponty, 1963, p. 13).

9. Because of the confined space inside an MRI scanner, most neuroimaging studies of human cognition and behavior do not allow natural behavior, and virtually none involve behavior that leads to self-generated sensory input.

10. Humans, on average, perform 2–3 saccadic eye movements per second, more than 100,000 per day.

11. Variations in eye movements during the execution of different cognitive tasks were first demonstrated by Alfred Yarbus (Yarbus, 1967).

12. Importantly, this gain in information is the result of an action initiated and controlled by the agent. This allows a more complete internal model of the resulting sensory inputs since their causes are partially known. In general, since agents can control and thus predict the actions of their bodies, self-generated movement plays a central role in defining the boundaries of the autonomous self.

13. A paradigm termed "hyperscanning" (Montague et al., 2002) allows the study of interactions among individual participants with fMRI by relaying the behavioral outputs of an individual in one scanner as inputs to another individual in a second scanner. While technically challenging and not easily conducive to natural behavior, simultaneous MRI of two or multiple individuals promises to reveal additional neural substrates of social interaction.

14. The extent of the differences between human and nonhuman minds, particularly those of our closest primate relatives and ancestors, continues to be a matter of much debate (Penn et al., 2008; Bolhuis and Wynne, 2009). Evolutionary relationships notwithstanding, functional discontinuities can arise as a result of sharp shifts, akin to phase transitions, in morphology and behavior. These discontinuities may become further magnified by the extraordinary ability of humans to extend their cognitive capacities by drawing on resources in their environment and by cultural transmission of knowledge. Abstractly, at least some of these capacities rely on achieving high levels of autonomy, the creation of causal links between actions and inputs.

References

Achacoso TB, Yamamoto WS. 1992. *AY's Neuroanatomy of C. elegans for Computation*. Boca Raton: CRC Press.

Achard S, Salvador R, Whitcher B, Suckling J, Bullmore ET. 2006. A resilient, low-frequency, small-world human brain functional network with highly connected association cortical hubs. *J Neurosci* 26: 63–72.

Achard S, Bullmore E. 2007. Efficiency and cost of economical brain functional networks. *PLOS Comput Biol* 3: e17.

Achlioptas D, D'Souza RM, Spencer J. 2009. Explosive percolation in random networks. *Science* 323: 1453–1455.

Adami C, Ofria C, Collier T. 2000. Evolution of biological complexity. *Proc Natl Acad Sci USA* 97: 4463–4468.

Adami C, Cerf NJ. 2000. Physical complexity of symbolic sequences. *Physica D* 137: 62–69.

Adami C. 2002. What is complexity? *Bioessays* 24: 1085–1094.

Addis DR, Wong AT, Schacter DL. 2007. Remembering the past and imagining the future: Common and distinct neural substrates during event construction and elaboration. *Neuropsychologia* 45: 1363–1377.

Adee S. 2008. Reverse engineering the brain. *IEEE Spectr* 45: 51–53.

Aertsen AM, Gerstein GL, Habib MK, Palm G. 1989. Dynamics of neuronal firing correlation: Modulation of "effective connectivity". *J Neurophysiol* 61: 900–917.

Aertsen A, Preissl H. 1991. Dynamics of activity and connectivity in physiological neuronal networks. In *Nonlinear Dynamics and Neuronal Networks*, Schuster HG (ed.), pp. 281–302, New York: VCH.

Afraimovich VS, Zhigulin VP, Rabinovich MI. 2004. On the origin of reproducible sequential activity in neural circuits. *Chaos* 14: 1123–1129.

Aharonov R, Segev L, Meilijson I, Ruppin E. 2003. Localization of function via lesion analysis. *Neural Comput* 15: 885–913.

Ahissar E, Arieli A. 2001. Figuring space by time. *Neuron* 32: 185–201.

Ahn YY, Jeong H, Kim BJ. 2006. Wiring cost in the organization of a biological neuronal network. *Physica A* 367: 531–537.

Aiello LC, Wheeler P. 1995. The expensive-tissue hypothesis: The brain and the digestive system in human and primate evolution. *Curr Anthropol* 36: 199–221.

Alava MJ, Dorogovtsev SN. 2005. Complex networks created by aggregation. *Phys Rev E Stat Nonlin Soft Matter Phys* 71: 036107.

Albert R, Jeong H, Barabási AL. 2000. Error and attack tolerance of complex networks. *Nature* 406: 378–382.

Albert R, Barabási AL. 2002. Statistical mechanics of complex networks. *Rev Mod Phys* 74: 47–97.

Alexander WH, Sporns O. 2002. An embodied model of learning, plasticity, and reward. *Adapt Behav* 10: 143–159.

Alexanderson GL. 2006. Euler and Königsberg's bridges: A historical view. *Bull Am Math Soc* 43: 567–573.

Allison T, Puce A, McCarthy G. 2000. Social perception from visual cues: Role of the STS region. *Trends Cogn Sci* 4: 267–278.

Almassy N, Edelman GM, Sporns O. 1998. Behavioral constraints in the development of neuronal properties: A cortical model embedded in a real world device. *Cereb Cortex* 8: 346–361.

Alstott J, Breakspear M, Hagmann P, Cammoun L, Sporns O. 2009. Modeling the impact of lesions in the human brain. *PLoS Comput Biol* 5: e1000408.

Altieri DC. 2008. Survivin, cancer networks and pathway-directed drug discovery. *Nat Rev Cancer* 8: 61–70.

Alvarez VA, Sabatini BL. 2007. Anatomical and physiological plasticity of dendritic spines. *Annu Rev Neurosci* 30: 79–97.

Alzheimer A. 1906. Über einen eigenartigen, schweren Erkrankungsprozess der Hirnrinde. *Neurol Zbl* 25: 1134.

Amaral LAN, Scala A, Barthelemy M, Stanley HE. 2000. Classes of small-world networks. *Proc Natl Acad Sci USA* 97: 11149–11152.

Amaral LAN, Ottino JM. 2004. Complex networks: Augmenting the framework for the study of complex systems. *Eur Phys J B* 38: 147–162.

Amunts K, Zilles K. 2001. Advances in cytoarchitectonic mapping of the human cerebral cortex. *Neuroimaging Clin N Am* 11: 151–169.

Amunts K, Zilles K. 2006a. Atlases of the human brain: Tools for functional neuroimaging. In *Neuroanatomical Tract Tracing 3: Molecules Neurons, and Systems*, Zaborsky L, Wouterlood FG, Lanciego JL (eds.), pp. 566–603, New York: Springer.

Amunts K, Zilles K. 2006b. A multimodal analysis of structure and function in Broca's region. In *Broca's Region*, Grodzinski Y, Amunts K (eds.), pp. 17–30, Oxford: Oxford University Press.

Ananthanarayanan R, Esser SK, Simon HD, Modha DS. 2009. The cat is out the bag: Cortical simulations with 109 neurons, 1013 synapses. In *Proceedings of the Conference on High Performance Computing Networking, Storage and Analysis.* Article 63.

Anderson JR, Jones BW, Yang JH, Shaw MV, Watt CB, et al. 2009. A computational framework for ultrastructural mapping of neural circuitry. *PLoS Biol* 7: e1000074.

Anderson P. 1999. Complexity theory and organization science. *Organ Sci* 10: 216–232.

Andrews-Hanna JR, Snyder AZ, Vincent JL, Lustig C, Head D, et al. 2007. Disruption of large-scale brain systems in advanced aging. *Neuron* 56: 924–935.

Angelucci A, Lebitt JB, Walton EJS, Hipe JM, Bullier J, et al. 2002. Circuits for local and global signal integration in primary visual cortex. *J Neurosci* 22: 8633–8646.

Anwander A, Tittgemeyer M, von Cramon DY, Friederici AD, Knösche TR. 2007. Connectivity-based parcellation of Broca's area. *Cereb Cortex* 17: 816–825.

Arenkiel BR, Ehlers MD. 2009. Molecular genetics and imaging technologies for circuit-based neuroanatomy. *Nature* 461: 900–907.

Arieli A, Shoham D, Hildesheim R, Grinvald A. 1995. Coherent spatiotemporal patterns of ongoing activity revealed by real-time optical imaging coupled with single-unit recording in the cat visual cortex. *J Neurophysiol* 73: 2072–2093.

Arieli A, Sterkin A, Grinvald A, Aertsen A. 1996. Dynamics of ongoing activity: Explanation of the large variability in evoked cortical responses. *Science* 273: 1868–1871.

Artzy-Randrup Y, Fleishman SJ, Ben-Tal N, Stone L. 2004. Comment on "Network motifs: Simple building blocks of complex networks" and "Superfamilies of evolved and designed networks." *Science* 305: 1107c.

Ascoli GA. 1999. Progress and perspectives in computational neuroanatomy. *Anat Rec* 257: 195–207.

Ashby WR. 1958. Requisite variety and its implications for the control of complex systems. *Cybernetica* 1: 83–99.

Ashby WR. 1960. *Design for a Brain*. London: John Wiley.

Auffray C, Chen Z, Hood L. 2009. Systems medicine: The future of medical genomics and healthcare. *Genome Med* 1: 2.

Averbeck BB, Seo M. 2008. The statistical neuroanatomy of frontal networks in the macaque. *PLoS Comput Biol* 4: e1000050.

Axelrod R, Cohen MD. 1999. *Harnessing Complexity: Organizational Implications of a Scientific Frontier*. New York: The Free Press.

Axer H, Leunert M, Murkoster M, Grassel D, Larsen L, et al. 2002. A 3D fiber model of the human brainstem. *Comput Med Imaging Graph* 26: 439–444.

Ay N, Bertschinger N, Der R, Güttler F, Olbrich E. 2008. Predictive information and explorative behavior of autonomous robots. *Eur Phys J B* 63: 329–339.

Baars B. 2005. Global workspace theory of consciousness: Toward a cognitive neuroscience of human experience. *Prog Brain Res* 150: 45–53.

Bailey P, De Barenne JCD, Garol HW, McCulloch WS. 1940. Sensory cortex of chimpanzee. *J Neurophysiol* 3: 469–485.

Bailey P, von Bonin G. 1951. *The Isocortex of Man*. Urbana: University of Illinois Press.

Bajcsy R. 1988. Active perception. *Proc IEEE* 76: 996–1005.

Bak P, Tang C, Wiesenfeld K. 1987. Self-organized criticality: An explanation of the 1/f noise. *Phys Rev Lett* 59: 381–384.

Bak P. 1996. *How Nature Works: The Science of Self-Organized Criticality*. New York: Copernicus Press.

Bak P, Chialvo DR. 2001. Adaptive learning by extremal dynamics and negative feedback. *Phys Rev E Stat Nonlin Soft Matter Phys* 63: 031912.

Balcan D, Colizza V, Gonçalves B, Hu H, Ramasco JJ, et al. 2009. Multiscale mobility networks and the spatial spreading of infectious diseases. *Proc Natl Acad Sci USA* 106: 21484–21489.

Balduzzi D, Tononi G. 2008. Integrated information in discrete dynamical systems: Motivation and theoretical framework. *PLoS Comput Biol* 4: e1000091.

Ball P. 1999. *The Self-Made Tapestry: Pattern Formation in Nature*. New York: Oxford University Press.

Ballard DH. 1991. Animate vision. *Artif Intell* 48: 57–86.

Bang-Jensen J, Gutin G. 2001. *Digraphs: Theory, Algorithms and Applications*. London: Springer.

Barabási AL, Albert R. 1999. Emergence of scaling in random networks. *Science* 286: 509–512.

Barabási AL, Albert R, Jeong H. 2000. Scale-free charachteristics of random networks: The topology of the World-Wide Web. *Physica A* 281: 69–77.

Barabási AL. 2002. *Linked: The New Science of Networks*. Cambridge: Perseus.

Barabási AL, Oltvai ZN. 2004. Network biology: Understanding the cell's functional organization. *Nat Rev Genet* 5: 101–111.

Barabási AL. 2009. Scale-free networks: A decade and beyond. *Science* 325: 412–413.

Barahona M, Pecora L. 2002. Synchronization in small-world systems. *Phys Rev Lett* 89: 054101.

Barbas H, Rempel-Clower N. 1997. Cortical structure predicts the pattern of corticocortical connections. *Cereb Cortex* 7: 635–646.

Barbas H, Hilgetag CC. 2002. Rules relating connections to cortical structure in primate prefrontal cortex. *Neurocomputing* 44–46: 301–308.

Barnett L, Buckley CL, Bullock S. 2009. Neural complexity and structural connectivity. *Phys Rev E Stat Nonlin Soft Matter Phys* 79: 051914.

Barraclough NE, Xiao D, Baker CI, Oram MW, Perrett DI. 2005. Integration of visual and auditory information by superior temporal sulcus neurons responsive to the sight of actions. *J Cogn Neurosci* 17: 377–391.

Barrat A, Barthélemy M, Vespignani A. 2008. *Dynamical Processes on Complex Networks.* Cambridge: Cambridge University Press.

Bar-Yam Y. 2004. Multiscale variety in complex systems. *Complexity* 9: 37–45.

Bassett DS, Bullmore ET. 2006. Small world brain networks. *Neuroscientist* 12: 512–523.

Bassett DS, Meyer-Lindenberg A, Achard S, Duke T, Bullmore ET. 2006. Adaptive reconfiguration of fractal small-world human brain functional networks. *Proc Natl Acad Sci USA* 103: 19518–19523.

Bassett DS, Bullmore ET, Verchinksi BA, Mattay VS, Weinberger DR, et al. 2008. Hierarchical organization of human cortical networks in health and schizophrenia. *J Neurosci* 28: 9239–9248.

Bassett DS, Bullmore ET, Meyer-Lindenberg A, Apud JA, Weinberger DR, et al. 2009. Cognitive fitness of cost-efficient brain functional networks. *Proc Natl Acad Sci USA* 106: 11747–11752.

Bassett DS, Bullmore ET. 2009. Human brain networks in health and disease. *Curr Opin Neurol* 22: 340–347.

Batagelj B, Mrvar A. 1998. Pajek—Program for large network analysis. *Connections* 21: 47–57.

Beckmann CF, DeLuca M, Devlin JT, Smith SM. 2005. Investigations into resting-state connectivity using independent component analysis. *Philos Trans R Soc Lond, B* 360: 1001–1013.

Beckmann M, Johansen-Berg H, Rushworth MFS. 2009. Connectivity-based parcellation of human cingulate cortex and its relation to functional specialization. *J Neurosci* 29: 1175–1190.

Bédard C, Kröger H, Destexhe A. 2006. Does the 1/f frequency scaling of brain signals reflect self-organized critical states? *Phys Rev Lett* 97: 118102.

Beer RD. 2000. Dynamical approaches to cognitive science. *Trends Cogn Sci* 4: 91–99.

Beggs JM, Plenz D. 2003. Neuronal avalanches in neocortical circuits. *J Neurosci* 23: 11167–11177.

Beggs JM, Plenz D. 2004. Neuronal avalanches are diverse and precise activity patterns that are stable for many hours in cortical slice cultures. *J Neurosci* 24: 5216–5229.

Beggs JM. 2007. Neuronal avalanche. *Scholarpedia* 2: 1344.

Behrens TEJ, Johansen-Berg H, Woolrich MW, Smith SM, Wheeler-Kingshott CAM, et al. 2003. Non-invasive mapping of connections between human thalamus and cortex using diffusion imaging. *Nat Neurosci* 6: 750–757.

Bekoff A. 2001. Spontaneous embryonic motility: An enduring legacy. *Int J Dev Neurosci* 19: 155–160.

Bell AJ. 2003. The co-information lattice. In *Proceedings of the Fifth International Workshop on Independent Component Analysis and Blind Signal Separation: ICA 2003,* Amari S, Cichocki A, Makino S, Murata N (eds.), pp. 921–926, Nara, Japan.

Belmonte MK, Allen G, Beckel-Mitchener A, Boulanger LM, Carper RA, et al. 2004. Autism and abnormal development of brain connectivity. *J Neurosci* 24: 9224–9231.

Bennett CH. 1988. Logical depth and physical complexity. In *The Universal Turing Machine: A Half-Century Survey*, Herken R (ed.), pp. 227–257, Oxford: Oxford University Press.

Bertschinger N, Natschläger T. 2004. Real-time computation at the edge of chaos in recurrent neural networks. *Neural Comput* 16: 1413–1436.

Bertschinger N, Olbrich E, Ay N, Jost J. 2008. Autonomy: An information theoretic perspective. *Biosystems* 91: 331–345.

Betsch BY, Einhäuser W, Körding KP, König P. 2004. The world from a cat's perspective—Statistics of natural videos. *Biol Cybern* 90: 41–50.

Beurle RL. 1956. Properties of a mass of cells capable of regenerating pulses. *Philos Trans R Soc Lond, B* 240: 55–94.

Biggs N, Lloyd E, Wilson R. 1976. *Graph Theory: 1736–1936*. Oxford: Clarendon Press.

Binzegger T, Douglas RJ, Martin KAC. 2009. Topology and dynamics of the canonical circuit of cat V1. *Neural Networks* 22: 1071–1078.

Biswal B, Yetkin FZ, Haughton VM, Hyde JS. 1995. Functional connectivity in the motor cortex of resting human brain using echo-planar MRI. *Magn Reson Med* 34: 537–541.

Biswal BB, Mennes M, Zuo XN, Gohel S, Kelly C, et al. 2010. Toward discovery science of human brain function. *Proc Natl Acad Sci USA* 107: 4734–4739.

Bleuler E. 1908. Die Prognose der Dementia praecox (Schizophreniegruppe). *Allg Z Psychiatr* 65: 436–464.

Bleuler E. 1950. *Dementia Praecox or the Group of Schizophrenias*. New York: International Universities Press.

Blondel VD, Guillaume JL, Lambiotte R, Lefebvre E. 2008. Fast unfolding of communities in large networks. *J Stat Mech Theor Exp* 10: 10008.

Boccaletti S, Latora V, Moreno Y, Chavez M, Hwang DU. 2006. Complex networks: Structure and dynamics. *Phys Rep* 424: 175–308.

Bohland JW, Wu C, Barbas H, Bokil H, Bota M, et al. 2009. A proposal for a coordinated effort for the determination of brainwide neuroanatomical connectivity in model organisms at a mesoscopic scale. *PLoS Comput Biol* 5: e1000334.

Bolhuis JJ, Wynne CDL. 2009. Can evolution explain how minds work? *Nature* 458: 832–833.

Bollobás B. 1979. *Graph Theory: An Introductory Course*. New York: Springer.

Bonanich P. 1972. Factoring and weighting approaches to clique identification. *J Math Sociol* 2: 113–120.

Bonacich P. 2007. Some unique properties of eigenvector centrality. *Soc Networks* 29: 555–564.

Bonchev D, Rouvray DH. 1990. *Chemical Graph Theory, Vol. 1 (Introduction and Fundamentals)*. New York: Gordon and Breach.

Bonifazi P, Goldin M, Picardo MA, Jorquera I, Cattani A, et al. 2009. GABAergic hub neurons orchestrate synchrony in developing hippocampal networks. *Science* 326: 1419–1424.

Bonner JT. 1988. *The Evolution of Complexity, by Means of Natural Selection*. Princeton: Princeton University Press.

Bonner JT. 2006. *Why Size Matters*. Princeton: Princeton University Press.

Börner K, Sanyal S, Vespignani A. 2007. Network science. *Annu Rev Inform Sci Tech* 41: 537–607.

Boorman ED, O'Shea J, Sebastian C, Rushworth MFS, Johansen-Berg H. 2007. Individual differences in white-matter microstructure reflect variation in functional connectivity during choice. *Curr Biol* 17: 1426–1431.

Borgatti SP. 2005. Centrality and network flow. *Soc Networks* 27: 55–71.

Borgatti SP, Mehra A, Brass DJ, Labianca G. 2009. Network analysis in the social sciences. *Science* 323: 892–895.

Borges JL. 2000. *The Aleph and Other Stories*. London: Penguin.

Bornholdt S, Rohlf T. 2000. Topological evolution of dynamical networks: Global criticality from local dynamics. *Phys Rev Lett* 84: 6114–6117.

Bornholdt S, Röhl T. 2003. Self-organized critical neural networks. *Phys Rev E Stat Nonlin Soft Matter Phys* 67: 066118.

Bota M, Dong HW, Swanson LW. 2005. Brain architecture management system. *Neuroinformatics* 3: 15–48.

Bota M, Swanson LW. 2007. Online workbenches for neural network connections. *J Comp Neurol* 500: 807–814.

Braitenberg V. 1974. Thoughts on the cerebral cortex. *J Theor Biol* 46: 421–447.

Braitenberg V. 1984. *Vehicles: Experiments in Synthetic Psychology*. Cambridge: MIT Press.

Braitenberg V, Schüz A. 1998. *Statistics and Geometry of Neuronal Connectivity*. Berlin: Springer.

Brandes U, Delling D, Gaertler M, Görke R, Hoefer M, et al. 2008. On modularity clustering. *IEEE Trans Knowl Data Eng* 20: 172–188.

Braun J. 2003. Natural scenes upset the visual applecart. *Trends Cogn Sci* 7: 7–9.

Breakspear M, Terry J, Friston K. 2003. Modulation of excitatory synaptic coupling facilitates synchronization and complex dynamics in a biophysical model of neuronal dynamics. *Network Comput Neural Syst* 14: 703–732.

Breakspear M, Stam CJ. 2005. Dynamics of a neural system with a multiscale architecture. *Phil Trans Roy Soc B* 360: 1051–1074.

Breakspear M, Jirsa VK. 2007. Neuronal dynamics and brain connectivity. In *Handbook of Brain Connectivity*, Jirsa VK, McIntosh AR (eds.), pp. 3–64, Springer: Berlin.

Brenner S. 2008. An interview with Sydney Brenner. *Nat Rev Mol Cell Biol* 9: 8–9.

Bressler SL, Coppola R, Nakamura R. 1993. Episodic multiregional cortical coherence at multiple frequencies during visual task performance. *Nature* 366: 153–156.

Bressler SL. 1995. Large-scale cortical networks and cognition. *Brain Res Brain Res Rev* 20: 288–304.

Bressler SL, Kelso JAS. 2001. Cortical coordination dynamics and cognition. *Trends Cogn Sci* 5: 26–36.

Bressler SL. 2004. Inferential constraint sets in the organization of visual expectation. *Neuroinformatics* 2: 227–237.

Bressler SL, Tognoli E. 2006. Operational principles of neurocognitive networks. *Int J Psychophysiol* 60: 139–148.

Bressler SL, McIntosh AR. 2007. The role of neural context in large-scale neurocognitive network operations. In *Handbook of Brain Connectivity*, Jirsa V, McIntosh AR (eds.), pp. 403–420, New York: Springer.

Bressler SL, Tang W, Sylvester CM, Shulman GL, Corbetta M. 2008. Top-down control of human visual cortex by frontal and parietal cortex in anticipatory visual spatial attention. *J Neurosci* 28: 10056–10061.

Briggman KL, Denk W. 2006. Towards neural circuit reconstruction with volume electron microscopy techniques. *Curr Opin Neurobiol* 16: 562–570.

Broca P. 1861a. Remarques sur le siége de la faculté du langage articulé, suivies d'une observation d'aphémie (perte de la parole). *Bulletin de la Société Anatomique de Paris* 6: 330–357.

Broca P. 1861b. Nouvelle observation d'aphémie produite par une lesion de la troisième circonvolution frontale. *Bulletin de la Société Anatomique de Paris* 6: 398–407.

Brodmann K. 1909. *Vergleichende Lokalisationslehre der Grosshirnrinde in ihren Prinzipien dargestellt auf Grund des Zellenbaues.* Leipzig: J.A. Barth.

Brooks RA. 1991. New approaches to robotics. *Science* 253: 1227–1232.

Brooks RA, Breazeal C, Marjanovic M, Scassellati B. 1999. The Cog project: Building a humanoid robot. *Lect Notes Comput Sci* 1562: 52–87.

Brovelli A, Ding M, Ledberg A, Chen Y, Nakamura R, et al. 2004. Beta oscillations in a large-scale sensorimotor cortical network: Directional influences revealed by Granger causality. *Proc Natl Acad Sci USA* 101: 9849–9854.

Bruno RM, Sakmann B. 2006. Cortex is driven by weak but synchronously active thalamocortical synapses. *Science* 312: 1622–1627.

Buchanan M. 2002. *Nexus: Small Worlds and the Groundbreaking Science of Networks.* New York: Norton.

Buckner RL, Snyder AZ, Shannon BJ, LaRossa G, Sachs R, et al. 2005. Molecular, structural and functional characterization of Alzheimer's disease: Evidence for a relationship between default activity, amyloid and memory. *J Neurosci* 25: 7709–7717.

Buckner RL, Vincent JL. 2007. Unrest at rest: Default activity and spontaneous network correlations. *Neuroimage* 37: 1091–1096.

Buckner RL, Andrews-Hanna JR, Schacter DL. 2008. The brain's default network: Anatomy, function, and relevance to disease. *Ann NY Acad Sci* 1124: 1–38.

Buckner RL, Sepulcre J, Talukdar T, Krienen FM, Liu H, et al. 2009. Cortical hubs revealed by intrinsic functional connectivity: Mapping, assessment of stability, and relation to Alzheimer's disease. *J Neurosci* 29: 1860–1873.

Büchel C, Friston KJ. 1997. Modulation of connectivity in visual pathways by attention: Cortical interactions evaluated with structural equation modelling and fMRI. *Cereb Cortex* 7: 768–778.

Büchel C, Coull JT, Friston KJ. 1999. The predictive value of changes in effective connectivity for human learning. *Science* 283: 1538–1541.

Büchel C, Friston K. 2000. Assessing interactions among neuronal systems using functional neuroimaging. *Neural Netw* 13: 871–882.

Bullmore E, Sporns O. 2009. Complex brain networks: Graph theoretical analysis of structural and functional systems. *Nat Rev Neurosci* 10: 186–198.

Bullock TH, Bennett MVL, Johnston D, Josephson R, Marder E, et al. 2005. The neuron doctrine, redux. *Science* 310: 791–793.

Buonomano DV, Maass W. 2009. State-dependent computations: Spatiotemporal processing in cortical networks. *Nat Rev Neurosci* 10: 113–125.

Butts CT. 2009. Revisiting the foundations of network analysis. *Science* 325: 414–416.

Butz M, Wörgötter F, van Ooyen A. 2009. Activity-dependent structural plasticity. *Brain Res Brain Res Rev* 60: 287–305.

Buzsáki G, Geisler C, Henze DA, Wang XJ. 2004. Interneuron diversity series: Circuit complexity and axon wiring economy of cortical interneurons. *Trends Neurosci* 27: 186–193.

Buzsáki G. 2006. *Rhythms of the Brain.* New York: Oxford University Press.

Cajal SR. 1995. *Histology of the Nervous System of Man and Vertebrates.* New York: Oxford University Press.

Cajal SR. 1999. *Advice for a Young Investigator.* Cambridge: MIT Press.

Calhoun VD, Adali T, McGinty VB, Pekar JJ, Watson TD, et al. 2001. fMRI activation in a visual-perception task: Network of areas detected using the general linear model and independent components analysis. *Neuroimage* 14: 1080–1088.

Calhoun VD, Eichele T, Pearlson G. 2009. Functional brain networks in schizophrenia: A review. *Frontiers Hum Neurosci* 3: 17.

Campbell AW. 1905. *Histological Studies on the Localisation of Cerebral Functions.* Cambridge: University Press.

Canals S, Beyerlein M, Merkle H, Logothetis NK. 2009. Functional MRI evidence for LTP-induced neural network reorganization. *Curr Biol* 19: 398–403.

Cang J, Renteria RC, Kaneko M, Liu X, Copenhagen DR, et al. 2005. Development of precise maps in visual cortex requires patterned spontaneous activity in the retina. *Neuron* 48: 797–809.

Carroll SB. 2005. *Endless Forms Most Beautiful: The New Science of Evo Devo and the Making of the Animal Kingdom.* New York: Norton.

Casey BJ, Giedd JN, Thomas KM. 2000. Structural and functional brain development and its relation to cognitive development. *Biol Psychol* 54: 241–257.

Casey BJ, Tottenham N, Liston C, Durston S. 2005. Imaging the developing brain: What have we learned about cognitive development? *Trends Cogn Sci* 9: 104–110.

Caspers S, Geyer S, Schleicher A, Mohlberg H, Amunts K, Zilles K. 2006. The human inferior parietal cortex: Cytoarchitectonic parcellation and interindividual variability. *Neuroimage* 33: 430–448.

Castellanos FX, Margulies DS, Kelly AMC, Uddin LQ, Ghaffari M, et al. 2008. Cingulate–precuneus interactions: A new locus of dysfunction in adult attention-deficit/hyperactivity disorder. *Biol Psychiatry* 63: 332–337.

Catani M, ffytche DH. 2005. The rises and falls of disconnection syndromes. *Brain* 128: 2224–2239.

Catani M. 2006. Diffusion tensor magnetic resonance imaging tractography in cognitive disorders. *Curr Opin Neurol* 19: 599–606.

Catani M, Mesulam M. 2008. What is a disconnection syndrome? *Cortex* 44: 911–913.

Cavanna AE, Trimble MR. 2006. The precuneus: A review of its functional anatomy and behavioural correlates. *Brain* 129: 564–583.

Chaitin GJ. 1977. Algorithmic information theory. *IBM J Res Develop* 21: 350–359.

Chartrand G. 1985. *Introductory Graph Theory.* New York: Dover.

Chartrand G, Lesniak L. 1996. *Graphs and Digraphs.* Boca Raton: Chapman and Hall.

Chen BL, Hall DH, Chklovskii DB. 2006. Wiring optimization can relate neuronal structure and function. *Proc Natl Acad Sci USA* 103: 4723–4728.

Chen ZJ, He Y, Rosa-Neto P, Germann J, Evans AC. 2008. Revealing modular architecture of human brain structural networks by using cortical thickness from MRI. *Cereb Cortex* 18: 2374–2381.

Cherkassky VL, Kana RK, Keller TA, Just MA. 2006. Functional connectivity in a baseline resting-state network in autism. *Neuroreport* 17: 1687–1690.

Cherniak C. 1992. Local optimization of neuron arbors. *Biol Cybern* 66: 503–510.

Cherniak C. 1994. Component placement optimization in the brain. *J Neurosci* 14: 2418–2427.

Cherniak C. 1995. Neural component placement. *Trends Neurosci* 18: 522–527.

Cherniak C, Mokhtarzada Z, Rodriguez-Esteban R, Changizi K. 2004. Global optimization of cerebral cortex layout. *Proc Natl Acad Sci USA* 101: 1081–1086.

Chialvo DR, Bak P. 1999. Learning from mistakes. *Neuroscience* 90: 1137–1148.

Chiang MC, Barysheva M, Shattuck DW, Lee AD, Madsen SK, et al. 2009. Genetics of brain fiber architecture and intellectual performance. *J Neurosci* 29: 2212–2224.

Chiel H, Beer R. 1997. The brain has a body: Adaptive behavior emerges from interactions of nervous system, body, and environment. *Trends Neurosci* 20: 553–557.

Chiel HJ, Ting LH, Ekeberg O, Hartmann MJZ. 2009. The brain in its body: Motor control and sensing in a biomechanical context. *J Neurosci* 29: 12807–12814.

Chklovskii DB, Schikorski T, Stevens CF. 2002. Wiring optimization in cortical circuits. *Neuron* 34: 341–347.

Chklovskii DB, Koulakov AA. 2004. Maps in the brain: What can we learn from them? *Annu Rev Neurosci* 27: 369–392.

Chklovskii DB, Mel BW, Svoboda K. 2004. Cortical rewiring and information storage. *Nature* 431: 782–788.

Chuang HY, Lee E, Liu YT, Lee D, Ideker T. 2007. Network-based classification of breast cancer metastasis. *Mol Syst Biol* 3: 140.

Clark A. 1997. *Being There: Putting Brain, Body, and the World Together Again.* Cambridge: MIT Press.

Clark A. 2008. *Supersizing the Mind: Embodiment, Action, and Cognitive Extension.* New York: Oxford University Press.

Clauset A, Shalizi CS, Newman MEJ. 2009. Power-law distributions in empirical data. *SIAM Rev* 51: 661–703.

Cohen JE. 1988. Threshold phenomena in random structures. *Discrete Appl Math* 19: 113–128.

Cohen AL, Fair DA, Dosenbach NUF, Miezin FM, Dierker D, et al. 2008. Defining functional areas in individual human brains using resting state functional connectivity MRI. *Neuroimage* 41: 45–57.

Colizza V, Barrat A, Barthélemy M, Vespignani A, et al. 2006. The role of the airline transportation network in the prediction and predictability of global epidemics. *Proc Natl Acad Sci USA* 103: 2015–2020.

Colizza V, Pastor-Satorras R, Vespignani A. 2007. Reaction–diffusion processes and metapopulation models in heterogeneous networks. *Nat Phys* 2: 110–115.

Colizza V, Vespignani A. 2008. Epidemic modeling in metapopulation systems with heterogeneous coupling pattern: Theory and simulations. *J Theor Biol* 251: 450–457.

Compte A, Sanchez-Vives MV, McCormick DA, Wang XJ. 2003. Cellular and network mechanisms of slow oscillatory activity (<1 Hz) and wave propagations in a cortical network model. *J Neurophysiol* 89: 2707–2725.

Conway F, Siegelman J. 2005. *Dark Hero of the Information Age: In Search of Norbert Wiener, the Father of Cybernetics.* New York: Basic Books.

Cossart R, Aronov D, Yuste R. 2003. Attractor dynamics of network UP states in the neocortex. *Nature* 423: 283–288.

Costa LF, Sporns O. 2005. Hierarchical features of large-scale cortical connectivity. *Eur J Phys B* 48: 567–573.

Costa LF, Rodrigues FA, Travieso G, Boas PRV. 2007. Characterization of complex networks: A survey of measurements. *Adv Phys* 56: 167–242.

Cover TM, Thomas JA. 1991. *Elements of Information Theory.* New York: Wiley.

Crick F. 1984. Neurobiology: Memory and molecular turnover. *Nature* 312: 101.

Crick F, Jones E. 1993. Backwardness of human neuroanatomy. *Nature* 361: 109–110.

Crick F. 1994. *The Astonishing Hypothesis: The Scientific Search for the Soul.* New York: Scribner's.

Crick F, Koch C. 1998a. Constraints on cortical and thalamic projections: The no-strong-loops hypothesis. *Nature* 391: 245–250.

Crick F, Koch C. 1998b. Consciousness and neuroscience. *Cereb Cortex* 8: 97–107.

Crofts JJ, Higham DJ. 2009. A weighted communicability measure applied to complex brain networks. *J R Soc Interface* 6: 411–414.

Cruse H, Duerr V, Schmitz J. 2007. Insect walking is based on a decentralized architecture revealing a simple and robust controller. *Philos Trans R Soc Lond A* 365: 221–250.

Crutchfield JP, Feldman DP. 2003. Regularities unseen, randomness observed: Levels of entropy convergence. *Chaos* 13: 25.

Cuntz H, Borst A, Segev I. 2007. Optimization principles of dendritic structure. *Theor Biol Med Model* 4: 21.

Cusick ME, Klitgord N, Vidal M, Hill DE. 2005. Interactome: Gateway into systems biology. *Hum Mol Genet* 14: R171–R181.

Dauguet J, Peled S, Berezovskii V, Delzescaux T, Warfield SK, et al. 2007. Comparison of fiber tracts derived from in-vivo DTI tractography with 3D histological neural tract tracer reconstruction on a macaque brain. *Neuroimage* 27: 530–538.

Damasio H, Damasio AR. 1989. *Lesion Analysis in Neuropsychology*. New York: Oxford University Press.

Damasio AR. 1989. Time-locked multiregional retroactivation: A systems-level proposal for the neural substrates of recall and recognition. *Cognition* 33: 25–62.

Damasio AR. 1994. *Descartes' Error: Emotion, Reason, and the Human Brain*. New York: Putnam.

Damasio A. 1999. *The Feeling of What Happens*. New York: Harcourt Brace.

Damoiseaux JS, Beckmann CF, Arigita E, Sanz EJ, Barkhof F, et al. 2008. Reduced resting-state brain activity in the "default network" in normal aging. *Cereb Cortex* 18: 1856–1864.

Damoiseaux JS, Smith SJ, Witter MP, Sanz-Arigita EJ, Barkhof F, et al. 2009. White matter tract integrity in aging and Alzheimer's disease. *Hum Brain Mapp* 30: 1051–1059.

Damoiseaux JS, Greicius MD. 2009. Greater than the sum of its parts: A review of studies combining structural connectivity and resting-state functional connectivity. *Brain Struct Funct* 213: 525–533.

Danon L, Diaz-Giulera A, Duch J, Arenas A. 2005. Comparing community structure identification. *J Stat Mech* P09008.

David O, Guillemain I, Saillet S, Reyt S, Deransart C, et al. 2009. Identifying neural drivers with functional MRI: An electrophysiological validation. *PLoS Biol* 6: e315.

Dawkins R. 1996. *Climbing Mount Improbable*. New York: Norton.

Dayan P, Abbott LF. 2001. *Theoretical Neuroscience: Computational and Mathematical Modeling of Neural Systems*. Cambridge: MIT Press.

Deacon TW. 1990. Rethinking mammalian brain evolution. *Am Zool* 30: 629–705.

Deco G, Jirsa VK, Robinson PA, Breakspear M, Friston K. 2008. The dynamic brain: From spiking neurons to neural masses and cortical fields. *PLoS Comput Biol* 4: e1000092.

Deco G, Jirsa V, McIntosh AR, Sporns O, Kötter R. 2009. Key role of coupling, delay, and noise in resting brain fluctuations. *Proc Natl Acad Sci USA* 106: 10302–10307.

Dehaene S, Sergent C, Changeux JP. 2003. A neuronal network model linking subjective reports and objective physiological data during conscious perception. *Proc Natl Acad Sci USA* 100: 8520–8525.

Deheane S, Changeux JP, Naccache L, Sackur J, Sergent C. 2006. Conscious, preconscious, and subliminal processing: A testable taxonomy. *Trends Cogn Sci* 10: 204–211.

Delbeuck X, Van der Linden M, Collette F. 2003. Alzheimer's disease as a disconnection syndrome? *Neuropsychol Rev* 13: 79–92.

DeLisi C. 2008. Santa Fe 1986: Human genome baby-steps. *Nature* 455: 876–877.

De Luca M, Beckmann CF, De Stefano N, Matthews PM, Smith SM. 2006. fMRI resting state networks define distinct modes of long-distance interactions in the human brain. *Neuroimage* 29: 1359–1367.

Denk W, Horstmann H. 2004. Serial block-face scanning electron microscopy to reconstruct three-dimensional tissue nanostructure. *PLoS Biol* 2: e329.

de Ridder A, Postma F, Hoedemaker S, Koene R, van Pelt J, et al. 2009. Simulated networks with realistic neuronal morphologies show small-world connectivity. *BMC Neurosci* 10(Suppl 1): 5.

D'Esposito M, Deouell LY, Gazzaley A. 2003. Alterations in the BOLD fMRI signal with ageing and disease: A challenge for neuroimaging. *Nat Rev Neurosci* 4: 863–872.

Dhawale A, Bhalla US. 2008. The network and the synapse: 100 years after Cajal. *HFSP J* 2: 12–16.

D'Huys O, Vicente R, Erneux T, Danckaert J, Fischer I. 2008. Synchronization properties of network motifs: Influence of coupling delay and symmetry. *Chaos* 18: 037116.

Dickson BJ. 2002. Molecular mechanisms of axon guidance. *Science* 298: 1959–1964.

Ding M, Chen Y, Bressler S. 2006. Granger causality: Basic theory and application to neuroscience. In *Handbook of Time Series Analysis: Recent Theoretical Developments and Applications*, Schelter B, Winterhalder M, Timmer J (eds.), pp. 437–459, Berlin: Wiley-VCH, Berlin.

Djurfeldt M, Lundqvist M, Johannson C, Rehn M, Ekeberg O, Lansner A. 2008. Brain-scale simulation of the neocortex on the IBM Blue Gene/L supercomputer. *IBM J Res Dev* 52: 31–41.

Dosenbach NU, Visscher KM, Palmer ED, Miezin FM, Wenger KK, et al. 2006. A core system for the implementation of task sets. *Neuron* 50: 799–812.

Dosenbach NU, Fair DA, Miezin FM, Cohen AL, Wenger KK, et al. 2007. Distinct brain networks for adaptive and stable task control in humans. *Proc Natl Acad Sci USA* 104: 11073–11078.

Dosenbach NU, Fair DA, Cohen AL, Schlaggar BL, Petersen SE. 2008. A dual-networks architecture of top-down control. *Trends Cogn Sci* 12: 99–105.

Douglas RJ, Koch C, Mahowald M, Martin KA, Suarez HH. 1995. Recurrent excitation in neocortical circuits. *Science* 269: 981–985.

Douglas RJ, Martin KAC. 2004. Neuronal circuits of the neocortex. *Annu Rev Neurosci* 27: 419–451.

Dronkers NF, Plaisant O, Iba-Zizen MT, Cabanis EA. 2007. Paul Broca's historic cases: High resolution MR imaging of the brains of Leborgne and Lelong. *Brain* 130: 1432–1441.

Dubois J, Hertz-Pannier L, Dehaene-Lambertz G, Cointepas Y, Le Bihan D. 2006. Assessment of the early organization and maturation of infants' cerebral white matter fiber bundles: A feasibility study using quantitative diffusion tensor imaging and tractography. *Neuroimage* 30: 1121–1132.

Duncan J, Seitz RJ, Kolodny J, Bor D, Herzog H, et al. 2000. A neural basis for general intelligence. *Science* 289: 457–460.

Dusser de Barenne JG, McCulloch WS. 1938. Functional organization in the sensory cortex of the monkey (*Macaca mulatta*). *J Neurophysiol* 1: 69–85.

Dusser de Barenne JG, McCulloch WS. 1939. Physiological delimitation of neurones in the central nervous system. *Am J Physiol* 127: 620–628.

Duyn JH, von Gelderen P, Li TQ, de Zwart JA, Koretsky AP, et al. 2007. High-field MRI of brain cortical substructure based on signal phase. *Proc Natl Acad Sci USA* 104: 11796–11801.

Edelman GM. 1978. Group selection and phasic re-entrant signalling: A theory of higher brain function. In *The Mindful Brain*, Edelman GM, Mountcastle VB (eds.), pp. 51–100, Cambridge: MIT Press.

Edelman GM. 1987. *Neural Darwinism*. New York: Basic Books.

Edelman GM. 1989. *The Remembered Present*. New York: Basic Books.

Edelman GM, Reeke GN, Gall WE, Tononi G, Williams D, et al. 1992. Synthetic neural modeling applied to a real-world artifact. *Proc Natl Acad Sci USA* 89: 7267–7271.

Edelman GM, Tononi G. 2000. *A Universe of Consciousness: How Matter Becomes Imagination*. New York: Basic Books.

Edelman GM, Gally JA. 2001. Degeneracy and complexity in biological systems. *Proc Natl Acad Sci USA* 98: 13763–13768.

Eguíluz VM, Chialvo DR, Cecchi GA, Baliki M, Apkarian AV. 2005. Scale-free brain functional networks. *Phys Rev Lett* 94: 018102.

Eisenstein M. 2009. Putting neurons on the map. *Nature* 461: 1149–1152.

Elman JL, Bates EA, Johnson MH, Karmiloff-Smith A, Parisi D, Plunkett K, eds. 1996. *Rethinking Innateness: A Connectionist Perspective on Development*. Cambridge: MIT Press.

Elman JL. 2005. Connectionist models of cognitive development: Where next? *Trends Cogn Sci* 9: 111–117.

Engel AK, König P, Kreiter AK, Singer W. 1991. Interhemispheric synchronization of oscillatory neuronal responses in cat visual cortex. *Science* 252: 1177–1179.

Epstein JM. 2009. Modelling to contain pandemics. *Nature* 460: 687.

Erdös P, Rényi A. 1960. On the evolution of random graphs. *Publ Math Inst Hung Acad Sci* 5: 17–61.

Ergün A, Lawrence CA, Kohanski MA, Brennan TA, Collins JJ. 2007. A network biology approach to prostate cancer. *Mol Syst Biol* 3: 82.

Estrada E, Hatano N. 2008. Communicability in complex networks. *Phys Rev E Stat Nonlin Soft Matter Phys* 77: 036111.

Euler L. 1736. Solutio problematis ad geometriam situs pertinentis. *Commentarii Academiae Scientiarum Imperialis Petropolitanae* 8: 128–140.

Fagiolo G. 2007. Clustering in complex directed networks. *Phys Rev E Stat Nonlin Soft Matter Phys* 76: 026107.

Fair DA, Dosenbach NUF, Church JA, Cohen AL, Brahmbhatt S, et al. 2007. Development of distinct control networks through segregation and integration. *Proc Natl Acad Sci USA* 104: 13507–13512.

Fair DA, Cohen AL, Dosenbach NU, Church JA, Miezin FM, et al. 2008. The maturing architecture of the brain's default network. *Proc Natl Acad Sci USA* 105: 4028–4032.

Fair DA, Cohen AL, Power JD, Dosenbach NUF, Church JA, et al. 2009. Functional brain networks develop from a "local to distributed" organization. *PLOS Comput Biol* 5: e1000381.

Fairén A. 2007. Cajal and Lorente de Nó on cortical interneurons: Coincidences and progress. *Brain Res Brain Res Rev* 55: 430–444.

Faisal AA, Selen LPJ, Wolpert DM. 2008. Noise in the nervous system. *Nat Rev Neurosci* 9: 292–303.

Felleman DJ, van Essen DC. 1991. Distributed hierarchical processing in the primate cerebral cortex. *Cereb Cortex* 1: 1–47.

Feller MB. 1999. Spontaneous correlated activity in developing neural circuits. *Neuron* 22: 653–656.

Ferrarini L, Veer IM, Baerends E, van Tol MJ, Renken RJ, et al. 2008. Hierarchical modularity in the resting-state human brain. *Hum Brain Mapp* 30: 2220–2231.

ffytche, DH, Catani, M. 2005. Beyond localization: From hodology to function. *Phil Trans R Soc B* 360: 767–779.

Finger S. 1994. *Origins of Neuroscience: A History of Explorations into Brain Function*. New York: Oxford University Press.

Finkel LH, Edelman GM. 1989. Integration of distributed cortical systems by reentry: A computer simulation of interactive functionally segregated visual areas. *J Neurosci* 9: 3188–3208.

Finlay BL, Darlington RB. 1995. Linked regularities in the development and evolution of mammalian brains. *Science* 268: 1578–1584.

Fiser J, Chiu C, Weliky M. 2004. Small modulation of ongoing cortical dynamics by sensory input during natural vision. *Nature* 431: 573–578.

Fiset P, Paus T, Daloze T, Plourde G, Meuret P, et al. 1999. Brain mechanisms of propofol-induced loss of consciousness in humans: A positron emission tomographic study. *J Neurosci* 19: 5506–5513.

Fitzpatrick P, Needham A, Natale L, Metta G. 2008. Shared challenges in object perception for robots and infants. *Infant Child Dev* 17: 7–24.

Floreano D, Suzuki M, Mattiussi C. 2005. Active vision and receptive field development in evolutionary robots. *Evol Comput* 13: 527–544.

Flourens P. 1846. *Phrenology Examined*. Philadelphia: Hogan and Thompson.

Fodor JA. 1983. *The Modularity of Mind*. Cambridge: MIT Press.

Fontanini A, Katz DB. 2008. Behavioral states, network states, and sensory response variability. *J Neurophysiol* 100: 1160–1168.

Fortunato S, Barthélemy M. 2007. Resolution limit in community detection. *Proc Natl Acad Sci USA* 104: 36–41.

Fox MD, Snyder AZ, Vincent JL, Corbetta M, Van Essen DC, et al. 2005. The human brain is intrinsically organized into dynamic, anticorrelated functional networks. *Proc Natl Acad Sci USA* 102: 9673–9678.

Fox MD, Snyder AZ, Zacks JM, Raichle ME. 2006. Coherent spontaneous activity accounts for trial-to-trial variability in human evoked brain responses. *Nat Neurosci* 9: 23–25.

Fox MD, Snyder AZ, Vincent JL, Raichle ME. 2007. Intrinsic fluctuations within cortical systems account for intertribal variability in human behavior. *Neuron* 56: 171–184.

Fox MD, Raichle M. 2007. Spontaneous fluctuations in brain activity observed with functional magnetic resonance imaging. *Nat Rev Neurosci* 8: 700–711.

Fraimann D, Balenzuela P, Foss J, Chialvo DR. 2009. Ising-like dynamics in large-scale functional brain networks. *Phys Rev E Stat Nonlin Soft Matter Phys* 79: 061922.

Franz SI. 1912. New phrenology. *Science* 35: 321–328.

Fransson P. 2006. How default is the default mode of brain function? Further evidence from intrinsic BOLD signal fluctuations. *Neuropsychologia* 44: 2836–2845.

Fransson P, Skiold B, Horsch S, Nordell A, Blennow M, et al. 2007. Resting-state networks in the infant brain. *Proc Natl Acad Sci USA* 104: 15531–15536.

Fransson P, Marrelec G. 2008. The precuneus/posterior cingulate cortex plays a pivotal role in the default mode network: Evidence from a partial correlation network analysis. *Neuroimage* 42: 1178–1184.

Freeman LC. 1977. A set of measures of centrality based on betweenness. *Sociometry* 40: 35–41.

Freeman LC. 1978. Centrality in social networks: Conceptual clarification. *Soc Networks* 1: 215–239.

Freeman WJ. 2003. Evidence from human scalp electroencephalograms of global chaotic itinerancy. *Chaos* 13: 1067–1077.

Freeman WJ, Homes MD, West GA, Vanhatalo S. 2006. Fine spatiotemporal structure of phase in human intracranial EEG. *Clin Neurophysiol* 117: 1228–1243.

Freeman WJ. 2007. Scale-free neocortical dynamics. *Scholarpedia* 2: 1357.

Fries P. 2005. A mechanism for cognitive dynamics: Neuronal communication through neuronal coherence. *Trends Cogn Sci* 9: 474–480.

Fries P. 2009. Neuronal gamma-band synchronization as a fundamental process in cortical computation. *Annu Rev Neurosci* 32: 209–224.

Friston KJ. 1993. Functional connectivity: The principal-component analysis of large (PET) data sets. *J Cereb Blood Flow Metab* 13: 5–14.

Friston KJ. 1994. Functional and effective connectivity in neuroimaging: A synthesis. *Hum Brain Mapp* 2: 56–78.

Friston KJ, Frith CD. 1995. Schizophrenia: A disconnection syndrome? *Clin Neurosci* 3: 89–97.

Friston KJ, Price CJ, Fletcher P, Moore C, Frackowiak RSJ, et al. 1996. The trouble with cognitive subtraction. *Neuroimage* 4: 97–104.

Friston KJ. 1997. Transients, metastability, and neuronal dynamics. *Neuroimage* 5: 164–171.

Friston KJ. 1998a. Imaging neuroscience: Principles or maps? *Proc Natl Acad Sci USA* 95: 796–802.

Friston KJ. 1998b. The disconnection hypothesis. *Schizophr Res* 30: 115–125.

Friston KJ. 2000. The labile brain. I. Neuronal transients and nonlinear coupling. *Philos Trans R Soc Lond B Biol Sci* 355: 215–236.

Friston KJ. 2002. Beyond phrenology: What can neuroimaging tell us about distributed circuitry? *Annu Rev Neurosci* 25: 221–250.

Friston KJ, Harrison L, Penny W. 2003. Dynamic causal modelling. *Neuroimage* 19: 1273–1302.

Friston KJ. 2004. Models of brain function in neuroimaging. *Annu Rev Psychol* 56: 57–87.

Friston KJ. 2005a. Models of brain function in neuroimaging. *Annu Rev Psychol* 56: 57–87.

Friston KJ. 2005b. A theory of cortical responses. *Phil Trans R Soc B* 360: 815–836.

Friston KJ. 2009a. Causal modeling and brain connectivity in functional magnetic resonance imaging. *PLoS Biol* 7: e1000033.

Friston KJ. 2009b. Modalities, modes, and models in functional neuroimaging. *Science* 326: 399–403.

Friston KJ. 2010. The free-energy principle: A unified brain theory? *Nat Rev Neurosci* 11: 127–138.

Fuster JM. 1980. *The Prefrontal Cortex*. New York: Raven.

Galán RF. 2008. On how network architecture determines the dominant patterns of spontaneous neural activity. *PLoS ONE* 3: e2148.

Galbraith JR. 1973. *Designing Complex Organizations*. Boston: Addison-Wesley Longman.

Gall FJ. 1835. *On the Organ of the Moral Qualities and Intellectual Faculties, and the Plurality of the Cerebral Organs*. Boston: Marsh, Capen and Lyon.

Gallagher JC, Beer RD, Espenschied KS, Quinn RD. 1996. Application of evolved locomotion controllers to a hexapod robot. *Robot Auton Syst* 19: 95–103.

Gallant JL, Connor CE, Van Essen DC. 1998. Neural activity in areas V1, V2 and V4 during free viewing of natural scenes compared to controlled viewing. *Neuroreport* 9: 2153–2158.

Gao W, Zhu H, Giovanello KS, Smith JK, Shen D, et al. 2009. Evidence on the emergence of the brain's default network from 2-week-old to 2-year-old healthy pediatric subjects. *Proc Natl Acad Sci USA* 106: 6790–6795.

Garey LJ. 1994. *Brodmann's Localization in the Cerebral Cortex*. London: Smith-Gordon.

Garrido MI, Kilner JM, Kiebel SJ, Friston KJ. 2007. Evoked brain responses are generated by feedback loops. *Proc Natl Acad Sci USA* 104: 20961–20966.

Gell-Mann M. 1995. What Is complexity? *Complexity* 1: 16–19.

Gerstein GL, Perkel DH. 1969. Simultaneously recorded trains of action potentials: Analysis and functional interpretation. *Science* 164: 828–830.

Geschwind N. 1965. Disconnexion syndromes in animals and man: Part I. *Brain* 88: 237–294.

Geschwind N. 1985. Mechanisms of change after brain lesions. *Ann N Y Acad Sci* 457: 1–11.

Ghazanfar AA, Maier JX, Hoffman KL, Logothetis NK. 2005. Multisensory integration of dynamic faces and voices in rhesus monkey auditory cortex. *J Neurosci* 25: 5004–5012.

Ghazanfar AA, Nielsen K, Logothetis NK. 2006. Eye movements of monkey observers viewing vocalizing conspecifics. *Cognition* 101: 515–529.

Ghazanfar AA, Schroeder CE. 2006. Is neocortex essentially multisensory? *Trends Cogn Sci* 10: 278–285.

Ghosh A, Rho Y, McIntosh AR, Kötter R, Jirsa VK. 2008a. Cortical network dynamics with time delays reveals functional connectivity in the resting brain. *Cogn Neurodyn* 2: 115–120.

Ghosh A, Rho Y, McIntosh AR, Kötter R, Jirsa VK. 2008b. Noise during rest enables the exploration of the brain's dynamic repertoire. *PLoS Comput Biol* 4: e1000196.

Gierer A, Meinhardt H. 1972. A theory of biological pattern formation. *Kybernetik* 12: 30.

Gilbert CD, Wiesel TN. 1989. Columnar specificity of intrinsic horizontal and corticocortical connections in cat visual cortex. *J Neurosci* 9: 2432–2442.

Girvan M, Newman MEJ. 2002. Community structure in social and biological networks. *Proc Natl Acad Sci USA* 99: 7821–7826.

Glahn DC, Winkler AM, Kochunov P, Almasy L, Duggirala R, et al. 2010. Genetic control over the resting brain. *Proc Natl Acad Sci USA* 107: 1223–1228.

Glickstein M. 2006. Golgi and Cajal: The neuron doctrine and the 100th anniversary of the 1906 Nobel Prize. *Curr Biol* 16: R147–R151.

Goebel R, Roebroek A, Kim D, Formisano E. 2003. Investigating directed cortical interactions in time-resolved fMRI data using vector autoregressive modeling and Granger causality mapping. *Magn Reson Imaging* 21: 1251–1261.

Goehler H, Lalowski M, Stelzl U, Waelter S, Stroedicke M, et al. 2004. A protein interaction network links GIT1, an enhancer of Huntingtin aggregation, to Huntington's disease. *Mol Cell* 15: 853–865.

Goldman-Rakic PS. 1988. Topography of cognition: Parallel distributed networks in primate association cortex. *Annu Rev Neurosci* 11: 137–156.

Goldman-Rakic PS. 1995. Architecture of the prefrontal cortex and the central executive. *Ann N Y Acad Sci* 769: 71–84.

Golland Y, Bentin S, Gelbard H, Benjamini Y, Heller R, et al. 2007. Extrinsic and intrinsic systems in the posterior cortex of the human brain revealed during natural sensory stimulation. *Cereb Cortex* 17: 766–777.

Golland Y, Golland P, Bentin S, Malach R. 2008. Data-driven clustering reveals a fundamental subdivision of the human cortex into two global systems. *Neuropsychologia* 46: 540–553.

Gómez-Gardeñes Y, Moreno Y, Arenas A. 2007a. Paths to synchronization on complex networks. *Phys Rev Lett* 98: 034101.

Gómez-Gardeñes J, Moreno Y, Arenas A. 2007b. Synchronizability determined by coupling strengths and topology on complex networks. *Phys Rev E Stat Nonlin Soft Matter Phys* 75: 066106.

Gong G, He Y, Concha L, Lebel C, Gross DW, et al. 2009. Mapping anatomical connectivity patterns of human cerebral cortex using in vivo diffusion tensor imaging tractography. *Cereb Cortex* 19: 524–536.

Gong P, Nikolaev AR, van Leeuwen C. 2003. Scale-invariant fluctuations of the dynamical synchronization in human brain electrical activity. *Neurosci Lett* 336: 33–36.

Gong P, van Leeuwen C. 2004. Evolution to a small-world network with chaotic units. *Europhys Lett* 67: 328–333.

Goodman MB, Hall DH, Avery L, Lockery SR. 1998. Active currents regulate sensitivity and dynamic range in *C. elegans* neurons. *Neuron* 20: 763–772.

Gould SJ. 1975. Allometry in primates, with emphasis on scaling and the evolution of the brain. *Contrib Primatol* 5: 244–292.

Gould SJ, Lewontin RC. 1979. The spandrels of San Marco and the Panglossian paradigm: A critique of the adaptationist programme. *Proc R Soc Lond B Biol Sci* 205: 581–598.

Gould SJ. 1996. *Full House*. New York: Harmony Books.

Grady CL, Furey ML, Pietrini P, Horwitz B, Rapoport SI. 2001. Altered brain functional connectivity and impaired short-term memory in Alzheimer's disease. *Brain* 124: 739–756.

Grady CL, Springer MV, Hongwanishkul D, McIntosh AR, Winocur G. 2006. Age-related changes in brain activity across the adult lifespan. *J Cogn Neurosci* 18: 227–241.

Grady CL. 2008. Cognitive neuroscience of aging. *Ann N Y Acad Sci* 1124: 127–144.

Granger CWJ. 1969. Investigating causal relations by econometric models and cross-spectral methods. *Econometrica* 37: 424–438.

Granovetter MS. 1973. The strength of weak ties. *Am J Sociol* 78: 1360–1380.

Gray CM, König P, Engel AK, Singer W. 1989. Oscillatory responses in cat visual cortex exhibit inter-columnar synchronization which reflects global stimulus properties. *Nature* 338: 334–337.

Gray CM, Singer W. 1989. Stimulus-specific neuronal oscillations in orientation columns of cat visual cortex. *Proc Natl Acad Sci USA* 86: 1698–1702.

Greicius MD, Krasnow B, Reiss AL, Menon V. 2003. Functional connectivity in the resting brain: A network analysis of the default mode hypothesis. *Proc Natl Acad Sci USA* 100: 253–258.

Greicius MD, Srivastava G, Reiss AL, Menon V. 2004. Default-mode network activity distinguishes Alzheimer's disease from healthy aging: Evidence from functional MRI. *Proc Natl Acad Sci USA* 101: 4637–4642.

Greicius M. 2008. Resting-state functional connectivity in neuropsychiatric disorders. *Curr Opin Neurol* 21: 424–430.

Greicius M, Kiviniemi V, Tervonen O, Vainionpää V, Alahuhta S, et al. 2008. Persistent default-mode network connectivity during light sedation. *Hum Brain Mapp* 29: 839–847.

Greicius MD, Supekar K, Menon V, Dougherty RF. 2009. Resting state functional connectivity reflects structural connectivity in the default mode network. *Cereb Cortex* 19: 72–78.

Gros C. 2009. Cognitive computation with autonomously active neural networks: An emerging field. *Cogn Comput* 1: 77–90.

Gross T, Blasius B. 2008. Adaptive coevolutionary networks: A review. *J R Soc Interface* 5: 259–271.

Guimerà R, Amaral LAN. 2005. Functional cartography of complex metabolic networks. *Nature* 433: 895–900.

Guimerà R, Mossa S, Turtschi A, Amaral LA. 2005. The worldwide air transportation network: Anomalous centrality, community structure and cities' global roles. *Proc Natl Acad Sci USA* 102: 7794–7799.

Guimerà R, Sales-Pardo M, Amaral LA. 2007. Classes of complex networks defined by role-to-role connectivity profiles. *Nat Phys* 3: 63–69.

Gusnard DA, Raichle ME. 2001. Searching for a baseline: Functional imaging and the resting human brain. *Nat Rev Neurosci* 2: 685–694.

Haeusler S, Schuch K, Maass W. 2009. Motif distribution, dynamical properties, and computational performance of two data-based cortical microcircuit templates. *J Physiol (Paris)* 103: 73–87.

Hagmann P. 2005. *From Diffusion MRI to Brain Connectomics: PhD Thesis.* Lausanne: Ecole Polytechnique Fédérale de Lausanne.

Hagmann P, Kurant M, Gigandet X, Thiran P, Wedeen VJ, et al. 2007. Mapping human whole-brain structural networks with diffusion MRI. *PLoS ONE* 2: e597.

Hagmann P, Cammoun L, Gigandet X, Meuli R, Honey CJ, et al. 2008. Mapping the structural core of human cerebral cortex. *PLoS Biol* 6: e159.

Haier RJ, Jung RE, Yeo RA, Head K, Alkire MT. 2004. Structural brain variation and general intelligence. *Neuroimage* 23: 425–433.

Haldeman C, Beggs JM. 2005. Critical branching captures activity in living neural networks and maximizes the number of metastable states. *Phys Rev Lett* 94: 058101.

Hampson M, Peterson BS, Skudlarski P, Gatenby JC, Gore JC. 2002. Detection of functional connectivity using temporal correlations in MR images. *Hum Brain Mapp* 15: 247–262.

Hampson M, Olson IR, Leung HC, Skudlarski P, Gore JC. 2004. Changes in functional connectivity of human MT/V5 with visual motion input. *Neuroreport* 15: 1315–1319.

Hampson M, Driesen NR, Skudlarski P, Gore JC, Constable RT. 2006a. Brain connectivity related to working memory performance. *J Neurosci* 26: 13338–13343.

Hampson M, Tokoglu F, Sun Z, Schafer RJ, Skudlarski P, et al. 2006b. Connectivity-behavior analysis reveals that functional connectivity between left BA39 and Broca's area varies with reading ability. *Neuroimage* 31: 513–519.

Hanahan D, Weinberg RA. 2000. The hallmarks of cancer. *Cell* 100: 57–70.

Happé F, Frith U. 2006. The weak coherence account: Detail-focused cognitive style in autism spectrum disorders. *J Autism Dev Disord* 36: 5–25.

Harary F. 1969. *Graph Theory.* Reading: Perseus Books.

Hari R, Kujala MV. 2009. Brain basis of human social interaction: From concepts to brain imaging. *Physiol Rev* 89: 453–479.

Harman KL, Humphrey GK, Goodale MA. 1999. Active manual control of object views facilitates visual recognition. *Curr Biol* 9: 1315–1318.

Hasson U, Yang E, Vallines I, Heeger DJ, Rubin N. 2008. A hierarchy of temporal receptive windows in human cortex. *J Neurosci* 28: 2539–2550.

He BJ, Snyder AZ, Vincent JL, Epstein A, Shulman GL, et al. 2007a. Breakdown of functional connectivity in frontoparietal networks underlies behavioral deficits in spatial neglect. *Neuron* 53: 905–918.

He BJ, Shulman GL, Snyder AZ, Corbetta M. 2007b. The role of impaired neuronal communication in neurological disorders. *Curr Opin Neurol* 20: 655–660.

He BJ, Snyder AZ, Zempel JM, Smyth MD, Raichle ME. 2008. Electrophysiological correlates of the brain's intrinsic large-scale functional architecture. *Proc Natl Acad Sci USA* 105: 16039–16044.

He Y, Chen ZJ, Evans AC. 2007c. Small-world anatomical networks in the human brain revealed by cortical thickness from MRI. *Cereb Cortex* 17: 2407–2419.

He Y, Wang J, Wang L, Chen ZJ, Yan C, et al. 2009. Uncovering intrinsic modular organization of spontaneous brain activity in humans. *PLoS ONE* 4: e5226.

Hebb DO. 1949. *The Organization of Behavior.* New York: Wiley.

Hedden T, Van Dijk KRA, Becker JA, Mehta A, Sperling RA, et al. 2009. Disruption of functional connectivity in clinically normal older adults harboring amyloid burden. *J Neurosci* 29: 12686–12694.

Hegdé J, Felleman DJ. 2007. Reappraising the functional implications of the primate visual anatomical hierarchy. *Neuroscientist* 13: 416–421.

Heisenberg M, Heusipp M, Wanke C. 1995. Structural plasticity in the Drosophila brain. *J Neurosci* 15: 1951–1960.

Hellwig B. 2000. A quantitative analysis of the local connectivity between pyramidal neurons in layers 2/3 of the rat visual cortex. *Biol Cybern* 82: 111–121.

Helmstaedter M, de Kock CPJ, Feldmeyer D, Bruno RM, Sakmann B. 2007. Reconstruction of an average cortical column *in silico*. *Brain Res Brain Res Rev* 55: 193–203.

Helmstaedter M, Briggman KL, Denk W. 2008. 3D structural imaging of the brain with photons and electrons. *Curr Opin Neurobiol* 18: 633–641.

Hilgetag CC, O'Neill MA, Young MP. 1996. Indeterminate organization of the visual system. *Science* 271: 776–777.

Hilgetag CC, Burns GA, O'Neill MA, Scannell JW, Young MP. 2000. Anatomical connectivity defines the organization of clusters of cortical areas in the macaque monkey and the cat. *Phil Trans R Soc B* 355: 91–110.

Hilgetag CC, Kaiser M. 2004. Clustered organization of cortical connectivity. *Neuroinformatics* 2: 353–360.

Hilgetag CC, Barbas H. 2005. Developmental mechanics of the primate cerebral cortex. *Anat Embryol (Berl)* 210: 411–417.

Hilgetag CC, Barbas H. 2006. Role of mechanical factors in the morphology of the primate cerebral cortex. *PLOS Comput Biol* 2: e22.

Hill S, Tononi G. 2005. Modeling sleep and wakefulness in the thalamocortical system. *J Neurophysiol* 93: 1671–1698.

Hodges A. 1983. *Alan Turing: The Enigma*. New York: Simon and Schuster.

Hodgkin AL, Huxley AF. 1952. A quantitative description of membrane current and its application to conduction and excitation in nerve. *J Phyiol* 117: 500–544.

Hofstadter D. 2007. *I Am a Strange Loop*. New York: Basic Books.

Honey CJ, Kötter R, Breakspear M, Sporns O. 2007. Network structure of cerebral cortex shapes functional connectivity on multiple time scales. *Proc Natl Acad Sci USA* 104: 10240–10245.

Honey CJ, Sporns O. 2008. Dynamical consequences of lesions in cortical networks. *Hum Brain Mapp* 29: 802–809.

Honey CJ, Sporns O, Cammoun L, Gigandet X, Thiran JP, et al. 2009. Predicting human resting-state functional connectivity from structural connectivity. *Proc Natl Acad Sci USA* 106: 2035–2040.

Honey CJ, Thivierge JP, Sporns O. 2010. Can structure predict function in the human brain? *Neuroimage*. In press.

Honey GD, Suckling J, Zelaya F, Long C, Routledge C, et al. 2003. Dopaminergic drug effects on physiological connectivity in a human cortico–striato–thalamic system. *Brain* 126: 1767–1781.

Honey G, Bullmore E. 2004. Human pharmacological MRI. *Trends Pharmacol Sci* 25: 366–374.

Horgan J. 1995. From complexity to perplexity. *Sci Am* 272(6): 104–109.

Horwitz B, Grady CL, Haxby JV, Schapiro MB, Rapoport SI, et al. 1992. Functional associations among human posterior extrastriate brain regions during object and spatial vision. *J Cogn Neurosci* 4: 311–322.

Horwitz B, Sporns O. 1994. Neural modeling and functional neuroimaging. *Hum Brain Mapp* 1: 269–283.

Horwitz B, Rumsey JM, Donohue BC. 1998. Functional connectivity of the angular gyrus in normal reading and dyslexia. *Proc Natl Acad Sci USA* 95: 8939–8944.

Horwitz B, Tagamets MA, McIntosh AR. 1999. Neural modeling, functional brain imaging, and cognition. *Trends Cogn Sci* 3: 91–98.

Horwitz B, Friston KJ, Taylor JG. 2000. Neural modeling and functional brain imaging: An overview. *Neural Netw* 13: 829–846.

Horwitz B. 2003. The elusive concept of brain connectivity. *Neuroimage* 19: 466–470.

Horwitz B, Warner B, Fitzer J, Tagamets MA, Husain FT, et al. 2005. Investigating the neural basis for functional and effective connectivity: Applications to fMRI. *Phil Trans R Soc B* 360: 1093–1108.

Hsu D, Beggs JM. 2006. Neuronal avalanches and criticality: A dynamical model for homeostasis. *Neurocomputing* 69: 1134–1136.

Hubel DH, Wiesel TN. 1962. Receptive fields, binocular interaction and functional architecture in the cat's visual cortex. *J Physiol* 160: 106–154.

Huberman BA, Hogg T. 1986. Complexity and adaptation. *Physica D* 22: 376–384.

Huerta MF, Koslow SH. 1996. Neuroinformatics: Opportunities across disciplinary and national borders. *Neuroimage* 4: S4–S6.

Hughlings Jackson J. 1879. On affections of speech from disease of the brain. *Brain* 2: 323–356.

Hughlings Jackson J. 1884. The Croonian lectures on evolution and dissolution of the nervous system. Lecture III. *BMJ* 1: 703–707.

Humphries MD, Gurney K, Prescott TJ. 2006. The brainstem reticular formation is a small-world, not scale-free, network. *Proc Biol Sci* 273: 503–511.

Humphries MD, Gurney K. 2008. Network "small-world-ness": A quantitative method for determining canonical network equivalence. *PLoS ONE* 3: e2051.

Husain FT, Tagamets MA, Fromm SJ, Braun AR, Horwitz B. 2004. Relating neuronal dynamics for auditory object processing to neuroimaging activity: A computational modeling and an fMRI study. *Neuroimage* 21: 1701–1720.

Huttenlocher PR. 1990. Morphometric study of human cerebral cortex development. *Neuropsychologia* 28: 517–527.

Ideker T, Sharan R. 2008. Protein networks in disease. *Genome Res* 18: 644–652.

Iida F, Pfeifer R, Steels L, Kuniyoshi Y, eds. 2004. *Embodied Artificial Intelligence*. Berlin: Springer.

Ijspeert AJ, Crespi A, Ryczko D, Cabelguen JM. 2007. From swimming to walking with a salamander robot driven by a spinal cord model. *Science* 315: 1416–1420.

Im K, Lee JM, Lyttleton O, Kim SH, Evans AC, Kim SI. 2008. Brain size and cortical structure in the adult human brain. *Cereb Cortex* 18: 2181–2191.

Ingram PJ, Stumpf MPH, Stark J. 2006. Network motifs: Structure does not determine function. *BMC Genomics* 7: 108.

Insel TR, Volkow ND, Li TK, Battey JF, Landis SC. 2003. Neuroscience networks. *PLoS Biol* 1: e17.

Ioannides AA. 2007. Dynamic functional connectivity. *Curr Opin Neurobiol* 17: 161–170.

Iturria-Medina Y, Canales-Rodriguez EJ, Melie-Garcia L, Valdes-Hernandez PA, Martinez-Montes E, et al. 2007. Characterizing brain anatomical connections using diffusion weighted MRI and graph theory. *Neuroimage* 36: 645–660.

Iturria-Medina Y, Sotero RC, Canales-Rodriguez EJ, Aleman-Gomez Y, Melie-Garcia L. 2008. Studying the human brain anatomical network via diffusion-weighted MRI and graph theory. *Neuroimage* 40: 1064–1076.

Izhikevich EM, Edelman GM. 2008. Large-scale model of mammalian thalamocortical systems. *Proc Natl Acad Sci USA* 105: 3593–3598.

Jacobs RA, Jordan MI. 1992. Computational consequences of a bias toward short connections. *J Cogn Neurosci* 4: 323–336.

James KH, Humphrey GH, Goodale MA. 2001. Manipulating and recognizing virtual objects: Where the action is. *Can J Exp Psychol* 55: 113–122.

James W. 1890. *The Principles of Psychology*. New York: Henry Holt.

Jeong H, Mason SP, Barabasi AL, Oltvai ZN. 2001. Lethality and centrality in protein networks. *Nature* 411: 41–42.

Jerison HJ. 1973. *Evolution of the Brain and Intelligence*. New York: Academic Press.

Jiang T, Liu Y, Shi F, Shu N, Liu B, et al. 2008. Multimodal magnetic resonance imaging for brain disorders: Advances and perspectives. *Brain Imaging Behav* 2: 249–257.

Jirsa VK, Kelso JAS. 2000. Spatiotemporal pattern formation in continuous systems with heterogeneous connection topologies. *Phys Rev E Stat Phys Plasmas Fluids Relat Interdiscip Topics* 62: 8462–8465.

Jirsa VK. 2004. Connectivity and dynamics of neural information processing. *Neuroinformatics* 2: 183–204.

Jirsa VK, McIntosh AR. 2007. *Handbook of Brain Connectivity*. New York: Springer.

Johansen-Berg H, Behrens TE, Robson MD, Drobnjak I, Rushworth MF, et al. 2004. Changes in connectivity profiles define functionally distinct regions in human medial frontal cortex. *Proc Natl Acad Sci USA* 101: 13335–13340.

Johansen-Berg H, Rushworth MFS. 2009. Using diffusion imaging to study human connectional anatomy. *Annu Rev Neurosci* 32: 75–94.

Johansen-Berg H, Behrens TEJ, eds. 2009. *Diffusion MRI: From Quantitative Measurement to in Vivo Neuroanatomy*. Amsterdam: Academic Press.

John ER, Schwartz E. 1978. The neurophysiology of information processing and cognition. *Annu Rev Psychol* 29: 1–29.

Johnson MB, Kawasawa YI, Mason CE, Krsnik Z, Coppola G, et al. 2009. Functional and evolutionary insights into human brain development through global transcriptome analysis. *Neuron* 62: 494–509.

Johnson MH. 2001. Functional brain development in humans. *Nat Rev Neurosci* 2: 475–483.

Johnston JM, Vaishnavi SN, Smyth MD, Zhang D, He BJ, et al. 2008. Loss of resting interhemispheric functional connectivity after complete section of the corpus callosum. *J Neurosci* 28: 6453–6458.

Jones AR, Overly CC, Sunkin SM. 2009. The Allen brain atlas: 5 years and beyond. *Nat Rev Neurosci* 10: 821–828.

Jontes JD, Smith SJ. 2000. Filopodia, spines, and the generation of synaptic diversity. *Neuron* 27: 11–14.

Just MA, Cherkassky VL, Keller TA, Kana RK, Minshew NJ. 2007. Functional and anatomical cortical underconnectivity in autism: Evidence from an FMRI study of an executive function task and corpus callosum morphometry. *Cereb Cortex* 17: 951–961.

Kaiser M, Hilgetag CC. 2004a. Modelling the development of cortical networks. *Neurocomputing* 58–60: 297–302.

Kaiser M, Hilgetag CC. 2004b. Spatial growth of real-world networks. *Phys Rev E Stat Nonlin Soft Matter Phys* 69: 036103.

Kaiser M, Hilgetag CC. 2004c. Edge vulnerability in neural and metabolic networks. *Biol Cybern* 90: 311–317.

Kaiser M, Hilgetag CC. 2006. Nonoptimal component placement, but short processing paths, due to long-distance projections in neural systems. *PLoS Comput Biol* 2: e95.

Kaiser M, Hilgetag CC. 2007. Development of multi-cluster cortical networks by time windows for spatial growth. *Neurocomputing* 70: 1829–1832.

Kaiser M, Görner M, Hilgetag CC. 2007a. Criticality of spreading dynamics in hierarchical cluster networks without inhibition. *N J Phys* 9: 110.

Kaiser M, Robert M, Andras P, Young MP. 2007b. Simulation of robustness against lesions of cortical networks. *Eur J Neurosci* 25: 3185–3192.

Kaiser M, Hilgetag CC, van Ooyen A. 2009. A simple rule for axon outgrowth and synaptic competition generates realistic connection lengths and filling fractions. *Cereb Cortex* 19: 3001–3010.

Kaisti KK, Metsähonkala L, Teräs M, Oikonen V, Aalto S, et al. 2002. Effects of surgical levels of propofol and sevoflurane anesthesia on cerebral blood flow in healthy subjects studied with positron emission tomography. *Anesthesiology* 96: 1358–1370.

Kaminski M, Ding M, Truccolo WA, Bressler SL. 2001. Evaluating causal relations in neural systems: Granger causality, directed transfer function and statistical assessment of significance. *Biol Cybern* 85: 145–157.

Kaneko K, Tsuda I. 2003. Chaotic itinerancy. *Chaos* 13: 926–936.

Kashtan N, Alon U. 2005. Spontaneous evolution of modularity and network motifs. *Proc Natl Acad Sci USA* 102: 13773–13778.

Kasthuri N, Lichtman JW. 2007. The rise of the "projectome." *Nat Methods* 4: 307–308.

Katz LC, Shatz CJ. 1996. Synaptic activity and the construction of cortical circuits. *Science* 274: 1133–1138.

Kauffman SA. 1993. *The Origins of Order: Self-Organization and Selection in Evolution.* New York: Oxford University Press.

Kauffman SA. 2000. *Investigations.* New York: Oxford University Press.

Kayser C, Salazar RF, König P. 2003. Responses to natural scenes in cat V1. *J Neurophysiol* 90: 1910–1920.

Keller TA, Kana RK, Just MA. 2007. A developmental study of the structural integrity of white matter in autism. *Neuroreport* 18: 23–27.

Kello CT, Beltz BC, Holden JG, Van Orden GC. 2007. The emergent coordination of cognitive function. *J Exp Psychol Gen* 136: 551–568.

Kello CT, Anderson GG, Holden JG, Van Orden GC. 2008. The pervasiveness of 1/f scaling in speech reflects the metastable basis of cognition. *Cogn Sci* 32: 1217–1231.

Kelso JAS. 1995. *Dynamic Patterns: The Self-Organization of Brain and Behavior.* Cambridge: MIT Press.

Kelso JAS, Tognoli E. 2007. Toward a complementary neuroscience: Metastable coordination dynamics of the brain. In *Downward Causation and the Neurobiology of Free Will,* Murphy N, Ellis GFR, O'Connor T (eds.), pp. 103–124, Berlin: Springer.

Kemmotsu N, Villalobos ME, Gaffrey MS, Courchesne E, Müller RA. 2005. Activity and functional connectivity of inferior frontal cortex associated with response conflict. *Brain Res Cogn Brain Res* 24: 335–342.

Kenet T, Bibitchkov D, Tsodyks M, Grinvald A, Arieli A. 2003. Spontaneously emerging cortical representations of visual attributes. *Nature* 425: 954–956.

Kennedy DP, Redcay E, Courchesne E. 2006. Failing to deactivate: Resting functional abnormalities in autism. *Proc Natl Acad Sci USA* 103: 8275–8280.

Kiebel SJ, Daunizeau J, Friston KJ. 2008. A hierarchy of time-scales and the brain. *PLoS Comput Biol* 4: e1000209.

Kim DI, Manoach DS, Mathalon DH, Turner JA, Mannell M, et al. 2009. Dysregulation of working memory and default-mode networks in schizophrenia using independent components analysis, an fBIRN and MCIC study. *Hum Brain Mapp* 30: 3795–3811.

Kinouchi O, Copelli M. 2006. Optimal dynamical range of excitable networks at criticality. *Nat Phys* 2: 348–351.

Kirschner M, Gerhart J. 1998. Evolvability. *Proc Natl Acad Sci USA* 95: 8420–8427.

Kirschner M, Gerhart J. 2005. *The Plausibility of Life: Resolving Darwin's Dilemma.* New Haven: Yale University Press.

Kitano H. 2002. Systems biology: A brief overview. *Science* 295: 1662–1664.

Kitano H. 2004. Biological robustness. *Nat Rev Genet* 5: 826–837.

Kitzbichler MG, Smith ML, Christensen DR, Bullmore E. 2009. Broadband criticality of human brain network synchronization. *PLoS Comput Biol* 5: e1000314.

Kleinberg J. 2000. Navigation in a small world. *Nature* 406: 845.

Kleinfeld D, Ahissar E, Diamond ME. 2006. Active sensation: Insights from the rodent vibrissa sensorimotor system. *Curr Opin Neurobiol* 16: 435–444.

Klyachko VA, Stevens CF. 2003. Connectivity optimization and the positioning of cortical areas. *Proc Natl Acad Sci USA* 100: 7937–7941.

Klyubin AS, Polani D, Nehaniv CL. 2008. Keep your options open: An information-based driving principle for sensorimotor systems. *PLoS ONE* 3: e4018.

Knoll AH, Bambach RK. 2000. Directionality in the history of life: Diffusion from the left wall or repeated scaling of the right? *Paleobiology* 26: 1–14.

Koch C, Laurent G. 1999. Complexity and the nervous system. *Science* 284: 96–98.

Koch C, Tononi G. 2008. Can machines be conscious? *IEEE Spectr* 45(6): 55–59.

Koch MA, Norris DG, Hund-Georgiadis M. 2002. An investigation of functional and anatomical connectivity using magnetic resonance imaging. *Neuroimage* 16: 241–250.

Koene RA, Tijms B, van Hees P, Postma F, de Ridder A, et al. 2009. A framework for the stochastic generation of large scale neuronal networks with realistic neuron morphologies. *Neuroinformatics* 7: 195–210.

König P, Engel AK, Singer W. 1996. Integrator or coincidence detector? The role of the cortical neuron revisited. *Trends Neurosci* 19: 130–137.

Körner E, Matsumoto G. 2002. Cortical architecture and self-referential control for brain-like computation. *IEEE Eng Med Biol Mag* 21: 121–133.

Kötter R, Sommer F. 2000. Global relationship between anatomical connectivity and activity propagation in the cerebral cortex. *Phil Trans R Soc B* 355: 127–134.

Kötter R, Stephan KE, Palomero-Gallagher N, Geyer S, Schleicher A, Zilles K. 2001. Multimodal characterisation of cortical areas by multivariate analyses of receptor binding and connectivity data. *Anat Embryol (Berl)* 204: 333–350.

Kötter R, Stephan KE. 2003. Network participation indices: Characterizing component roles for information processing in neural networks. *Neural Netw* 16: 1261–1275.

Kötter R. 2004. Online retrieval, processing, and visualization of primate connectivity data from the CoCoMac database. *Neuroinformatics* 2: 127–144.

Kötter R. 2007. Anatomical concepts of brain connectivity. In *Handbook of Brain Connectivity*, Jirsa VK, McIntosh AR (eds.), pp. 149–167, Springer: Berlin.

Kötter R, Reid AT, Krumnack A, Wanke E, Sporns O. 2007. Shapley ratings in brain networks. *Front Neuroinformatics* 1: 2.

Konrad A, Winterer G. 2008. Disturbed structural connectivity in schizophrenia—Primary factor in pathology or epiphenomenon? *Schizophr Bull* 34: 72–92.

Krebs VE. 2002. Mapping networks of terrorist cells. *Connections* 24: 43–52.

Kubicki M, McCarley R, Westin CF, Park HJ, Maier S, et al. 2005a. A review of diffusion tensor imaging studies in schizophrenia. *J Psychiatr Res* 41: 15–30.

Kubicki M, McCarley RW, Shenton ME. 2005b. Evidence for white matter abnormalities in schizophrenia. *Curr Opin Psychiatry* 18: 121–134.

Kwok HF, Jurica P, Raffone A, Van Leeuwen C. 2007. Robust emergence of small-world structure in networks of spiking neurons. *Cogn Neurodyn* 1: 39–51.

Lakoff G, Johnson M. 1999. *Philosophy in the Flesh: The Embodied Mind and its Challenge to Western Thought*. New York: Basic Books.

Langton CG. 1990. Computation at the edge of chaos. *Physica D* 42: 12–37.

Larson-Prior LJ, Zempel JM, Nolan TS, Prior FW, Snyder AZ, et al. 2009. Cortical network functional connectivity in the descent to sleep. *Proc Natl Acad Sci USA* 106: 4489–4494.

Lashley KS. 1929. *Brain Mechanisms and Intelligence: A Quantitative Study of Injuries to the Brain*. Chicago: University of Chicago Press.

Lashley KS. 1931. Mass action in cerebral function. *Science* 73: 245–254.

Lashley KS, Clark G. 1946. The cytoarchitectonic structure of the cerebral cortex of Ateles: A critical examination of architectonic studies. *J Comp Neurol* 85: 223–306.

Lashley KS. 1947. Structural variation in the nervous system in relation to behavior. *Psychol Rev* 54: 325–334.

Latora V, Marchiori M. 2001. Efficient behavior of small-world networks. *Phys Rev Lett* 87: 198701.

Latora V, Marchiori M. 2003. Economic small-world behavior in weighted networks. *Eur Phys J B* 32: 249–263.

Laughlin SB, Sejnowski TJ. 2003. Communication in neuronal networks. *Science* 301: 1870–1874.

Laureys S, Owen AM, Schiff ND. 2004. Brain function in coma, vegetative state, and related disorders. *Lancet Neurol* 3: 537–546.

Lee L, Harrison LM, Mechelli A. 2003. A report of the functional connectivity workshop, Düsseldorf 2002. *Neuroimage* 19: 457–465.

Legenstein R, Maass W. 2007. Edge of chaos and prediction of computational performance for neural microcircuit models. *Neural Netw* 20: 323–333.

Lein ES, Hawrylycz MJ, Ao N, Ayres M, Bensinger A, et al. 2007. Genome-wide atlas of gene expression in the adult mouse brain. *Nature* 445: 168–176.

Lenartowicz A, McIntosh AR. 2005. The role of anterior cingulate cortex in working memory is shaped by functional connectivity. *J Cogn Neurosci* 17: 1026–1042.

Lennie P. 2003. The cost of cortical computation. *Curr Biol* 13: 493–497.

Leopold DA, Murayama Y, Logothetis NK. 2003. Very slow activity fluctuations in monkey visual cortex: Implications for functional brain imaging. *Cereb Cortex* 13: 422–433.

Lewontin RC. 1983. The organism as the subject and object of evolution. *Scientia* 118: 63–82.

Levina A, Herrmann J, Geisel T. 2007. Dynamical synapses causing self-organized criticality in neural networks. *Nat Phys* 3: 857–860.

Li Y, Liu Y, Li J, Qin W, Li K, et al. 2009. Brain anatomical network and intelligence. *PLoS Comput Biol* 5: e1000395.

Liang H, Bressler SL, Ding M, Truccolo WA, Nakamura R. 2002. Synchronized activity in prefrontal cortex during anticipation of visuomotor processing. *Neuroreport* 13: 2011–2015.

Liang M, Zhou Y, Jiang T, Liu Z, Tian L, et al. 2006. Widespread functional disconnectivity in schizophrenia with resting-state functional magnetic resonance imaging. *Neuroreport* 17: 209–213.

Lichtheim L. 1885. On aphasia. *Brain* 7: 433–484.

Lichtman JW, Livet J, Sanes JR. 2008. A technicolour approach to the connectome. *Nat Rev Neurosci* 9: 417–422.

Lichtman JW, Sanes JR. 2008. Ome sweet ome: What can the genome tell us about the connectome? *Curr Opin Neurobiol* 18: 346–353.

Liley DTJ, Wright JJ. 1994. Intracortical connectivity of pyramidal and stellate cells: Estimates of synaptic densities and coupling symmetry. *Network Comp Neural Syst* 5: 175–189.

Lin W, Zhu Q, Gao W, Chen Y, Toh CH, et al. 2008. Functional connectivity MR imaging reveals cortical functional connectivity in the developing brain. *AJNR Am J Neuroradiol* 29: 1883–1889.

Linkenkaer-Hansen K, Nikouline VV, Palva JM, Ilmoniemi RJ. 2001. Long-range temporal correlations and scaling behavior in human brain oscillations. *J Neurosci* 21: 1370–1377.

Linkenkaer-Hansen K, Nikulin VV, Palva JM, Kaila K, Ilmoniemi RJ. 2004. Stimulus-induced change in long-range temporal correlations and scaling behaviour of sensorimotor oscillations. *Eur J Neurosci* 19: 203–211.

Lipson H, Pollack JB, Suh NP. 2002. On the origin of modular variation. *Evolution* 56: 1549–1556.

Liu Y, Liang M, Zhou Y, He Y, Hao Y, et al. 2008. Disrupted small-world networks in schizophrenia. *Brain* 131: 945–961.

Livet J, Weissman TA, Kang H, Draft RW, Lu J, et al. 2007. Transgenic strategies for combinatorial expression of fluorescent proteins in the nervous system. *Nature* 450: 56–62.

Lizier JT, Piraveenan M, Pradhana D, Prokopenko M, Yaeger LS. 2009. Functional and structural topologies in evolved neural networks In *Advances in Artificial Life: Proceedings of the Tenth European Conference on Artificial Life (ECAL2009)*, Kampis G, Szathmáry E, Fernando C, Jelasity M, Jordan F, et al. (eds.), Springer: Heidelberg.

Llinás RR. 1988. The intrinsic electrophysiological properties of mammalian neurons: Insights into central system function. *Science* 242: 1654–1664.

Llinás RR. 2001. *I of the Vortex*. Cambridge: MIT Press.

Lloyd S, Pagels H. 1988. Complexity as thermodynamic depth. *Ann Phys* 188: 186–213.

Lloyd S. 2001. Measures of complexity: A nonexhaustive list. *IEEE Contr Syst Mag* 21: 7–8.

Logothetis NK, Pauls J, Augath M, Trinath T, Oeltermann A. 2001. Neurophysiological investigation of the basis of the fMRI signal. *Nature* 412: 150–157.

Logothetis NK, Wandell BA. 2004. Interpreting the BOLD signal. *Annu Rev Physiol* 66: 735–769.

Lombardo MV, Barnes JL, Wheelwright SJ, Baron-Cohen S. 2007. Self-referential cognition and empathy in autism. *PLoS ONE* 2: e883.

Lorente de Nó R. 1938. Analysis of the activity of the chains of internuncial neurons. *J Neurophysiol* 1: 207–244.

Lu J, Tapia JC, White OL, Lichtman JW. 2009. The interscutularis muscle connectome. *PLoS Biol* 7: e1000032.

Luczak A, Barthó P, Marguet SL, Buzsáki G, Harris KD. 2007. Sequential structure of neocortical spontaneous activity in vivo. *Proc Natl Acad Sci USA* 104: 347–352.

Luczak A, Barthó P, Harris KD. 2009. Spontaneous events outline the realm of possible sensory responses in neocortical populations. *Neuron* 62: 413–425.

Ludwig E, Klingler L. 1956. *Atlas Cerebri Humani*. Boston: Little, Brown and Company.

Lungarella M, Pegors T, Bulwinkle D, Sporns O. 2005. Methods for quantifying the informational structure of sensory and motor data. *Neuroinformatics* 3: 243–262.

Lungarella M, Sporns O. 2006. Mapping information flow in sensorimotor networks. *PLoS Comput Biol* 2: e144.

Lungarella M, Ishiguro K, Kuniyoshi Y, Otsu N. 2007. Methods for quantifying the causal structure of bivariate time series. *Int J Bifurcat Chaos* 17: 903–921.

Lux T, Westerhoff F. 2009. Economic crisis. *Nat Phys* 5: 2–3.

Maass W, Natschläger T, Markram H. 2002. Real-time computing without stable states: A new framework for neural computation based on perturbations. *Neural Comput* 14: 2531–2560.

Macagno ER, Levinthal C, Sobel I. 1979. Three-dimensional computer reconstruction of neurons and neuronal assemblies. *Annu Rev Biophys Bioeng* 8: 323–351.

MacEvoy SP, Hanks TD, Paradiso MA. 2008. Macaque V1 activity during natural vision: Effects of natural scenes and saccades. *J Neurophysiol* 99: 460–472.

MacLean JN, Watson BO, Aaron GB, Yuste R. 2005. Internal dynamics determine the cortical response to thalamic stimulation. *Neuron* 48: 811–823.

Maffei A, Fontanini A. 2009. Network homeostasis: A matter of coordination. *Curr Opin Neurobiol* 19: 1–6.

Mantini D, Perruci MG, Del Gratta C, Romani GL, Corbetta M. 2007. Electrophysiological signatures of resting state networks in the human brain. *Proc Natl Acad Sci USA* 104: 13170–13175.

Mao BQ, Hamzei-Sichani F, Aronov D, Froemke RC, Yuste R. 2001. Dynamics of spontaneous activity in neocortical slices. *Neuron* 32: 883–898.

Marcus GF. 2001. *The Algebraic Mind: Integrating Connectionism and Cognitive Science.* Cambridge: MIT Press.

Marder E, Prinz AA. 2002. Modeling stability in neuron and network function: The role of activity in homeostasis. *Bioessays* 24: 1145–1154.

Marder E, Goaillard JM. 2006. Variability, compensation and homeostasis in neuron and network function. *Nat Rev Neurosci* 7: 563–574.

Mason MF, Norton MI, Van Horn JD, Wegner DM, Grafton ST, et al. 2007. Wandering minds: The default network and stimulus-independent thought. *Science* 315: 393–395.

Massimini M, Ferrarelli F, Huber R, Esser SK, Singh H, et al. 2005. Breakdown of cortical effective connectivity during sleep. *Science* 309: 2228–2232.

Masuda N, Aihara K. 2004. Global and local synchrony of coupled neurons in small-world networks. *Biol Cybern* 90: 302–309.

Maturana HR, Varela FJ. 1980. *Autopoiesis and Cognition.* Dordrecht: Reidel.

Maye A, Hsieh CH, Sugihara G, Brembs B. 2007. Order in spontaneous behavior. *PLoS ONE* 2: e443.

Mayr E. 1959. Darwin and the evolutionary theory in biology. In *Evolution and Anthropology: A Centennial Appraisal*, Meggers BJ (ed.), pp. 1–10, Washington, DC: The Anthropological Society of Washington.

McCulloch WS. 1945. A heterarchy of values determined by the topology of nervous nets. *Bull Math Biophys* 7: 89–93.

McEwen BS. 2007. Physiology and neurobiology of stress and adaptation: Central role of the brain. *Physiol Rev* 87: 873–904.

McGill W. 1954. Multivariate information transmission. *Psychometrika* 19: 97–116.

McGuffie K, Henderson-Sellers A. 2001. Forty years of numerical climate modeling. *Int J Climatol* 21: 1067–1109.

McIntosh AR, Gonzalez-Lima F. 1994. Structural equation modeling and its application to network analysis in functional brain imaging. *Hum Brain Mapp* 2: 2–22.

McIntosh AR, Grady CL, Ungerleider LG, Haxby JV, Rapoport SI, et al. 1994. Network analysis of cortical visual pathways mapped with PET. *J Neurosci* 14: 655–666.

McIntosh AR, Grady CL, Haxby JV, Ungerleider LG, Horwitz B. 1996. Changes in limbic and prefrontal functional interactions in a working memory task for faces. *Cereb Cortex* 6: 571–584.

McIntosh AR, Nyberg L, Bookstein FL, Tulving E. 1997. Differential functional connectivity of prefrontal and medial temporal cortices during episodic memory retrieval. *Hum Brain Mapp* 5: 323–327.

McIntosh AR. 1999. Mapping cognition to the brain through neural interactions. *Memory* 7: 523–548.

McIntosh AR, Rajah MN, Lobaugh NJ. 1999. Interactions of prefrontal cortex related to awareness in sensory learning. *Science* 284: 1531–1533.

McIntosh AR. 2000. Towards a network theory of cognition. *Neural Netw* 13: 861–870.

McIntosh AR, Rajah MN, Lobaugh NJ. 2003. Functional connectivity of the medial temporal lobe relates to learning and awareness. *J Neurosci* 23: 6520–6528.

McIntosh AR. 2004. Contexts and catalysts. *Neuroinformatics* 2: 175–181.

McIntosh AR. 2008. Large-scale network dynamics in neurocognitive function. In *Coordination: Neural, Behavioral and Social Dynamics*, Jirsa VK, Richardson MJ (eds.), pp. 183–204, Springer: Berlin.

McIntosh AR, Kovacevic N, Itier R. 2008. Increased brain signal variability accompanies lower behavioral variability in development. *PLoS Comput Biol* 4: e1000106.

Meinhardt H. 2009. *The Algorithmic Beauty of Sea Shells*. Fourth Edition. Berlin: Springer.

Melloni L, Schwiedrzik CM, Rodriguez E, Singer W. 2009. (Micro)Saccades, corollary activity and cortical oscillations. *Trends Cogn Sci* 13: 239–245.

Meltzoff AN, Kuhl PK, Movellan J, Sejnowski TJ. 2009. Foundations for a new science of learning. *Science* 325: 284–288.

Merleau-Ponty M. 1963. *The Structure of Behaviour*. Boston: Beacon Press.

Mesulam MM. 1990. Large-scale neurocognitive networks and distributed processing for attention, language, and memory. *Ann Neurol* 28: 597–613.

Mesulam MM. 1998. From sensation to cognition. *Brain* 121: 1013–1052.

Mesulam MM. 2000. *Principles of Behavioral and Cognitive Neurology*. Oxford: Oxford University Press.

Mesulam M. 2005. Imaging connectivity in the human cerebral cortex: The next frontier? *Ann Neurol* 57: 5–7.

Mesulam M. 2009. Defining neurocognitive networks in the BOLD new world of computed connectivity. *Neuron* 62: 1–3.

Metta G, Fitzpatrick P. 2003. Better vision through manipulation. *Adapt Behav* 11: 109–128.

Meunier D, Achard S, Morcom A, Bullmore E. 2009a. Age-related changes in modular organization of human brain functional networks. *Neuroimage* 44: 715–723.

Meunier D, Lambiotte R, Fornito A, Ersche KD, Bullmore ET. 2009b. Hierarchical modularity in human brain functional networks. *Front Neuroinformatics* 3: 37.

Meyer K, Damasio A. 2009. Convergence and divergence in a neural architecture for recognition and memory. *Trends Neurosci* 32: 376–382.

Micheloyannis S, Pachou E, Stam CJ, Breakspear M, Bitsios P, et al. 2006. Small-world networks and disturbed functional connectivity in schizophrenia. *Schizophr Res* 87: 60–66.

Micheva KD, Smith SK. 2007. Array tomography: A new tool for imaging the molecular architecture and ultrastructure of neural circuits. *Neuron* 55: 25–36.

Milh M, Kaminska A, Huon C, Lapillonne A, Ben-Ari Y, et al. 2007. Rapid cortical oscillations and early motor activity in premature human neonate. *Cereb Cortex* 17: 1582–1594.

Miller FJ, Weaver KE, Ojemann JG. 2009. Direct electrophysiological measurement of human default network areas. *Proc Natl Acad Sci USA* 106: 12174–12177.

Milo R, Shen-Orr S, Itzkovitz S, Kashtan N, Chklovskii D, et al. 2002. Network motifs: Simple building blocks of complex networks. *Science* 298: 824–827.

Milo R, Itzkovitz S, Kashtan N, Levitt R, Shen-Orr S, et al. 2004a. Superfamilies of evolved and designed networks. *Science* 303: 1538–1542.

Milo R, Itzkovitz S, Kashtan N, Levitt R, Alon U. 2004b. Response to Comment on "Network motifs: Simple building blocks of complex networks" and "Superfamilies of evolved and designed networks." *Science* 305: 1107d.

Milstein J, Mormann F, Fried I, Koch C. 2009. Neuronal shot noise and Brownian $1/f^2$ behavior in the local field potential. *PLoS ONE* 4: e4338.

Minerbi A, Kahana R, Goldfeld L, Kaufman M, Marom S, et al. 2009. Long-term relationships between synaptic tenacity, synaptic remodeling, and network activity. *PLoS Biol* 7: e1000136.

Minoshima S, Giordani B, Berent S, Frey KA, Foster NL, Kuhl DE. 1997. Metabolic reduction in the posterior cingulate cortex in very early Alzheimer's disease. *Ann Neurol* 42: 85–94.

Mitchell M, Hraber PT, Crutchfield JP. 1993. Revisiting the edge of chaos: Evolving cellular automata to perform computations. *Complex Systems* 7: 89–130.

Mitchell M. 2009. *Complexity: A Guided Tour*. New York: Oxford University Press.

Mitchison G. 1991. Neuronal branching patterns and the economy of cortical wiring. *Proc Biol Sci* 245: 151–158.

Mitchison G. 1992. Axonal trees and cortical architecture. *Trends Neurosci* 15: 122–126.

Mobbs PG. 1982. The brain of the honeybee *Apis mellifera*. I. The connections and spatial organization of the mushroom bodies. *Phil Trans R Soc B* 298: 309–354.

Möller R. 2000. Insect visual homing strategies in a robot with analog processing. *Biol Cybern* 83: 231–243.

Montague PR, Berns GS, Cohen JD, McClure SM, Pagnoni G, et al. 2002. Hyperscanning: Simultaneous fMRI during linked social interactions. *Neuroimage* 16: 1159–1164.

Morcom AM, Fletcher PC. 2007. Does the brain have a baseline? Why we should be resisting a rest. *Neuroimage* 37: 1073–1082.

Moreno JL, Jennings HH. 1938. Statistics of social configurations. *Sociometry* 1: 342–374.

Moreno Y, Pacheco AF. 2004. Synchronization of Kuramoto oscillators in scale-free networks. *Europhys Lett* 68: 603–609.

Morgan RJ, Soltesz I. 2008. Nonrandom connectivity of the epileptic dentate gyrus predicts a major role for neuronal hubs in seizures. *Proc Natl Acad Sci USA* 105: 6179–6184.

Morosan P, Rademacher J, Schleicher A, Amunts K, Schormann T, et al. 2001. Human primary auditory cortex: Cytoarchitectonic subdivisions and mapping into a spatial reference system. *Neuroimage* 13: 684–701.

Morosan P, Schleicher A, Amunts K, Zilles K. 2005. Multimodal architectonic mapping of human superior temporal gyrus. *Anat Embryol (Berl)* 210: 401–406.

Morris R. 2001. *The Evolutionists: The Struggle for Darwin's Soul*. New York: Freeman.

Motter AE, Toroczkai Z. 2007. Introduction: Optimization in networks. *Chaos* 17: 026101.

Mountcastle VB. 1978. An organizing principle for cerebral function. In *The Mindful Brain*, Edelman GM, Mountcastle VB (eds.), pp. 7–50, Cambridge: MIT Press.

Mountcastle VB. 1998. *Perceptual Neuroscience: The Cerebral Cortex*. Cambridge: Harvard University Press.

Müller-Linow M, Hilgetag CC, Hütt MT. 2008. Organization of excitable dynamics in hierarchical biological networks. *PLoS Comput Biol* 4: e1000190.

Murre JM, Sturdy DP. 1995. The connectivity of the brain: Multi-level quantitative analysis. *Biol Cybern* 73: 529–545.

Nelson ME, Bower JM. 1990. Brain maps and parallel computers. *Trends Neurosci* 13: 403–408.

Netoff TI, Clewley R, Arno S, Keck T, White JA. 2004. Epilepsy in small-world networks. *J Neurosci* 24: 8075–8083.

Newman MEJ. 2002. Assortative mixing in networks. *Phys Rev Lett* 89: 208701.

Newman MEJ. 2003. The structure and function of complex networks. *SIAM Rev* 45: 167–256.

Newman MEJ, Girvan M. 2004. Finding and evaluating community structure in networks. *Phys Rev E Stat Nonlin Soft Matter Phys* 69: 026113.

Newman MEJ. 2005. Power laws, Pareto distributions and Zipf's law. *Contemp Phys* 46: 323–351.

Newman MEJ. 2006. Modularity and community structure in networks. *Proc Natl Acad Sci USA* 103: 8577–8582.

Newman MEJ, Barabási AL, Watts DJ. 2006. *The Structure and Dynamics of Networks*. Princeton: Princeton University Press.

Nir Y, Hasson U, Levy I, Yeshurun Y, Malach R. 2006. Widespread functional connectivity and fMRI fluctuations in human visual cortex in the absence of visual stimulation. *Neuroimage* 30: 1313–1324.

Nir Y, Mukamel R, Dinstein I, Privman E, Harel M, et al. 2008. Interhemispheric correlations of slow spontaneous neuronal fluctuations revealed in human sensory cortex. *Nat Neurosci* 11: 1100–1108.

Nisbach F, Kaiser M. 2007. Time domains for spatial network development generate multiple-cluster small-world networks. *Eur Phys J B* 58: 185–191.

Nishikawa T, Motter AE, Lai YC, Hoppensteadt FC. 2003. Heterogeneity in oscillator networks: Are smaller worlds easier to synchronize? *Phys Rev Lett* 91: 014101.

Niven JE, Laughlin SB. 2008. Energy limitation as a selective pressure on the evolution of sensory systems. *J Exp Biol* 211: 1792–1804.

Nunez PL. 2000. Toward a quantitative description of large-scale neocortical dynamic function and EEG. *Behav Brain Sci* 23: 371–398.

O'Donovan MJ, Chub N, Wenner P. 1998. Mechanisms of spontaneous activity in developing spinal networks. *J Neurobiol* 37: 131–145.

Ohki K, Chung S, Ch'ng YH, Kara P, Reid RC. 2005. Functional imaging with cellular resolution reveals precise micro-architecture in visual cortex. *Nature* 433: 597–603.

Olbrich E, Bertschinger N, Ay N, Jost J. 2008. How should complexity scale with system size? *Eur Phys J B* 63: 407–415.

Onnela JP, Saramaki J, Kertesz J, Kaski K. 2005. Intensity and coherence of motifs in weighted complex networks. *Phys Rev E Stat Nonlin Soft Matter Phys* 71: 065103.

Pajevic S, Plenz D. 2009. Efficient network reconstruction from dynamical cascades identifies small-world topology of neuronal avalanches. *PLoS Comput Biol* 5: e1000271.

Palla G, Derenyi I, Farkas I, Vicsek T. 2005. Uncovering the overlapping community structure of complex networks in nature and society. *Nature* 435: 814–818.

Palm C, Axer M, Grässel D, Dammers J, Lindemeyer J, et al. 2010. Towards ultra-high resolution fibre tract mapping of the human brain—registration of polarized light images and reorientation of fibre vectors. *Front Hum Neurosci* 4: 9.

Paninski L. 2003. Estimation of entropy and mutual information. *Neural Comput* 15: 1191–1254.

Parkhurst DJ, Niebur E. 2003. Scene content selected by active vision. *Spat Vis* 16: 125–154.

Parvizi J, Van Hoesen GW, Buckwalter J, Damasio A. 2006. Neural connections of the posteromedial cortex in the macaque. *Proc Natl Acad Sci USA* 103: 1563–1568.

Pascual-Leone A, Walsh V, Rothwell J. 2000. Transcranial magnetic stimulation in cognitive neuroscience—Virtual lesion, chronometry, and functional connectivity. *Curr Opin Neurobiol* 10: 232–237.

Passingham RE, Stephan KE, Kötter R. 2002. The anatomical basis of functional localization in the cortex. *Nat Rev Neurosci* 3: 606–616.

Pastor-Satorras R, Vespignani A. 2004. *Evolution and Structure of the Internet*. Cambridge: Cambridge University Press.

Paus T. 1999. Imaging the brain before, during, and after transcranial magnetic stimulation. *Neuropsychologia* 37: 219–224.

Paus T, Collins DL, Evans AC, Leonard G, Pike B, et al. 2001. Maturation of white matter in the human brain: A review of magnetic resonance studies. *Brain Res Bull* 54: 255–266.

Pearlmutter BA, Houghton CJ. 2009. A new hypothesis for sleep: Tuning for criticality. *Neural Comput* 21: 1622–1641.

Pearson KG, Goodman CS. 1979. Correlation of variability in structure with variability in synaptic connections of an identified interneuron in locusts. *J Comp Neurol* 184: 141–166.

Pechura CM, Martin JB, eds. 1991. *Mapping the Brain and Its Functions: Integrating Enabling Technologies into Neuroscience Research*. Washington, DC: National Academy Press.

Penn DC, Holyoak KJ, Povinelli DJ. 2008. Darwin's mistake: Explaining the discontinuity between human and nonhuman minds. *Behav Brain Sci* 31: 109–130.

Pennisi E. 2007. Working the (gene count) numbers: Finally, a firm answer? *Science* 316: 1113.

Penny WD, Stephan KE, Mechelli A, Friston KJ. 2004. Comparing dynamic causal models. *Neuroimage* 22: 1157–1172.

Pereira AF, Smith LB. 2009. Developemental changes in visual object recognition between 18 and 24 months of age. *Dev Sci* 12: 67–80.

Perlbarg V, Marrelec G. 2008. Contribution of exploratory methods to the investigation of extended large-scale brain networks in functional MRI: Methodologies, results, and challenges. *Int J Biomed Imaging* 2008: 218519.

Pfeifer R, Scheier C. 1999. *Understanding Intelligence*. Cambridge: MIT Press.

Pfeifer R, Bongard JC. 2007. *How the Body Shapes the Way We Think—A New View of Intelligence*. Cambridge: MIT Press.

Pfeifer R, Lungarella M, Iida F. 2007. Self-organization, embodiment, and biologically inspired robotics. *Science* 318: 1088–1093.

Pfeifer R, Lungarella M, Sporns O. 2008. The synthetic approach to embodied cognition: A primer. In *Handbook of Cognitive Science: An Embodied Approach*, Calvo O, Gomila, A (eds.), pp. 121–137, Elsevier, Amsterdam.

Phillips CG, Zeki S, Barlow HB. 1984. Localization of function in the cerebral cortex: Past, present and future. *Brain* 107: 328–361.

Phillips WA, Singer W. 1997. In search of common foundations for cortical computation. *Behav Brain Sci* 20: 657–722.

Plenz D, Thiagarajan TC. 2007. The organizing principles of neuronal avalanches: Cell assemblies in the cortex? *Trends Neurosci* 30: 101–110.

Poil SS, van Ooyen A, Linkenkaer-Hansen K. 2008. Avalanche dynamics of human brain oscillations: Relation to critical branching processes and temporal correlations. *Hum Brain Mapp* 29: 770–777.

Polani S. 2009. Information: Currency of life? *HFSP J* 3: 307–316.

Pomarol-Clotet E, Salvador R, Sarró S, Gomar J, Vila F, et al. 2008. Failure to deactivate in the prefrontal cortex in schizophrenia: Dysfunction of the default mode network? *Psychol Med* 38: 1185–1193.

Pool IS, Kochen M. 1978. Contacts and influence. *Soc Networks* 1: 5–51.

Price CJ, Friston KJ. 2002. Degeneracy and cognitive anatomy. *Trends Cogn Sci* 6: 416–421.

Prill RJ, Iglesias PA, Levchenko A. 2005. Dynamic properties of network motifs contribute to biological network organization. *PLoS Biol* 3: e343.

Prinz AA, Bucher D, Marder E. 2004. Similar network activity from disparate circuit parameters. *Nat Neurosci* 7: 1345–1352.

Puce A, Perrett D. 2003. Electrophysiology and brain imaging of biological motion. *Philos Trans R Soc Lond B Biol Sci* 358: 435–445.

Quiroga RQ, Reddy L, Kreiman G, Koch C, Fried I. 2005. Invariant visual representation by single neurons in the human brain. *Nature* 435: 1102–1107.

Rabinovich MI, Varona P, Selverston AI, Abarbanel HDI. 2006. Dynamical principles in neuroscience. *Rev Mod Phys* 78: 1213–1265.

Rabinovich MI, Huerta R, Varona P, Afraimovich VS. 2008a. Transient cognitive dynamics, metastability, and decision making. *PLoS Comput Biol* 4: e1000072.

Rabinovich M, Huerta R, Laurent G. 2008b. Transient dynamics for neural processing. *Science* 321: 48–50.

Raff RA. 1996. *The Shape of Life: Genes, Development, and the Evolution of Animal Form.* Chicago: University of Chicago Press.

Raffone A, van Leeuwen C. 2003. Dynamic synchronization and chaos in an associative neural network with multiple active memories. *Chaos* 13: 1090–1104.

Raichle ME, MacLeod AM, Snyder AZ, Powers WJ, Gusnard DA, Shulman GL. 2001. A default mode of brain function. *Proc Natl Acad Sci USA* 98: 676–682.

Raichle ME, Mintun MA. 2006. Brain work and brain imaging. *Annu Rev Neurosci* 29: 449–476.

Raichle ME, Snyder AZ. 2007. A default mode of brain function: A brief history of an evolving idea. *Neuroimage* 37: 1083–1090.

Raichle ME. 2009. A paradigm shift in functional brain imaging. *J Neurosci* 29: 12729–12734.

Raichle ME. 2010. Two views of brain function. *Trends Cogn Sci* 14: 180–190.

Rajkowska G, Goldman-Rakic PS. 1995. Cytoarchitectonic definition of prefrontal areas in the normal human cortex. II. Variability in locations of areas 9 and 46 and relationship to the Talairach coordinate system. *Cereb Cortex* 5: 323–337.

Rao RPN, Ballard DH. 1999. Predictive coding in the visual cortex: A functional interpretation of some extra-classical receptive-field effects. *Nat Neurosci* 2: 79–87.

Ravasz E, Barabási AL. 2003. Hierarchical organization in complex networks. *Phys Rev E Stat Nonlin Soft Matter Phys* 67: 026112.

Rees G, Kreiman G, Koch C. 2002. Neural correlates of consciousness in humans. *Nat Rev Neurosci* 3: 261–270.

Reid AT, Krumnack A, Wanke E, Kötter R. 2009. Optimization of cortical hierarchies with continuous scales and ranges. *Neuroimage* 47: 611–617.

Reigl M, Alon U, Chklovskii DB. 2004. Search for computational modules in the *C. elegans* brain. *BMC Biol* 2: 25.

Reijneveld JC, Ponten SC, Berendse HW, Stam CJ. 2007. The application of graph theoretical analysis to complex networks in the brain. *Clin Neurophysiol* 118: 2317–2331.

Riesenhuber M, Poggio T. 1999. Hierarchical models of object recognition in cortex. *Nat Neurosci* 2: 1019–1025.

Riesenhuber M, Poggio T. 2000. Models of object recognition. *Nat Neurosci* 3: 1199–1204.

Rilling JK, Glasser MF, Preuss TM, Ma X, Zhao T, et al. 2008. The evolution of the arcuate fasciculus revealed with comparative DTI. *Nat Neurosci* 11: 426–428.

Ringo JL. 1991. Neuronal interconnection as a function of brain size. *Brain Behav Evol* 38: 1–6.

Robinson PA, Rennie CJ, Rowe DL, O'Connor SC, Gordon E. 2005. Multiscale brain modeling. *Phil Trans R Soc B* 360: 1043–1050.

Rodriguez E, George N, Lachaux JP, Martinerie J, Renault B, et al. 1999. Perception's shadow: Long-distance synchronization of human brain activity. *Nature* 397: 430–433.

Roebroeck A, Formisano E, Goebel R. 2005. Mapping directed influence over the brain using Granger causality and fMRI. *Neuroimage* 25: 230–242.

Roelfsema PR, Engel AK, König P, Singer W. 1997. Visuomotor integration is associated with zero time-lag synchronization among cortical areas. *Nature* 385: 157–161.

Roxin A, Riecke H, Solla SA. 2004. Self-sustained activity in a small-world network of excitable neurons. *Phys Rev Lett* 92: 198101.

Rubinov M, Knock SA, Stam CJ, Micheloyannis S, Harris AWF, et al. 2009a. Small-world properties of nonlinear brain activity in schizophrenia. *Hum Brain Mapp* 30: 403–416.

Rubinov M, Sporns O, van Leeuwen C, Breakspear M. 2009b. Symbiotic relationship between brain structure and dynamics. *BMC Neurosci* 10: 55.

Rubinov M, Sporns O. 2010. Complex network measures of brain connectivity: Uses and interpretations. *Neuroimage*. In press.

Rudrauf D, Douiri A, Kovach C, Lachaux JP, Cosmelli D, et al. 2006. Frequency flows and the time-frequency dynamics of multivariate phase synchronization in brain signals. *Neuroimage* 31: 209–227.

Rumelhart DE, McClelland JL, and the PDP Research Group. 1986. *Parallel Distributed Processing: Explorations in the Microstructure of Cognition*. Cambridge: MIT Press.

Ruppin E, Schwartz EL, Yeshurun Y. 1993. Examining the volume efficiency of the cortical architecture in a multi-processor network model. *Biol Cybern* 70: 89–94.

Rushworth MFS, Behrens TEJ, Johansen-Berg H. 2006. Connection patterns distinguish 3 regions of human parietal cortex. *Cereb Cortex* 16: 1418–1430.

Salin PA, Bullier J. 1995. Corticocortical connections in the visual system: Structure and function. *Physiol Rev* 75: 107–154.

Salvador R, Suckling J, Coleman MR, Pickard JD, Menon D, et al. 2005. Neurophysiological architecture of functional magnetic resonance images of human brain. *Cereb Cortex* 15: 1332–1342.

Sanchez-Vives M, McCormick D. 2000. Cellular and network mechanisms of rhythmic recurrent activity in neocortex. *Nat Neurosci* 3: 1027–1034.

Sandberg A, Bostrom N. 2008. *Whole Brain Emulation: A Roadmap*, Technical Report #2008-3, Future of Humanity Institute, Oxford University.

Sauer U, Heinemann M, Zamboni N. 2007. Genetics: Getting closer to the whole picture. *Science* 316: 550–551.

Scannell JW, Blakemore C, Young MP. 1995. Analysis of connectivity in the cat cerebral cortex. *J Neurosci* 15: 1463–1483.

Scannell JW. 1997. Determining cortical landscapes. *Nature* 386: 452.

Scannell JW, Burns GAPC, Hilgetag CC, O'Neil MA, Young MP. 1999. The connectional organization of the cortico–thalamic system of the cat. *Cereb Cortex* 9: 277–299.

Schacter DL, Addis DR, Buckner RL. 2007. Remembering the past to imagine the future: The prospective brain. *Nat Rev Neurosci* 8: 657–661.

Scheperjans F, Hermann K, Eickhoff SB, Amunts K, Schleicher A, Zilles K. 2008. Observer-independent cytoarchitectonic mapping of the human superior parietal cortex. *Cereb Cortex* 18: 846–867.

Schilbach L, Eickhoff SB, Rotarska-Jagiela A, Fink GR, Vogeley K. 2008. Minds at rest? Social cognition as the default mode of cognizing and its putative relationship to the "default system" of the brain. *Conscious Cogn* 17: 457–467.

Schleicher A, Amunts K, Geyer S, Morosan P, Zilles K. 1999. Observer-independent method for microstructural parcellation of cerebral cortex: A quantitative approach to cytoarchitectonics. *Neuroimage* 9: 165–177.

Schleicher A, Palomero-Gallagher N, Morosan P, Eickhoff S, Kowalski T, et al. 2005. Quantitative architectonic analysis: A new approach to cortical mapping. *Anat Embryol (Berl)* 210: 373–386.

Schmahmann JD, Pandya DN. 2006. *Fiber Pathways of the Brain*. New York: Oxford University Press.

Schmahmann JD, Pandya DN. 2007. Cerebral white matter—Historical evolution of facts and notions concerning the organization of the fiber pathways of the brain. *J Hist Neurosci* 16: 237–267.

Schmahmann JD, Pandya DN, Wang R, Dai G, D'Arceuil HE, et al. 2007. Association fibre pathways of the brain: Parallel observations from diffusion spectrum imaging and autoradiography. *Brain* 130: 630–653.

Schmitt JE, Lenroot RK, Wallace GL, Ordaz S, Taylor KN, et al. 2008. Identification of genetically mediated cortical networks: A multivariate study of pediatric twins and siblings. *Cereb Cortex* 18: 1737–1747.

Schneidman E, Still S, Berry MJ, Bialek W. 2003. Network information and connected correlations. *Phys Rev Lett* 91: 238701.

Schnitzler A, Gross J. 2005. Normal and pathological oscillatory communication in the brain. *Nat Rev Neurosci* 6: 285–296.

Schölvinck ML, Maier A, Ye FQ, Dyun JH, Leopold DA. 2010. Neural basis of global resting-state fMRI activity. *Proc Natl Acad Sci USA* (in press).

Scholz J, Klein MC, Behrens TEJ, Johansen-Berg H. 2009. Training induces changes in white-matter architecture. *Nat Neurosci* 12: 1367–1368.

Schreiber T. 2000. Measuring information transfer. *Phys Rev Lett* 85: 461–464.

Schwarz AJ, Gozzi A, Reese T, Heidbreder CA, Bifone A. 2007. Pharmacological modulation of functional connectivity: The correlation structure underlying the phMRI response to d-amphetamine modified by selective dopamine D3 receptor antagonist SB277011A. *Magn Reson Imaging* 25: 811–820.

Seeley WW, Menon V, Schatzberg AF, Keller J, Glover GH, et al. 2007. Dissociable intrinsic connectivity networks for salience processing and executive control. *J Neurosci* 27: 2349–2356.

Seeley WW, Crawford RK, Zhou J, Miller BL, Greicius MD. 2009. Neurodegenerative diseases target large-scale human brain networks. *Neuron* 62: 42–52.

Sejnowski TJ, Paulsen O. 2006. Network oscillations: Emerging computational principles. *J Neurosci* 26: 1673–1676.

Seth A, Edelman GM. 2004. Environment and behavior influence the complexity of evolved neural networks. *Adapt Behav* 12: 5–20.

Seth AK, McKinstry JL, Edelman GM, Krichmar JL. 2004. Visual binding through reentrant connectivity and dynamic synchronization in a brain-based device. *Cereb Cortex* 14: 1185–1199.

Seth AK. 2005. Causal connectivity analysis of evolved neural networks during behavior. *Netw Comp Neural Syst* 16: 35–54.

Seth A. 2008. Causal networks in simulated neural systems. *Cogn Neurodyn* 2: 49–64.

Seung HS. 2009. Reading the book of memory: Sparse sampling versus dense mapping of connectomes. *Neuron* 62: 17–29.

Shanahan M. 2008. Dynamical complexity in small-world networks of spiking neurons. *Phys Rev E Stat Nonlin Soft Matter Phys* 78: 041924.

Shanahan M. 2010. *Embodiment and the Inner Life*. New York: Oxford University Press.

Shannon CE 1948. A mathematical theory of communication. *Bell Syst Tech J* 27: 379–423 and 623–656.

Sharan R, Ulitsky I, Shamir R. 2007. Network-based prediction of protein function. *Mol Syst Biol* 3: 88.

Shehzad Z, Kelly AMC, Reiss PT, Gee DG, Gotimer K, et al. 2009. The resting brain: Unconstrained yet reliable. *Cereb Cortex* 19: 2209–2229.

Shepard GM. 1991. *Foundations of the Neuron Doctrine*. New York: Oxford University Press.

Sherrington CS. 1940. *Man on His Nature*. Cambridge: University Press.

Shin CW, Kim S. 2006. Self-organized criticality and scale-free properties in emergent functional neural networks. *Phys Rev E Stat Nonlin Soft Matter Phys* 74: 045101.

Shmuel A, Leopold DA. 2008. Neuronal correlates of spontaneous fluctuations in fMRI signals in monkey visual cortex: Implications for functional connectivity at rest. *Hum Brain Mapp* 29: 751–761.

Shoham S, O'Connor DH, Segev R. 2006. How silent is the brain: Is there a "dark matter" problem in neuroscience. *J Comp Physiol A* 192: 777–784.

Sholl DA. 1953. Dendritic organization in the neurons of the visual and motor cortices of the cat. *J Anat* 87: 387–406.

Shulman GL, Fiez JA, Corbetta M, Buckner RL, Miezin FM, Raichle ME, Petersen SE. 1997. Common blood flow changes across visual tasks. II. Decreases in cerebral cortex. *J Cogn Neurosci* 9: 648–663.

Siegal ML, Promislow DEL, Bergman A. 2007. Functional and evolutionary inference in gene networks: Does topology matter? *Genetica* 129: 83–103.

Simon HA. 1955. On a class of skew distribution functions. *Biometrika* 42: 425–440.

Simon HA. 1962. The architecture of complexity. *Proc Am Philos Soc* 106: 467–482.

Simon HA. 1969. *The Sciences of the Artificial*. Cambridge: MIT Press.

Simon HA. 1996) *The Sciences of the Artificial*. Third Edition. Cambridge: MIT Press.

Singer W, Gray CM. 1995. Visual feature integration and the temporal correlation hypothesis. *Annu Rev Neurosci* 18: 555–586.

Singer W. 1999. Neuronal synchrony: A versatile code for the definition of relations? *Neuron* 24: 49–65.

Siri B, Berry H, Cessac B, Delord B, Quoy M. 2008. A mathematical analysis of the effects of Hebbian learning rules on the dynamics and structure of discrete-time random recurrent neural networks. *Neural Comput* 20: 2937–2966.

Skudlarski P, Jagannathan K, Calhoun VD, Hampson M, Skudlarska BA, et al. 2008. Measuring brain connectivity: Diffusion tensor imaging validates resting state temporal correlations. *Neuroimage* 43: 554–561.

Smit DJA, Stam CJ, Posthuma D, Boomsma DI, de Geus EJC. 2008. Heritability of "small-world" networks in the brain: A graph theoretical analysis of resting-state EEG functional connectivity. *Hum Brain Mapp* 29: 1368–1378.

Smith LB, Thelen E. 2003. Development as a dynamic system. *Trends Cogn Sci* 7: 343–348.

Smith LB, Breazeal C. 2007. The dynamic lift of developmental process. *Dev Sci* 10: 61–68.

Smith SJ. 2007. Circuit reconstruction tools today. *Curr Opin Neurobiol* 17: 601–608.

Smith SM, Fox PT, Miller KL, Glahn DC, Fox PM, et al. 2009. Correspondence of the brain's functional architecture during activation and rest. *Proc Natl Acad Sci USA* 106: 13040–13045.

Solé RV, Valverde S. 2004. Information theory of complex networks: On evolution and architectural constraints. *Lect Notes Phys* 650: 189–207.

Solé RV, Valverde S. 2006. Are network motifs the spandrels of cellular complexity? *Trends Ecol Evol* 21: 419–422.

Soltesz I. 2006. *Diversity in the Neuronal Machine: Order and Variability in Interneuronal Microcircuits*. New York: Oxford University Press.

Song M, Zhou Y, Li J, Liu Y, Tian L, et al. 2008. Brain spontaneous functional connectivity and intelligence. *Neuroimage* 41: 1168–1176.

Song S, Sjöström PJ, Reigl M, Nelson S, Chklovskii DB. 2005. Highly nonrandom features of synaptic connectivity in local cortical circuits. *PLoS Biol* 3: e68.

Sorg C, Riedl V, Mühlau M, Calhoun VD, Eichele T, et al. 2007. Selective changes of resting-state networks in individuals at risk for Alzheimer's disease. *Proc Natl Acad Sci USA* 104: 18760–18765.

Sperry RW. 1964. *Problems Outstanding in the Evolution of Brain Function.* New York: The American Museum of Natural History.

Sporns O, Gally JA, Reeke GN, Edelman GM. 1989. Reentrant signaling among simulated neuronal groups leads to coherency in their oscillatory activity. *Proc Natl Acad Sci USA* 86: 7265–7269.

Sporns O, Tononi G, Edelman GM. 1991. Modeling perceptual grouping and figure–ground segregation by means of active reentrant circuits. *Proc Natl Acad Sci USA* 88: 129–133.

Sporns O, Tononi G, Edelman GM. 2000a. Theoretical neuroanatomy: Relating anatomical and functional connectivity in graphs and cortical connection matrices. *Cereb Cortex* 10: 127–141.

Sporns O, Tononi G, Edelman GM. 2000b. Connectivity and complexity: The relationship between neuroanatomy and brain dynamics. *Neural Netw* 13: 909–922.

Sporns O, Tononi G. 2002. Classes of network connectivity and dynamics. *Complexity* 7: 28–38.

Sporns O. 2003. Graph theory methods for the analysis of neural connectivity patterns. In *Neuroscience Databases: A Practical Guide*, Kötter R (ed.), pp. 171–186, Boston: Klüwer.

Sporns O, Kötter R. 2004. Motifs in brain networks. *PLoS Biol* 2: 1910–1918.

Sporns O, Chialvo D, Kaiser M, Hilgetag CC. 2004. Organization, development and function of complex brain networks. *Trends Cogn Sci* 8: 418–425.

Sporns O, Zwi J. 2004. The small world of the cerebral cortex. *Neuroinformatics* 2: 145–162.

Sporns O. 2004. Complex neural dynamics. In *Coordination Dynamics: Issues and Trends*, Jirsa VK, Kelso JAS (eds.), pp. 197–215, Springer-Verlag, Berlin.

Sporns O, Tononi G, Kötter R. 2005. The human connectome: A structural description of the human brain. *PLoS Comput Biol* 1: 245–251.

Sporns O. 2006. Small-world connectivity, motif composition, and complexity of fractal neuronal connections. *Biosystems* 85: 55–64.

Sporns O, Lungarella M. 2006. Evolving coordinated behavior by maximizing information structure. In Rocha L et al. (eds.), *Artificial Life X*. Cambridge: MIT Press.

Sporns O. 2007. Complexity. *Scholarpedia* 2: 1623.

Sporns O, Honey CJ, Kötter R. 2007. Identification and classification of hubs in brain networks. *PLoS ONE* 2: e1049.

Srinivasan R, Russell DP, Edelman GM, Tononi G. 1999. Increased synchronization of neuromagnetic responses during conscious perception. *J Neurosci* 19: 5435–5448.

Stam CJ. 2004. Functional connectivity patterns of human magnetoencephalographic recordings: A "small-world" network? *Neurosci Lett* 355: 25–28.

Stam CJ, de Bruin EA. 2004. Scale-free dynamics of global functional connectivity in the human brain. *Hum Brain Mapp* 22: 97–109.

Stam CJ. 2006. *Nonlinear Brain Dynamics.* New York: Nova Science.

Stam CJ, Reijneveld JC. 2007. Graph theoretical analysis of complex networks in the brain. *Nonlinear Biomed Phys* 1: 3.

Stam CJ, Jones BF, Nolte G, Breakspear M, Scheltens P. 2007. Small-world networks and functional connectivity in Alzheimer's disease. *Cereb Cortex* 17: 92–99.

Stam CJ, de Haan W, Daffertshofer A, Jones BF, Manshanden I, et al. 2009. Graph theoretical analysis of magnetoencephalographic functional connectivity in Alzheimer's disease. *Brain* 132: 213–224.

Steno N. 1965. *Lecture on the Anatomy of the Brain*. Copenhagen: Nordisk Forlag Brusck.

Stepanyants A, Hof PR, Chklovskii DB. 2002. Geometry and structural plasticity of synaptic connectivity. *Neuron* 34: 275–288.

Stepanyants A, Chklovskii DB. 2005. Neurogeometry and potential synaptic connectivity. *Trends Neurosci* 28: 387–394.

Stephan KE, Hilgetag CC, Burns GAPC, O'Neill MA, Young MP, et al. 2000. Computational analysis of functional connectivity between areas of primate cerebral cortex. *Phil Trans R Soc B* 355: 111–126.

Stephan KE, Kamper L, Bozkurt A, Burns GAPC, Young MP, et al. 2001. Advanced database methodology for the collation of connectivity data on the macaque brain (CoCoMac). *Proc Trans R Soc B* 356: 1159–1186.

Stephan KE. 2004. On the role of general system theory for functional neuroimaging. *J Anat* 205: 443–470.

Stephan KE, Baldeweg T, Friston KJ. 2006. Synaptic plasticity and dysconnection in schizophrenia. *Biol Psychiatry* 59: 929–939.

Stephan KE, Friston KJ. 2007. Models of effective connectivity in neural systems. In *Handbook of Brain Connectivity*, Jirsa VK, McIntosh AR (eds.), pp. 303–325, Berlin: Springer.

Stephan KE, Kasper L, Harrison LM, Daunizeau J, de Ouden HEM, et al. 2008. Nonlinear dynamic causal models for fMRI. *Neuroimage* 42: 649–662.

Steriade M, Núñez A, Amzica F. 1993. A novel slow (<1 Hz) oscillation of neocortical neurons in vivo: Depolarizing and hyperpolarizing components. *J Neurosci* 13: 3252–3265.

Stern Y. 2002. What is cognitive reserve? Theory and research application of the reserve concept. *J Int Neuropsychol Soc* 8: 448–460.

Stevens CF. 1989. How cortical interconnecedness varies with network size. *Neural Comput* 1: 473–479.

Stiefel KM, Sejnowski TJ. 2007. Mapping function onto neuronal morphology. *J Neurophysiol* 98: 513–526.

Striedter GF. 2005. *Principles of Brain Evolution*. Sunderland: Sinauer.

Strogatz SH. 2001. Exploring complex networks. *Nature* 410: 268–277.

Stumpf MPH, Wiuf C, May RM. 2005. Subnets of scale-free networks are not scale-free: Sampling properties of networks. *Proc Natl Acad Sci USA* 102: 4221–4224.

Suckling J, Wink AM, Bernard FA, Barnes A, Bullmore E. 2008. Endogenous multifractal brain dynamics are modulated by age, cholinergic blockade and cognitive performance. *J Neurosci Methods* 174: 292–300.

Supekar K, Menon V, Rubin D, Musen M, Greicius MD. 2008. Network analysis of intrinsic functional brain connectivity in Alzheimer's disease. *PLoS Comput Biol* 4: e1000100.

Supekar K, Musen M, Menon V. 2009. Development of large-scale functional brain networks in children. *PLoS Biol* 7: e1000157.

Sur M, Rubenstein JLR. 2005. Patterning and plasticity of the cerebral cortex. *Science* 310: 805–810.

Suzuki M, Floreano D. 2008. Enactive robot vision. *Adapt Behav* 16: 122–128.

Swanson LW. 2003. *Brain Architecture*. Oxford: Oxford University Press.

Swanson LW. 2007. Quest for the basic plan of nervous system circuitry. *Brain Res Rev* 55: 356–372.

Szentágothai J. 1977. The Ferrier Lecture, 1977: The neuron network of the cerebral cortex: A functional interpretation. *Proc R Soc Lond B Biol Sci* 201: 219–248.

Tagamets MA, Horwitz B. 1998. Integrating electrophysiological and anatomical experimental data to create a large-scale model that simulates a delayed match-to-sample human brain imaging study. *Cereb Cortex* 8: 310–320.

Takahashi E, Dai G, Wang R, Ohki K, Rosen GD, et al. 2010. Development of cerebral fiber pathways in cats revealed by diffusion spectrum imaging. *Neuroimage* 49: 1231–1240.

Tanigawa H, Wang Q, Fuujita I. 2005. Organization of horizontal axons in the inferior temporal cortex and primary visual cortex of the macaque. *Cereb Cortex* 15: 1887–1899.

Thelen E, Smith LB. 1994. *A Dynamic Systems Approach to the Development of Cognition and Action.* Cambridge: MIT Press.

Thivierge JP, Marcus GF. 2007. The topographic brain: From neural connectivity to cognition. *Trends Neurosci* 30: 251–259.

Thompson PM, Cannon TD, Narr KL, van Erp T, Poutanen VP, et al. 2001. Genetic influences on brain structure. *Nat Neurosci* 4: 1253–1258.

Toga AW, Thompson PM. 2005. Genetics of brain structure and intelligence. *Annu Rev Neurosci* 28: 1–23.

Tognoli E, Lagarde J, De Guzman GC, Kelso JAS. 2007. The phi complex as a neuromarker of human social coordination. *Proc Natl Acad Sci USA* 104: 8190–8195.

Tognoli E. 2008. EEG coordination dynamics: Neuromarkers of social coordination. In *Coordination: Neural, Behavioral and Social Dynamics*, Jirsa VK, Richardson MJ (eds.), pp. 309–323, Berlin: Springer.

Tognoli E, Kelso JAS. 2009. Brain coordination dynamics: True and false faces of phase synchrony and metastability. *Prog Neurobiol* 87: 31–40.

Tomassini V, Jbabdi S, Klein JC, Behrens TEJ, Pozzilli C, et al. 2007. Diffusion-weighted imaging tractography-based parcellation of the human lateral premotor cortex identifies dorsal and ventral subregions with anatomical and functional specializations. *J Neurosci* 27: 10259–10269.

Tononi G, Sporns O, Edelman GM. 1992. Reentry and the problem of integrating multiple cortical areas: Simulation of dynamic integration in the visual system. *Cereb Cortex* 2: 310–335.

Tononi G, Sporns O, Edelman GM. 1994. A measure for brain complexity: Relating functional segregation and integration in the nervous system. *Proc Natl Acad Sci USA* 91: 5033–5037.

Tononi G, Sporns O, Edelman GM. 1996. A complexity measure for selective matching of signals by the brain. *Proc Natl Acad Sci USA* 93: 3422–3427.

Tononi G, Edelman GM. 1998. Consciousness and complexity. *Science* 282: 1846–1851.

Tononi G, Edelman GM, Sporns O. 1998. Complexity and coherency: Integrating information in the brain. *Trends Cogn Sci* 2: 474–484.

Tononi G, Sporns O, Edelman GM. 1999. Measures of degeneracy and redundancy in biological networks. *Proc Natl Acad Sci USA* 96: 3257–3262.

Tononi G, Edelman GM. 2000. Schizophrenia and the mechanisms of conscious integration. *Brain Res Brain Res Rev* 31: 391–400.

Tononi G, Sporns O. 2003. Measuring information integration. *BMC Neurosci* 4: 31.

Tononi G. 2004. An information integration theory of consciousness. *BMC Neurosci* 5: 42.

Tononi G. 2008. Consciousness as integrated information: A provisional manifesto. *Biol Bull* 215: 216–242.

Tononi G, Koch C. 2008. The neural correlates of consciousness: An update. *Ann N Y Acad Sci* 1124: 239–261.

Torborg CL, Feller MB. 2005. Spontaneous patterned retinal activity and the refinement of retinal projections. *Prog Neurobiol* 76: 213–235.

Toro R, Fox P, Paus T. 2008. Functional coactivation map of the human brain. *Cereb Cortex* 18: 2553–2559.

Traub RD, Miles R, Wong RK. 1989. Model of the origin of rhythmic population oscillations in the hippocampal slice. *Science* 243: 1319–1325.

Travers J, Milgram S. 1969. An experimental study of the small world problem. *Sociometry* 32: 425–443.

Treisman A. 1996. The binding problem. *Curr Opin Neurobiol* 6: 171–178.

Tsodyks M, Kenet T, Grinvald A, Arieli A. 1999. Linking spontaneous activity of single cortical neurons and the underlying functional architecture. *Science* 286: 1943–1946.

Tuch D, Reese TG, Wiegell MR, Makris N, Belliveau JW, et al. 2002. High angular resolution diffusion imaging reveals intravoxel white matter fiber heterogeneity. *Magn Reson Med* 48: 577–582.

Tuch DS, Reese TG, Wiegell MR, Wedeen VJ. 2003. Diffusion MRI of complex neural architecture. *Neuron* 40: 885–895.

Turing AM. 1948. Intelligent Machinery, National Physical Laboratory Report. In *Machine Intelligence,* Vol. 5, Meltzer B, Michie D (eds.), pp. 3–23, Edinburgh: Edinburgh University Press.

Turing A. 1952. The chemical basis of morphogenesis. *Phil Trans R Soc B* 237: 37–72.

Ungerleider LG, Mishkin M. 1982. Two cortical visual systems. In *Analysis of Visual Behaviour,* Ingle DG, Goodale MA, Mansfield RJQ (eds.), pp. 549–586, Cambridge: MIT Press.

Uttal WR. 2001. *The New Phrenology: The Limits of Localizing Cognitive Processes in the Brain.* Cambridge: MIT Press.

Uttley AM. 1955. The probability of neural connexions. *Proc R Soc Lond B Biol Sci* 144: 229–240.

Uylings HBM, Rajkowska G, Sanz-Arigita E, Amunts K, Zilles K. 2005. Consequences of large interindividual variability for human brain atlases: Converging macroscopical imaging and microscopical neuroanayomy. *Anat Embryol (Berl)* 210: 423–431.

Valencia M, Pastor MA, Fernández-Seara MA, Artieda J, Martinerie J, et al. 2009. Complex modular structure of large-scale brain networks. *Chaos* 19: 023119.

Van den Heuvel MP, Mandl RC, Luigjes J, Hulshoff Pol HE. 2008a. Microstructural organization of the cingulum tract and the level of default mode functional connectivity. *J Neurosci* 28: 10844–10851.

Van den Heuvel MP, Stam CJ, Boersma M, Hulshoff Pol HE. 2008b. Small-world and scale-free organization of voxel based resting-state functional connectivity in the human brain. *Neuroimage* 43: 528–539.

Van den Heuvel MP, Mandl RCW, Kahn RS, Hulshoff Pol HE. 2009a. Functionally linked resting-state networks reflect the underlying structural connectivity architecture of the human brain. *Hum Brain Mapp* 30: 3127–3141.

Van den Heuvel MP, Stam CJ, Kahn RS, Hulshoff Pol HE. 2009b. Efficiency of functional brain networks and intellectual performance. *J Neurosci* 29: 7619–7624.

Vanderwolf CH. 2000. Are neocortical gamma waves related to consciousness? *Brain Res* 855: 217–224.

van de Ven VG, Formisano E, Prvulovic D, Roeder CH, Linden DEJ. 2004. Functional connectivity as revealed by spatial independent component analysis of fMRI measurements during rest. *Hum Brain Mapp* 22: 165–178.

Van Essen DC, Maunsell JHR. 1983. Hierarchical organization and functional streams in the visual cortex. *Trends Neurosci* 6: 370–375.

Van Essen DC, Felleman DJ, DeYoe EA, Olavarria J, Knierim J. 1990. Modular and hierarchical organization of extrastriate visual cortex in the macaque monkey. *Cold Spring Harb Symp Quant Biol* 55: 679–696.

Van Essen DC, Anderson CH, Felleman DJ. 1992. Information processing in the primate visual system: An integrated systems perspective. *Science* 255: 419–423.

Van Essen DC. 1997. A tension-based theory of morphogenesis and compact wiring in the central nervous system. *Nature* 385: 313–318.

Van Essen DC, Dierker D. 2007. On navigating the human cerebral cortex: Response to "in praise of tedious anatomy." *Neuroimage* 37: 1050–1054.

Van Ooyen A. 2003. *Modeling Neural Development*. Cambridge: MIT Press.

Varela FJ, Thompson E, Rosch E. 1991. *The Embodied Mind: Cognitive Science and Human Experience*. Cambridge: MIT Press.

Varela FJ. 1995. Resonant cell assemblies: A new approach to cognitive functions and neuronal synchrony. *Biol Res* 28: 81–95.

Varela F, Lachaux JP, Rodriguez E, Martinerie J. 2001. The brainweb: Phase synchronization and large-scale integration. *Nat Rev Neurosci* 2: 229–239.

Variano EA, McCoy JH, Lipson H. 2004. Networks, dynamics, and modularity. *Phys Rev Lett* 92: 188701.

Varki A, Geschwind DH, Eichler EE. 2008. Explaining human uniqueness: Genome interactions with environment, behaviour and culture. *Nat Rev Genet* 9: 749–763.

Vatikiotis-Bateson E, Eigsti IM, Yano S, Munhall KG. 1998. Eye movement of perceivers during audiovisual speech perception. *Perception Psychophys* 60: 926–940.

Vazquez A, Flammini A, Maritan A, Vespignani A. 2003. Global protein function prediction from protein–protein interaction networks. *Nat Biotechnol* 21: 697–700.

Venter JC, Adams MD, Myers EW, Li PW, Mural RJ, et al. 2001. The sequence of the human genome. *Science* 291: 1304–1351.

Verschure PFMJ, Voegtlin T, Douglas RJ. 2003. Environmentally mediated synergy between perception and behaviour in mobile robots. *Nature* 425: 620–624.

Vespignani A. 2009. Predicting the behavior of techno-social systems. *Science* 325: 425–428.

Vicente R, Gollo LL, Mirasso CR, Fischer I, Pipa G. 2008. Dynamical relaying can yield zero time lag neuronal synchrony despite long conduction delays. *Proc Natl Acad Sci USA* 105: 17157–17162.

Vincent JL, Patel GH, Fox MD, Snyder AZ, Baker JT, et al. 2007. Intrinsic functional architecture in the anaesthetized monkey brain. *Nature* 447: 83–86.

Vinje WE, Gallant JL. 2000. Sparse coding and decorrelation in primary visual cortex during natural vision. *Science* 287: 1273–1276.

Vinje WE, Gallant JL. 2002. Natural stimulation of the nonclassical receptive field increases information transmission efficiency in V1. *J Neurosci* 22: 2904–2915.

Vogels TP, Rajan K, Abbott LF. 2005. Neural network dynamics. *Annu Rev Neurosci* 28: 357–376.

Vogelstein B, Lane D, Levine AJ. 2000. Surfing the p53 network. *Nature* 408: 307–310.

Volkow ND, Wolf AP, Brodie JD, Cancro R, Overall JE, et al. 1988. Brain interactions in chronic schizophrenics under resting and activation conditions. *Schizophr Res* 1: 47–53.

Von Bonin G. 1960. *Some Papers on the Cerebral Cortex*. Springfield: Charles C. Thomas.

Von der Malsburg, C. 1981. The correlation theory of brain function. Intern. Rep., 81–2, MPI Biophysikalische Chemie, Gottingen, Germany.

Von der Malsburg C, Schneider W. 1986. A neural cocktail-party processor. *Biol Cybern* 54: 29–40.

Von Economo C, Koskinas GN. 1925. *Die Cytoarchitektonik der Hirnrinde des erwachsenen Menschen*. Berlin: Springer.

Von Monakow C. 1969. Diaschisis. Excerpted and translated from "*Die Lokalisation im Grosshirn und der Abbau der Funktion durch kortikale Herde*," Wiesbaden, Bergmann, 1914. In *Brain and Behavior I: Mood States and Mind*, Pribram KH (ed.), pp. 27–36, Baltimore: Penguin.

Von Stein A, Rappelsberger P, Sarntheim J, Petsche H. 1999. Synchronization between temporal and parietal cortex during multimodal object processing in man. *Cereb Cortex* 9: 137–150.

Von Stein A, Chiang C, König P. 2000. Top-down processing mediated by interareal synchronization. *Proc Natl Acad Sci USA* 97: 14748–14753.

Wagner A. 2005. Robustness, evolvability, and neutrality. *FEBS Lett* 579: 1772–1778.

Wagner GP, Altenberg L. 1996. Perspective: Complex adaptations and the evolution of evolvability. *Evolution* 50: 967–976.

Wagner GP, Pavlicev M, Cheverud JM. 2007. The road to modularity. *Nat Rev Genet* 8: 921–931.

Walker EA. 1940. A cytoarchitectural study of the prefrontal area of macaque monkey. *J Comp Neurol* 73: 59–86.

Wang K, Liang M, Wang L, Tian L, Zhang X, et al. 2007. Altered functional connectivity in early Alzheimer's disease: A resting-state fMRI study. *Hum Brain Mapp* 28: 967–978.

Wang J, Wang L, Zang Y, Yang H, Tang H, et al. 2009a. Parcellation-dependent small-world brain functional networks: A resting-state fMRI study. *Hum Brain Mapp* 30: 1511–1523.

Wang L, Zhu C, Zang Y, Cao Q, Zhang H, et al. 2009b. Altered small-world brain functional networks in children with attention-deficit/hyperactivity disorder. *Hum Brain Mapp* 30: 638–649.

Ward LM. 2003. Synchronous neural oscillations and cognitive processes. *Trends Cogn Sci* 7: 553–559.

Wasserman S, Faust K. 1994. *Social Network Analysis: Methods and Applications.* Cambridge: Cambridge University Press.

Watson JD. 1990. The human genome project: Past, present, and future. *Science* 248: 44–49.

Watts DJ, Strogatz SH. 1998. Collective dynamics of "small-world" networks. *Nature* 393: 440–442.

Watts DJ. 1999. Networks, dynamics, and the small-world phenomenon. *Am J Sociol* 105: 493–527.

Watts DJ. 2003. *Six Degrees: The Science of a Connected Age.* New York: Norton.

Watts DJ. 2004. The "new" science of networks. *Annu Rev Sociol* 30: 243–270.

Webb B. 1995. Using robots to model animals: A cricket test. *Robot Auton Syst* 16: 117–134.

Wedeen VJ, Hagmann P, Tseng WY, Reese TG, Weisskoff RM. 2005. Mapping complex tissue architecture with diffusion spectrum magnetic resonance imaging. *Magn Reson Med* 54: 1377–1386.

Wedeen VJ, Wang R, Schmahmann JD, Takahashi E, Kaas JH, et al. 2009. Diffusion spectrum MRI in three mammals: Rat, monkey and human. *Frontiers Neurosci* 3: 74–77.

Weliky M, Katz LC. 1999. Correlational structure of spontaneous neuronal activity in the developing lateral geniculate nucleus in vivo. *Science* 285: 599–604.

Wen Q, Chklovskii DB. 2005. Segregation of the brain into gray and white matter: A design minimizing conduction delays. *PLoS Comput Biol* 1: e78.

Wen Q, Stepanyants A, Elston GN, Grosberg AY, Chklovskii DB. 2009. Maximization of the connectivity repertoire as a statistical principle governing the shapes of dendritic arbors. *Proc Natl Acad Sci USA* 106: 12536–12541.

Werner G. 2007. Metastability, criticality and phase transitions in brain and its models. *Biosystems* 90: 496–508.

Wernicke C. 1874. *Der aphasische Symptomenkomplex: Eine psychologische Studie auf anatomischer Basis.* Breslau: Cohn & Weigert.

Wernicke C. 1876. Das Urwindungssystem des menschlichen Genirns. *Eur Arch Psychiatry Clin Neurosci* 6: 298–326.

White JG. 1985. Neuronal connectivity in *Caenorhabditis elegans. Trends Neurosci* 8: 277–283.

White JG, Southgate E, Thomson JN, Brenner S. 1986. The structure of the nervous system of the nematode *Caenorhabditis elegans. Philos Trans R Soc Lond, B* 314: 1–340.

Whitfield-Gabrieli S, Thermenos HW, Milanovic S, Tsuang MT, Faraone SV, et al. 2009. Hyperactivity and hyperconnectivity of the default network in schizophrenia and in first-degree relatives of persons with schizophrenia. *Proc Natl Acad Sci USA* 106: 1279–1284.

Wiener N. 1948. *Cybernetics: Or Control and Communication in the Animal and the Machine*. Paris: Librairie Hermann & Cie, and Cambridge: MIT Press.

Wiener N. 1956. *I Am a Mathematician*. New York: Doubleday.

Williams GC. 1966. *Adaptation and Natural Selection: A Critique of Some Current Evolutionary Thought*. Princeton: Princeton University Press.

Williamson WR, Hiesinger PR. 2008. Synaptic patterning by morphogen signaling. *Sci Signal* 1: pe20.

Willinger W, Alderson D, Doyle JC. 2009. Mathematics and the Internet: A source of enormous confusion and great potential. *Not Am Math Soc* 56: 586–599.

Womelsdorf T, Schoffelen JM, Oostenveld R, Singer W, Desimone R, et al. 2007. Modulation of neuronal interactions through neuronal synchronization. *Science* 316: 1609–1612.

Woodruff PW, Wright IC, Shuriquie N, Russouw H, Rushe T, et al. 1997. Structural abnormalities in male schizophrenics reflect fronto–temporal dissociations. *Psychol Med* 27: 1257–1266.

Wu Y, Li P, Chen M, Xiao J, Kurths J. 2009. Response of scale-free networks with community structure to external stimuli. *Physica A* 388: 2987–2994.

Yacoub E, Harel N, Uğurbil K. 2008. High-field fMRI unveils orientation columns in humans. *Proc Natl Acad Sci USA* 105: 10607–10612.

Yaeger LS. 1994. Computational genetics, physiology, metabolism, neural systems, learning, vision, and behavior or Polyworld: Life in a new context. In *Artificial Life III: Proceedings*, Langton CG (ed.), pp. 263–298, Reading, MA: Addison-Wesley.

Yaeger LS, Sporns O. 2006. Evolution of neural structure and complexity in a computational ecology. In *Artificial Life X: Proceedings*, Rocha LM, Yaeger LS, Bedeau MA, Floreano D, Goldstone RL, et al. (eds.), pp. 330–336, Cambridge: MIT Press.

Yaeger LS, Griffith V, Sporns O. 2008. Passive and driven trends in the evolution of complexity. In *Artificial Life XI: Proceedings*, Bullock S, Noble J, Watson R, Bedau MA (eds.), pp. 725–732, Cambridge: MIT Press.

Yaeger LS. 2009. How evolution guides complexity. *HFSP J* 3: 328–339.

Yang G, Pan F, Gan WB. 2009. Stably maintained dendritic spines are associated with lifelong memories. *Nature* 462: 920–924.

Yarbus A. 1967. *Eye Movements and Vision*. New York: Plenum Press.

Yoshimura Y, Dantzker JLM, Callaway EM. 2005. Excitatory cortical neurons form fine-scale functional networks. *Nature* 433: 868–873.

Young MP. 1992. Objective analysis of the topological organization of the primate cortical visual system. *Nature* 358: 152–155.

Young MP. 1993. The organization of neural systems in the primate cerebral cortex. *Proc Biol Sci* 252: 13–18.

Young MP, Scannell JW. 1996. Component-placement optimization in the brain. *Trends Neurosci* 19: 413–414.

Young MP. 2000. The architecture of visual cortex and inferential processes in vision. *Spat Vis* 13: 137–146.

Young MP, Hilgetag CC, Scannell JW. 2000. On imputing function to structure from the behavioural effects of brain lesions. *Philos Trans R Soc Lond B Biol Sci* 355: 147–161.

Young RM. 1990. *Mind, Brain and Adaptation in the Nineteenth Century: Cerebral Localization and Its Biological Context from Gall to Ferrier*. Oxford: Clarendon Press.

Young JZ. 1951. Growth and plasticity in the nervous system. *Proc R Soc Lond B Biol Sci* 139: 18–37.

Yu S, Huang D, Singer W, Nikolić D. 2008. A small world of neuronal synchrony. *Cereb Cortex* 18: 2891–2901.

Yu YC, Bultje RS, Wang X, Shi SH. 2009. Specific synapses develop preferentially among sister excitatory neurons in the neocortex. *Nature* 458: 501–505.

Zeki S. 1978. Functional specialization in the visual cortex of the rhesus monkey. *Nature* 274: 423–428.

Zeki S, Shipp S. 1988. The functional logic of cortical connections. *Nature* 335: 311–317.

Zeki S. 1993. *A Vision of the Brain*. London: Blackwell.

Zeki S. 2005. Cerebral cartography 1905–2005. *Phil Trans R Soc B* 360: 651–652.

Zalesky A, Fornito A, Hardin IH, Cocchi L, Yücel M, et al. 2010. Whole-brain anatomical networks: Does the choice of nodes matter? *Neuroimage*. In press.

Zemanová L, Zhou C, Kurths J. 2006. Structural and functional clusters of complex brain networks. *Physica D* 224: 202–212.

Zhang D, Snyder AZ, Fox MD, Sansbury MW, Shimony JS, et al. 2008. Intrinsic functional relations between human cerebral cortex and thalamus. *J Neurophysiol* 100: 1740–1748.

Zhang D, Raichle M. 2010. Disease and the brain's dark energy. *Nat Rev* Neurology 6: 15–28.

Zhang K, Sejnowski TJ. 2000. A universal scaling law between gray matter and white matter of the cerebral cortex. *Proc Natl Acad Sci USA* 97: 5621–5626.

Zhigulin VP. 2004. Dynamical motifs: Building blocks of complex dynamics in sparsely connected random networks. *Phys Rev Lett* 92: 238701.

Zhou C, Zemanova L, Zamora G, Hilgetag CC, Kurths J. 2006. Hierarchical organization unveiled by functional connectivity in complex brain networks. *Phys Rev Lett* 97: 238103.

Zhou C, Kurths J. 2006. Hierarchical synchronization in complex networks with heterogeneous degrees. *Chaos* 16: 015104.

Zhou C, Zemanová L, Zamora G, Hilgetag CC, Kurths J. 2007a. Structure–function relationship in complex brain networks expressed by hierarchical synchronization. *N J Phys* 9: 178.

Zhou Y, Liang M, Tian L, Wang K, Hao Y, Liu H, et al. 2007b. Functional disintegration in paranoid schizophrenia using resting-state fMRI. *Schizophr Res* 97: 194–205.

Zilles K, Palomero-Gallagher N, Schleicher A. 2004. Transmitter receptors and functional anatomy of the cerebral cortex. *J Anat* 205: 417–432.

Zola-Morgan S. 1995. Localization of brain function: The legacy of Franz Joseph Gall (1758–1828). *Annu Rev Neurosci* 18: 359–383.

Zubler F, Douglas R. 2009. A framework for modeling the growth and development of neurons and networks. *Frontiers Comput Neurosci* 3: 25.

Index

Printed in the United States
by Baker & Taylor Publisher Services